Why People Go to Psychiatrists

Why People Go to Psychiatrists

CHARLES KADUSHIN

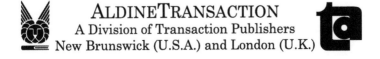
ALDINETRANSACTION
A Division of Transaction Publishers
New Brunswick (U.S.A.) and London (U.K.)

To My Parents

Second printing 2009
Copyright © 1969 by Charles Kadushin.

This book is printed on acid-free paper that meets the American National Standard for Permanence of Paper for Printed Library Materials.

Library of Congress Catalog Number: 2006045623
ISBN: 978-0-202-30903-3
Printed in the United States of America

Library of Congress Cataloging-in-Publication Data

Kadushin,, Charles.
    Why people go to psychiatrists / Charles Kadushin.
        p. cm.
    Originally published: New York: Atherton Press, 1969.
    Includes bibliographical references (p.   ).
    ISBN 0-202-30903-7 (pbk.: alk. paper)
        1. Mental illness   2. Psychotherapy.   I. Title.

RC480.5.K32   2006
616.89—dc22   2006045623

Contents

V ⚙ TOWARD BETTER COMMUNITY MENTAL-HEALTH PROGRAMS

Acknowledgments

All survey research is the product of the labors of many people. Because of the requirements of anonymity, my two most important debts can only be generally acknowledged. I am most indebted to more than 1,500 people who told the story of how they came to apply to a psychiatric clinic. I hope that their experiences can somehow lead to a better understanding of mental health treatment resources and thereby indirectly compensate them. I owe a special debt of gratitude to the directors and staff of the ten clinics that opened their doors and records to us, allowed us access to their patients, corrected our research instruments, helped us with data collection, and criticized parts of our final report. I hope that the point of view of someone from another professional background can in some way repay their many efforts on behalf of our research.

This study began as part of a program of research into religion and psychiatry at the Bureau of Applied Social Research under a grant from the American Foundation of Religion and Psychiatry. Samuel Z. Klausner was director of this program, and since its termination in 1961 he has remained adviser, critic, and friend. John Cotton, M.D., served as chairman of a research board for the American Foundation and helped us to gain access to the clinics we studied. Elena Padilla, then research director of the New York City Community Mental Health Board, helped in many ways. Hans L. Zetterberg contributed greatly as dissertation sponsor and adviser for an earlier work based on data that served as a pretest for this study. David L. Sills, Bernard Berelson, and Allen Barton were directors of the Bureau of Applied Social Research during the years in which this study was designed and analyzed, and each contributed his unique skills. Clara Shapiro was Administrative Director of the Bureau, and she and her staff facilitated the study in countless ways. The study could not have taken place without Vivian Biasotti Vallier, the field director; Jan Eckert Azumi, the coding supervisor; and Susan Flusser Tausig, who organized the analysis to which Richard Faust and Allan Lippman also contributed. To the several interviewers and many coders I owe special thanks. Helmut Guttenberg, Peter Graham, and the staff of the tabulation department of the Bureau helped to organize data processing. The analysis depended on computer programs designed by Kenneth King, director of the Columbia University Computer Center, and Philip Sidel of the Bureau. Raymond Boudon, Neil Henry, and David Elesh helped with the latent structure analysis. I am indebted to J. B. Kruskal and Bell Telephone Laboratories for the MDSCAL program and to Irving Silverman for his Tryon Clustering program.

I am grateful to Paul Goodman for permission to quote from his *Empire City* and to the *American Sociological Review* for permission to reprint portions of my article, "The Friends and Supporters of Psychotherapy: On Social Circles in Urban Life."

The study was supported by grants from the American Foundation of Religion and Psychiatry, the National Institute of Mental Health, and the New York City Health Research Council. The Columbia University Computer Center supported the computer work. Finally, I owe a special intellectual debt to Paul F. Lazarsfeld and Robert K. Merton. Though I am grateful to all the people and organizations that helped me, I alone am of course responsible for any errors of omission or commission.

THE STUDY AND THE CAST OF CHARACTERS

I

The Decision to Go to
a Psychiatrist

❄

1

If this is not the age of anxiety it is certainly the age of the recognition and treatment of anxiety through psychiatry. Traditionally rejected by the public, forgotten by philanthropists, and belittled by medical practice, the mentally disturbed and those who treat them are now elevated into positions not only of respectability but even of honor and prominence. Ours is the first generation in which a President of the United States has delivered to Congress a message on mental illness.[1] In the ten-year period from 1950 to 1960, voluntary contributions to mental health campaigns have increased fivefold.[2] And federal contributions to this field have sharply and continually risen since World War II both in the field of research and now more recently in the provision of facilities and personnel for community mental health centers.[3] The number of psychiatrists and neurologists has vastly increased, and the field itself has been gaining in medical prestige as more and more medical students have been given early training in modern psychiatry. The number of nonmedically trained professionals in the mental health field, including psychologists, social workers, and ministers, has also increased in the last twenty years. There is even evidence that the traditional reaction of the public to mental disorder—denial of its presence and rejection of those labeled ill—is undergoing considerable change.[4]

Although it is true that only 2 per cent of the adult American population will admit that they have ever consulted a psychiatrist or a psychologist for a personal problem,[5] the importance of the people who have actually received office therapy transcends the sheer numbers involved. The opinion leaders of the nation's culture—writers, artists, and people in the communications industry—together with those in the health professions, form at least one-third of those who have been in analytic office treatment. The college-educated are between six and twenty times as likely as others (depending on the particular locale) to go to psychiatrists. These educated persons have written, published, and read an enormous number of books and articles about psychotherapy and psychoanalysis. American fiction has been so affected by psychoanalytic material that one literary critic complained that the very style of the modern novel has been ruined by "our psychiatrically centered culture."[6]

As a result, though there are more patients in mental hospitals than there are in office treatment, when people think of psychiatrists they think of the couch rather than the hospital. In terms of the distribution of psychiatrists, at any rate, this stereotype is true, for the majority of psychiatrists spend most of their time with office patients rather than with those who are hospitalized.* Outpatient psychotherapy[7] is the most influential procedure in modern psychiatry and has contributed no less than have tranquilizers to a re-evaluation of our entire system of dealing with mental illness, crime, and other forms of social deviation.

❉ Do People Go to Psychiatrists Because They Are "Sick"?

The success and importance of outpatient psychotherapy depend on the supply of patients. Had not the right kind of patient come to him, Freud could not have made his contributions to psychiatry. This book examines the very basis of the doctor-patient relationship which is often taken for granted—the willingness of the patient to come to the healer.

---

* Since *all* the persons we have studied applied to a psychiatric facility (regardless of the professional affiliation of the person who actually did the intake or treatment), and since the overwhelming number of persons we studied who had prior treatment had been treated by a psychiatrist, this book generally follows popular usage and calls psychotherapists "psychiatrists," except when it is obviously inappropriate. It should be noted, however, that not all psychiatrists practice psychotherapy, and not all psychotherapists have been trained as psychiatrists. For a brief explanation of the differences between psychiatrists, psychologists, psychoanalysts, social workers, and clergymen, see footnote 7.

Why should better educated people in the United States seek psychiatric help? Are they more neurotic than others? For that matter, why should anyone go? Though psychoanalysis was developed as a technique for aiding middle-class neurotics,[8] contemporary community mental health centers offer some form of psychotherapy to all classes. For the psychotherapy movement aims not only to re-educate the intelligentsia but also to give insight to the masses. Re-education and insight available through psychotherapy require as a precondition that the potential patient, no matter what his background, recognize his need and be willing to endure an expenditure of time, money, and psychic pain. To the psychotherapist with his medical model firmly in mind, there seems to be only one logical reason for entering psychotherapy: people do so because they are "sick" and need treatment.

The distinguished psychoanalyst Lawrence S. Kubie is one of the few who has written on this topic.

> The so-called "neurotic" among adults is merely one in whom there are . . . those crystallized neurotic states which we call the psychoneuroses. These are self-diagnosing. Their recognition requires no skill or subtlety. Indeed, such patients come to us without urging, telling us that they have fears, depressions, compulsions, obsessions, etc. With few exceptions they seek help on their own initiative for the relief of their painful symptoms. . . . The cultural tolerance for overt neurotic symptoms may vary widely in different settings, as will the cultural tolerance for those personality quirks which manifest in concealed ways the subtle influence of the neurotic process. Therefore, culture is one of the forces which determine if and when a patient will look upon himself as ill or at least as needing help and whether he will seek help. Ultimately, however, what determines a patient's attitude toward his own neurotic process and neurotic symptoms is the amount of pain these cause him.[9]

This statement is ambiguous, however. Symptoms are viewed as automatically self-diagnosing and yet also dependent on "culture." In the end, just how "sick" the patient feels determines whether or not he will seek help, so that the ultimate answer remains: people go to psychiatrists because they feel sick.

But the fact is that a great many people who feel sick do not seek treatment. About 5 per cent of a national sample of American adults said they worried all the time.[10] This surely means that they feel "pain." Yet of these, less than one-quarter said they had actually used *some* form of professional help—usually not a psychiatrist. Another eighth of those who were worried all the time admitted that they *could* have used professional help. The rest did not want help at all from any professional source. Almost one-fifth of the entire sample said they had feelings of an impending nervous breakdown. This too seems to be an experience of psychic pain. Yet, of these, less than one-third actually sought professional help. Only a small part of the iceberg shows.

Perhaps the judgment of psychiatrists themselves should be introduced as evidence that even "sick" people fail to seek the help they need. A sample of midtown Manhattan was interviewed with a wide battery of questions about personal problems and emotional well-being. These protocols were then independently evaluated by two psychiatrists. They estimated that about one-quarter of the population was psychiatrically impaired. But only a little over one-quarter of those judged impaired had ever been to a psychotherapist.[11] In comparison, fewer than one out of ten who were judged *not* impaired went to a psychiatrist or psychologist. Although being "sick" thus accounts for some of the difference between those who went to a therapist and those who did not, there is obviously much more to the story.

What, then, does explain the decision to seek psychiatric help? This is the basic problem with which we are here concerned. In the first place, there is not one decision to go to a psychiatrist, there are many. Though not all people decide these matters in exactly the same sequence, there are several stages in the process of going to a psychiatrist: realizing a problem, consulting with relatives and friends, deciding upon the type of healer (minister, palm reader, doctor, or psychiatrist or other psychotherapist), and finally choosing an individual practitioner. Different factors affect each stage. To be sure, the first requirement for admission to a psychiatrist is having a "problem" and thus almost everybody who goes to a psychiatrist must decide that he has something the psychiatrist can "fix." In this sense, everybody who goes to a psychiatrist is "sick." Though all professionals believe that the client has an incorrect formulation of his problem, the stand taken by psychotherapists deserves further examination. One of Karen Horney's pupils reports Miss Horney's views of the initial psychiatric interview:

> The reasons the patient gives for coming to the initial interview may be quite different [from the deeper reasons]. His real reasons for coming may not always be clear to him, even after a year or two of analysis. Most patients come into analysis at a time of acute disturbance, although they may give a history of chronic suffering.[12]

In addition, "other patients may come for advice about others," though this may be only the surface desire. And "patients come for advice about analysis in general when they actually want advice about themselves." Finally, "even though there seems to be no real incentive, the patient is in the office for *some* reason. . . ."

There are several themes in this account. First, problems come in layers, ranging from the most immediate to the most basic and long-standing. Second, the patient is unlikely to present the "right" problem.

Third, no matter what the patient says, he must have some problem, that is, he is likely to be "sick." The import of these themes is that the patient's formulation of his "ticket of admission" is to be ignored or at least does not present serious data for understanding the reasons why he came. Yet a patient does have to give *some* account of his presence in the office. At the very least, then, some people come to psychotherapists while others do not because some people can formulate a "problem" they feel appropriate to take to a psychotherapist and about which they can talk; others either cannot condense their experience into a "problem," or do not feel free enough to talk about it, or cannot find a connection between their "problem" and a psychotherapist. For example, if I should feel a pain in my jaw, I might decide it was a toothache and go to a dentist. Others might not even notice such pain or, if they did, might be afraid to go to a dentist. In any case, upon my arrival at the dentist's office he might tell me that what is really wrong is that my sinus is inflamed. I came to the dentist for the "wrong" reasons. Nonetheless, anyone who wanted to know why I had gone to the dentist had at least better find out that I thought I had a toothache, that I think toothaches are something dentists can "fix," and that I knew how to find a dentist. At the level of "problems," then, the issue for research is what kinds of people formulate what kinds of problems— for no problem, no psychotherapist! Presenting problems are now seen not as "rationalizations" or the "wrong" problem or not the "real" problem but as indicators reflecting the complex process of the decision to seek psychiatric care.

✹ *Social Forces and Presenting Problems*

People do not go to psychiatrists because they are "really sick." They go because they *think* they are sick, and even this does not fully explain their action. Holding in abeyance the other factors which explain going to a psychiatrist, the question now becomes why do some people feel that they have problems suitable for psychiatric help, for we can assume that everyone has the *potential* to feel emotional distress. In particular, what is the *process* through which these problems come to the attention of people who go to a psychiatrist? Why do different people present different problems? A study of the differences between applicants for therapy affords us some perspective on the social forces that produce the chainlike development of problems. First there is stress, then the reaction to stress, and then the conceptualization of the reaction. In addition, the problems of people who go to psychotherapists are affected by everything that happens to them during the referral process. This chain suggests that we refine the question of why different people eventually present different problems by breaking it down into five separate but related questions:

Do people present different problems because they are under different pressures?

Do people present different problems because they have different socially and culturally defined ways of reacting to pressure?

Do people present different problems because they have different ways of expressing their feelings and emotions which result from their reaction to pressure?

Do people present different problems because they are differently affected by the recruitment and referral processes that led to the psychotherapist's office?

Do people present different problems because they have differing expectations of what therapists want to hear?

Beneath all these issues is the question of why some problems appear so devastating to some people that they must take them to a psychotherapist. In our culture there are basically two reactions people can have to a problem. In the first reaction—which for lack of a better name I shall call a Marxian reaction—one blames the situation or the environment: "The reason I cannot advance in my job is that the employer is prejudiced." The second type of reaction is Freudian: "The reason I cannot advance in my job is that I am inadequate to the task." One must see problems in some Freudian manner before they become fit material to take to a psychotherapist. Our contention is that social position has a good deal to do with the attitude of people to all these issues.[13]

This point will become clearer if we get down to some concrete cases. Here are two typical applicants for therapy, both of whom present some sort of physical symptom as a reason for seeking help, but who have strikingly different social positions.[14]

A 24-year-old single woman applied to a psychoanalytic clinic. She is now working as a social worker but will go back for her second year of social work school in the Fall. She comes from a lower-middle-class Jewish family, with whom she still lives in Brooklyn.

She is fairly well read in psychoanalytic theory. She had also received a fair amount of psychotherapy before applying, but she has not been in treatment for many years. She has discussed her problem with friends but was referred to this clinic by her social work supervisor during a discussion of her general problems. She is obviously quite sophisticated about therapy.

In answer to our questionnaire, she wrote as follows (our questions are italicized):

Please write a general description of your problem.

"Lack of confidence in myself. Free-floating anxiety. Psychosomatic symptoms."

What seem to be the main things about your problem that are bothering you now? Please list them in order of their importance to you.

"1. Lack of confidence in myself. Feeling that I am a failure.

2. Being frightened all the time but not being able to put my finger on exactly what bothers me.

3. Stomach pains."

How did you first notice the problem or become aware of it? What was it like then? When did it occur? Write a brief description.

"I first noticed this problem many years ago. I can't really recall exactly when I first became aware of it. I do know that as a child I was terribly frightened and was afraid to leave my mother's side. I used to be afraid of going to school and would vomit every morning before leaving the house."

The following case is quite different, although the man also presents a physical symptom and some problems with his job.

A 63-year-old airplane mechanic applied to a psychiatric clinic in a general hospital. He was born in Cuba, and his father was a captain in a South American army. He had about 10 or 12 years of schooling in South America. He is married and has three daughters who live at home; all are registered nurses.

In the beginning of the interview he was asked how he had come to go to the clinic.

"I happened to come for a physical checkup.. He said [the examining physician] that he was going to send me to the nervous doctor. [This had occurred just half an hour before. He had then briefly seen one of the psychiatrists in the distributing clinic who diagnosed him as having a reactive depression.] I came for a physical. I have trouble with my heart. I lose my voice."

What, briefly, seem to be the main problems that brought you here?

"The only problem was at work—I'm going to try to get an easy job. I was sick on Friday. I went to the doctor there and they said to go to a clinic."

Anything else?

"I had bronchitis six weeks ago."

He was then asked whether any of the problem areas read off from a check list bothered him. In addition to those problems already mentioned he added that his arm hurts, from time to time, that he suffers from fatigue, that he works too hard, that he fights with his sisters because "they tell me to go to a psychiatrist," that "I get disgusted and unhappy," that "I want to do things on my own—I'm too independent," and that "lately about a year ago I can't stay with my wife [cannot complete intercourse], but that don't worry me."

Which of these problems you have mentioned do you now consider the most important? Which is the next most important?

"I don't know. I don't worry about anything. Well . . . First, to stay on the job I have. A lot of fellows my age—they drop out because they feel sick. Second, to settle the social security."

How did you first come to decide that your problem was something you ought to think about seriously?

"I've been reading [newspapers and magazines. He can't remember any particular article.] Sometimes mental problems cause physical problems."

Later he was asked whether anyone noticed his problem or mentioned it to him without his first mentioning it. His daughters, sisters, and wife had urged him to see a psychiatrist for the last two years. His wife,

"She's a good woman, she says take it easy. She says . . . go see the doctor. [She says] she can't rest at nighttime because I jump—that I should go to the clinic."

As for his daughters and sisters,

"They are right. They see I need a psychiatrist. I take the dishes and I throw them. If I tell her [a daughter] to wash the dishes before she watches television and she doesn't . . . They don't like the way I want things to be done."

However, when presented with a check list and asked, *Which of the following describe how you feel about the cause of your problem,* he chose the alternative which was phrased, *If I could only change my surroundings or the situation I find myself in, everything would be all right.* He commented,

"Even tne same plant but different work . . . I think it's because I find that the kind of work I'm doing is too hard. I want to avoid heart trouble."

When asked whether he knew others with similar problems, he said, "Friends who are unhappy on the job."

What do they do about it?

"They change jobs."

While a clinician might approach these cases in one fashion, here is the sociological reaction to them. Different social structures can create different problems for their participants because these social structures subject them to different pressures. The nature of the airplane mechanic's job together with his age may place a considerable strain on his physical capabilities. In the other case, the strains of supervision of a beginning caseworker also lead to anxieties.

Given the same social pressures, there are different socially and culturally structured ways of reacting to them. The amount of straw that will break a camel's back depends on the type of camel, as well as on the kind of straw. The ambitious social worker does not wish to withdraw from her job, but the airplane mechanic does and hopes only for social security. Their actual physical symptoms are different, too. The girl has a disorder which she associates with anxiety, while the skilled worker has a potential "heart" condition which he believes to be connected with heavy manual labor. He constantly returns to the idea that he is physically ill, whereas the girl places her physical symptoms last on the list. So, the type of problem or situation that represents the "last straw" is likely to be different for different types of persons, though in both cases physical symptoms seem "legitimate" ways of reacting to pressure. The girl notes that she has done this before as a child. The man probably also has previously had this pattern. And both cultures—Jewish and Latin American—allow for anxiety to be translated into physical spheres.

Persons in dissimilar social positions may have different ways of verbally expressing their feelings or problems. The girl's sophistication is evident. She doesn't claim to have a "real" stomach disorder. She reports "psychosomatic symptoms." There is considerable evidence from the man's presentation of himself that he does suspect that his physical illnesses may not be the underlying cause of his difficulties. He may even perceive the sham in his pretense of applying only for a physical check-up. But aside from his obvious motivation—not to admit fully to this self-deception—he does not have an adequate conceptual framework in which to express the emotional nature of his difficulties: "I take the dishes and I throw them."

The socially structured pattern of recruitment to psychotherapy may affect the type of problems that actually appear on the psychotherapists' doorstep. This process of recruitment involves the gamut of selective referral processes and personal influences which constitute the subject matter of this book. The social worker's referral network includes both professionals and friends likely to emphasize the emotional aspects of her problem. They referred her to a psychoanalytic clinic. On the other hand, the airplane mechanic's network is mainly composed of persons knowledgeable about medicine rather than psychiatry. Only upon his arrival at the hospital is the switch from physical medicine to psychotherapy actually made. Working-class persons such as the airplane mechanic are likely to go to psychotherapists only if they have a physical symptom or pain that other doctors cannot cure. Professionals such as the social worker may go to psychotherapists for a variety of problems. Hence, among those who finally do come to psychotherapists, working-class persons more frequently present physical symptoms than do professional applicants who are better able to articulate their underlying emotional problems.

Persons in different social positions may have different expectations of what psychotherapy is like and what psychotherapists want to hear. The airplane mechanic is evidently afraid of psychiatry and feels more comfortable if he can say to himself that he is really going to the clinic because he is physically ill. His physical reaction is more acceptable not only to him but, he feels, to others as well: "A lot of people are ignorant—they think you're getting crazy or something like that [if you go to a psychiatrist]." On the other hand, the social worker "knows" that she had better not make too much of her physical symptoms. In her view, psychotherapists are interested in hearing about emotional problems, such as anxiety and insecurity. Besides, she may feel that only those with "irrational defenses" present physical symptoms. In both cases, an image of what psychotherapy might be like guides the formulation of the problem to be brought to the psychotherapist. In so doing, these applicants seek to protect their self-concept. The girl does not wish to appear unsophisticated. The man does not wish to appear "crazy."

Finally, although both applicants could have taken a Marxian position and blamed their work situation for their problems—and therefore tried to change that situation—only the airplane mechanic considered this. But neither the mechanic nor the social worker held to a Marxian position. What makes them see the flaw within themselves? Most probably, the influence of significant others is crucial—the social worker's milieu in general and her supervisor in particular, and the mechanic's quite forceful sisters.

❀ How People with Problems Become Psychiatric Patients

In studying why people who go to psychiatrists think they have problems, we must study the pressures upon them, the various forces that impel them to recognize and express their problems, and the circumstances that lead them to feel that their problems should be taken to a psychotherapist. The formulation of presenting problems represents both the beginning and the end of a long process of pressure, reaction, expression, referral, and anticipation. The decision to go to a psychiatrist consists of four separate but related stages: realization of a problem, discussion of the problem with friends and relatives, choice of the type of professional healer to attend (such as a doctor, a psychiatrist, a psychologist, or a faith healer), and selection of a particular practitioner. These stages may be repeated a number of times, especially if a person goes to more than one professional.

All but the first stage in this decision not only affect the way patients view their problems but also have an independent effect on their motivation. In both the cases just reviewed, there was informal consultation with friends and relatives. What sorts of persons engage in such consultation, and is it at their own behest or do others intervene to tell them they are "crazy"? There may be a variety of functions served by lay consultation. Do laymen really tell potential applicants for psychotherapy something new—do they exercise strong social control and force people to recognize their illness or do they merely reinforce and confirm what the potential patient already knows? In the case of the social worker, confirmation was the chief function of lay intervention; in the case of the mechanic, his relatives pointed out something new that he had not previously understood. In other words, how crucial is lay intervention in the formulation of a problem?

Realization of a problem is only half the battle. One must then decide that other laymen or oneself cannot help and that professional help must be sought. Most persons who apply for psychotherapy have made this decision not once but several times. Almost half have previously visited nonpsychiatrist physicians, and a majority of those applying to psychiatric clinics have previously talked to other psychotherapists, mostly to psychiatrists. Nothing so annoys a professional as having a patient "shop" from one professional to another. The shoppers are said to be poor patients, "crocks," or bargain hunters. Are they, really? Previous attempts to get help may be necessary "training" for psychotherapy, or merely painful concomitants of our inefficient system of recruiting patients. Mistakes or not, past decisions in any case have an important impact on current choices. In short, we need an assessment of the whole process of "shopping."

The number of different types of professionals who are ready and willing to counsel disturbed persons is far larger than most medically oriented persons realize. Besides ministers, physicians, psychiatrists, psychologists, and social workers who might practice psychotherapy there are faith healers, Christian Science practitioners, theosophists, chiropractors, and even bartenders. Not a few people consult the police as their first source for professional mental health advice. How do applicants for psychotherapy view these many alternatives? In particular, what is their "map" of the professions? Ministers could be seen as more like faith healers and palm readers or they could be associated with the liberal professions such as law or medicine. Psychiatrists might be seen as unique and like no other profession or they might be seen as allied with medicine or even to have some similarity to bartenders. The way people contemplating getting help for their problems view the professions must in part determine which profession they eventually select.

Finally, when it comes to the choice of an individual practitioner or therapist, applicants for psychotherapy face a unique problem. One of the striking characteristics of psychiatry is that it is a relatively invisible profession. All medical specialties are relatively distant from potential clients, but psychiatry is in a far more remote position. More than half of New York City's adult population can give the name of a surgeon when asked for one, but only 15 per cent can name a psychiatrist[15] and only 6 per cent can name a psychologist; 25 per cent could name a mental health clinic but most named Bellevue—a place whose image in New York City is not too different from that of Bethlehem ("Bedlam") in London of two hundred years ago. So the first problem for a person once he decides to go to a psychiatrist or other psychotherapist is to find one! In fact, the problem is sufficiently severe that merely accidentally hearing about a psychiatrist who sounds reliable is often sufficient to trigger the final decision to go.

Given the fact that some effort must be expended to find a therapist, how do people find one? What is the difference between those who undertake a systematic search for the names of psychiatrists and psychiatric clinics and those who wait until a name falls into their laps? And once they discover the name of a psychiatrist, psychiatric clinic, or other psychotherapist, how do prospective applicants rate or evaluate them? What criteria do they have in mind? What do they generally expect from therapy? Do most people view it as advice-giving on the part of the therapist or do they expect that they themselves will have to take an active part in the treatment? And finally, how long do they think it will take? These and other questions become immediately relevant once going to a psychotherapist is viewed as problematic rather than as an automatic result of illness.

Did he fall or was he pushed is the question most people ask when they hear that someone is going to a psychiatrist. Do people eventually go to a psychiatrist mainly because they are forced into it or do they go because they are really motivated to do so? This question has a two-part answer because there is a difference between being told that one has emotional problems and being told to go to a psychiatrist or to "get some help." It is quite possible for personal influence to be of paramount importance at one stage of the decision but not at another. And this brings up the matter of "referral." Who refers people to psychiatrists or to other psychotherapists? Are some channels preferred by some types of persons while others utilize quite different sources? These questions cannot be answered by the usual referral statistics kept by psychiatrists and psychiatric clinics, for various influences can intervene at any stage of the decision process. A physician may have told a patient that he has emotional problems, but a friend may have actually given him the name of a psychiatrist or other therapist. Who then has made the "referral"? All statistics kept by psychiatrists include the category of "self-referral." Yet unless a patient looks up the name of the psychiatrist in a directory, he cannot be "self-referred," for some *person* must have told him about the psychiatrist. Though the proportion usually listed by psychiatrists and psychiatric clinics as self-referred is fairly large, very few who seek help ever look up names in a directory. (Only 1 per cent of New York City's population would do so if they needed help,[16] only 15 per cent of our sample of applicants actually tried this, and only 2 per cent got the name of their current choice from such a service.) The concept of "self-referral" therefore confuses the *amount* of pressure placed upon a person to go to a psychiatrist with the *source* of the pressure. Only a thorough unraveling of the entire decision process can determine the role of other people in the final act of going to a psychiatrist.

❁ *Social Circles and Self-Concept*

Dividing the decision to go to a psychotherapist or psychiatrist into the stages of realizing a problem, consulting with friends and relatives, selecting a type of profession, and choosing an individual practitioner may give the impression that the decision is fragmented, a series of static steps. Though each stage may indeed involve different problems for the individual contemplating psychotherapy, two very important themes link each stage to the next.

First, the entire decision is a learning process, as are all depth decisions such as marriage, choosing a career, getting divorced, undertaking an operation, and so on.[17] The person who decided to go to a psychotherapist is not the same person after the decision that he was before. Though buying soap does not change a person's self-concept, going to a psychotherapist, even if no treatment at all takes place, changes a person's self-concept from that of a person who is by and large self-sufficient to that of a person who requires professional help to get through life. The very process of deciding to go to a psychiatrist or psychotherapist is "therapeutic" and much that must ultimately change as a result of therapy already begins to change during the decision to seek help.

Second, changing one's self-concept is very difficult and much help is needed. This help comes not from one or two personal influencers, though such help is certainly important, but from an entire circle of influencers—whom we call the "Friends and Supporters of Psychotherapy." This mythical but nonetheless very real social organization consists of a loose social circle of people knowledgeable about and interested in psychotherapy. Its structure intervenes at every point in the process of deciding to go to a psychotherapist, and its influence is more readily measurable than the inner and more subtle changes in individual self-concept. Persons affiliated with the Friends and Supporters of Psychotherapy have different problems from others; they are more likely to be supported than coerced into realizing they do have problems.

They also tend to receive different kinds of advice. They read different books about therapy, and even go about finding therapists in ways quite different from those not associated with the Friends and Supporters of Psychotherapy. In fact, "membership" in this circle is in many ways equivalent to considerable previous experience in psychotherapy in preparing applicants for further treatment. Other social position factors are of course also important, but none, not even level of education, transcends this social circle membership. For social circles are a basic phenomenon of modern urban life. Every member of a circle does not necessarily know every other member, but he may know a person who knows another person, who in turn knows him. One of the favorite party games in metropolitan areas is to ask a new face, "Do you know Mr. Jones?" If he does know Mr. Jones then the stranger is transformed into an acquaintance, for his location in a network of social circles is related to one's own position. Circles are important in "society," in the art and literary world, in science, in sports, and even in medicine. Freud, living in Vienna, a city which might be said to have invented the modern urban circle, knew this well enough when he gathered a group about him who were interested in psychoanalysis. Later this group became more formal, but psychoanalysis retained a social as well as a scientific base. Many of our findings, then, can be interpreted and explained in terms of the influence of an entire set of persons upon an individual who is attempting to change his basic self.

Despite its early development as a method of treating individuals, psychotherapy is not a contract exclusively between an individual patient and a healer; nor are families and social circles the only groups involved. Each person who applies for psychiatric treatment is a potential troublemaker for society: he is a deviant. The failure of the mentally ill to meet society's standards is obvious for the overtly psychotic. But the failure of the less severely disturbed to meet their own standards builds a reservoir of discontent which if left unrelieved and unattended can lead to serious social malaise. So the entire process of psychotherapy and the decision to apply for psychiatric treatment is not a matter of indifference to society. In fact, public expenditures for mental patients are about a billion dollars a year in the United States and are rapidly increasing.[18] This book will therefore not only consider the acts of individuals in undertaking psychotherapy but will also examine the structure of facilities for outpatient care and will consider the impact of the Friends and Supporters of Psychotherapy upon this structure. Despite the self-filtering of applicants, the outpatient system does not hang together very well: the requirements of community mental health and the needs of the Friends and Supporters of Psychotherapy are at odds, and neither is well served by the requirements for training new psychotherapists.

✿ How to Unravel Decisions

Now that the goals of the study are clear, where can one get evidence to bear on the issues? The best source is people who have actually applied for psychotherapy. By means of questionnaires, interviews, and clinic records, we have collected data on 1,452 applicants to ten New York City psychiatric clinics. A more complete account of our methods for gathering data is found in the next chapter. Here we will discuss some basic issues in the strategy of data-collection: why we studied applicants only, why clinics, and why New York City.

First, why not compare applicants to those who did not go to psychiatrists? Indeed, such comparisons can be valuable, and we have already cited some evidence about the population at large. But there are serious difficulties in attempting a comparative study of those who do and those who do not go to psychiatrists. By no means the least important obstacle is the very small number of persons who have been to psychotherapists that turns up in a net designed to catch a representative sample of an entire population.[19] The sheer infrequency with which psychiatric help is sought bars us from comparing, on a sound statistical basis, those who go with those who do not go to psychiatrists. For no amount of careful "matching" of those who do with some other sample of those who do not go to a therapist is entirely satisfactory. Suppose we get a list of names of people who go to psychiatrists and then ascertain their level of education. We then "match" them with a sample chosen in such a way that both groups have the same level of education. Have we not thrown out the baby with the bath? One of the main differences between those who go and those who do not go to psychiatrists is their level of education! Or suppose we match them on the basis of having similar problems. Here again we eliminate by this matching procedure a great deal of that which we wish to study. Finally, since we are interested in the very *process* of deciding to go to psychiatrists, questions pertaining to this process can be reasonably asked only of those who have actually undertaken it. Of those who have never even considered going to a psychiatrist it is obviously impossible to ask why they delayed going!

The basic data which can reveal why people go to psychiatrists must come from applicants themselves. For it is their *subjective* feelings that are involved in understanding the process. Even if the reasons they give are the "wrong" reasons, they are still extremely important, for without the reasons that people give to themselves and to others they cannot take the crucial step of going to a therapist. Unless they can find some formula to connect themselves with psychotherapy they cannot make the final step. This does not mean that all the information they give us is without foundation in reality, but that even if it is not well founded it is important. Or at least this is what Freud tried to teach us when he explained that everything a person says, even his slips of the tongue, has some meaning.

The method we use to collect and analyze much of the data is called "reason analysis," a system for analyzing the causes of action. A system and method are necessary, for it is easy to see that without careful planning, the analysis of subjective reasons could produce quite unreliable data.[20] Essentially, the idea is to construct in advance of data collection an "accounting scheme" that lists all the factors which, for the purposes of any one investigation, may be said to propel or inhibit a person from taking a particular action. Because the decision to undertake psychotherapy is composed of four different decisions (realizing a problem, consulting laymen, choosing a type of healer, and selecting an individual practitioner), a separate accounting scheme had to be constructed for each stage. A theory of action must guide the researcher's decision as to what he should include in the accounting scheme, for anything not included to begin with cannot later be analyzed. And some limitation on factors is essential if only to avoid an infinite causal regression.

Our selection of factors was guided by the considerations given in this chapter and by Parsons' "action frame of reference."[21] For each of the four decisions, information was obtained on the applicant's cognitive orientation—what he saw, knew, and had information about; his cathectic orientation—the amount and nature of the emotional energy he invested in a situation; and his valuational orientation—the weight he assigned to the various factors he saw and felt. In addition, information was obtained about the timing of each step and the way two key aspects of the situation—media and personal influence—impinged upon the decider. A good deal of background information about the applicant himself was also secured. We mention all this here not because the accounting scheme and the theory intrude upon the actual analysis of the data but because they are largely hidden.

❀ New York City Clinics as a Research Site

Because we want to talk about psychotherapy in general, why study clinics? This is mainly dictated by convenience. Good reason analysis must be undertaken with people who have been "caught in the act." The best way to discover the reasons why a person entered psychotherapy is *not* to ask him about it *after* he has already started with a given therapist but *directly at the time he is applying for treatment.* As we explain in greater detail in Chapter 2 on data-gathering, only clinics can supply a convenient stream of applicants who can be interviewed or be sent questionnaires. Psychotherapists' records simply are insufficient for the purposes of a sophisticated reason analysis, as the therapists are interested in treatment, not research into the social factors leading people to come to their offices. It is true that studying only clinic patients limits the generality of what we have to say, but not as much as it might appear. Five of the clinics in our study are psychoanalytic clinics connected with institutes for training psychoanalysts. These clinics attempt to replicate the conditions of private practice as much as they can. In fact, they draw from the same pool of patients as do private therapists. Most of their applicants have already been to at least one *private* psychotherapist, and these patients tend to have educational attainments and occupational characteristics similar to those of private patients. Since the clinics have scaled fees, their applicants do tend to be less wealthy than those in private treatment. But many fairly well-to-do people apply to clinics for a variety of reasons, including inability to find a reliable private therapist. The clinics do not generally *accept* such persons, preferring to refer them to private sources. Nevertheless, they are found in our sample of *applicants*. Analysis of the demographic characteristics of analytic clinic applicants does show that they tend to be younger members (and hence not as wealthy) of the *same* social groups that comprise the bulk of private analytic patients.

There are as many gains from a study of clinic patients as there are losses. A far wider range of patients can be studied. We have collected data on very poor patients who are completely unsophisticated about psychotherapy as well as on ultra-knowledgeable residents in psychiatry. We have religious Protestant White Anglo-Saxons and atheistic East European Jews. Because our clinics are of such varying nature (ranging from general hospital clinics, to a religio-psychiatric clinic a majority of whose therapists are ministers, to analytic clinics connected with major psychoanalytic institutes), we can extrapolate from our findings applications to community mental health problems in general, and so need not confine our analysis to the rather special case of private practice with upper-middle-class, not very sick patients.

New York City is special in far too many ways even to begin to enumerate. Because it is the capital of psychotherapy in the United States, if not of the world, phenomena that might be latent in other communities are prominent in New York City. A student of "bums" observed in the book *Subways Are for Sleeping* (later turned into a not very successful musical) that "New York attracts the most talented people in the world in the arts and professions. It also attracts them in other fields. Even the bums are talented."[22] One might add, so are the psychiatric patients, and their therapists. Certainly there are more of both in New York. In most communities there are a few psychotherapists and one mental health clinic, if there are any facilities at all. New York City had 61 adult outpatient clinics open to the general public around the time we gathered our data (1960), or about one clinic per 125,000 of the population. And New York City has more psychotherapists than has any city anywhere else in the world. There are about 3,550 physicians who practice as psychiatrists in New York City, of whom close to 2,000 are members of the American Psychiatric Association, and almost 300 are members of the American Psychoanalytic Association. There are also about 1,000 clinical psychologists and about 900 social workers who are employed in a psychiatric setting. Finally, though exact statistics are not available, there are also more members of the "Friends and Supporters of Psychotherapy" in New York City than anywhere else; and they create so large a demand for treatment that the facilities provided are none too numerous. In fact, all the clinics have long waiting lists and only about one in ten applicants can get more than ten sessions of therapy.

Size has consequences besides mere proliferation of facilities. Density of population or of organizations leads to a division of labor, either among people or among organizations. Just about every movement in psychotherapy is represented among the therapists in New York. Even the clinics tend to specialize in different types of therapies and different types of patients. There are clinics for working-class people and others for middle-class people and there are some for Adlerians and others for Freudians. The "magic" of the referral system generally sends people along to the clinic which best matches them. In communities that have only one or two clinics and only a few private therapists this process of self-selection cannot operate, and therefore the entire referral system is less visible and its "magic" harder to account for. There is one curious outcome of heterogeneity of facilities, however. The patients select the clinics, rather than the clinics the patients. Because applicants to the different types of clinics are already self-selected, and therefore within any one clinic fairly homogeneous, there is barely a relationship in most New York clinics between the social characteristics of patients or their presenting problems and their selection for treatment. This is not true of communities in which there are only a few clinics. In smaller communities, therapists tend to select patients who have middle-class characteristics. In New York City, however, there is little difference in most clinics between patients accepted and those rejected—at least in terms of their social characteristics.[23]

The complexity of New York City permits many problems to be explored that will only begin to appear in the psychiatric treatment systems of other communities. New York City has been a forerunner in the psychotherapy movement, and a study of the way its outpatient system operates can tell a great deal about what may happen in the rest of the United States over the next ten years.

The book is divided into five parts. The first part presents the cast of characters and devotes one chapter to the process of research and the researchers, another to the clinics and their patients, and a third to the Friends and Supporters of Psychotherapy. Once the actors have been introduced, the remaining parts of the book examine in detail the four stages of deciding to seek psychotherapy. Part Two discusses the first stage—the discovery of problems. After a chapter explaining how to describe and analyze problems from a sociological point of view and how they relate to the type of clinic to which patients apply, a chapter follows which shows why traditional psychiatric diagnoses are not related to the decision to undertake psychotherapy. The last chapter in Part Two shows how problems relate to an applicant's social position as well as to his knowledge about psychotherapy and suggests which problems are most likely to lead a person to seek psychotherapy. Part Three discusses several intermediate stages in the decision. Consultation with laymen about problems generally follows when a person becomes aware of his problem, and so the first chapter of the section is concerned with the two functions of lay advice—support and control. The next two chapters deal with the several previous attempts to get professional help that most applicants to clinics have already made, and their images of the healing professions. Part Four covers the decision to seek help at the clinic where we gathered our data, perforce the last step for those who participated in our research. Aspects of this decision are analyzed in three separate chapters. First comes the search for information and the acquisition of knowledge about clinics and other sources of treatment. Then comes an evaluation of the qualities of clinics and anticipation and evaluation of therapy itself. The personal influence of others is the last step in the process for many applicants. Part Five discusses the general implications for community mental health of our analyses of clinic structure and individual decision-making.

NOTES

1. Eighty-eighth Congress, 1st Session, House of Representatives Document No. 58, Message from the President of the United States Relative to Mental Illness and Mental Retardation.
2. Joint Commission on Mental Illness and Health, *Action for Mental Health* (New York: Basic Books, 1961), Table 2, p. 15.
3. U.S. Department of Health, Education and Welfare, Public Health Service, *Health Manpower Source Book, Section 14, Medical Specialists*, Public Health Service Publication Number 263 (1962), p. 11.

4. Paul V. Lemkau and Guido M. Crocetti, "An Urban Population's Opinion and Knowledge about Mental Illness," *The American Journal of Psychiatry* (February 1962), 118 : 8.
5. Gerald Gurin, Joseph Veroff, and Sheila Feld, *Americans View Their Mental Health* (New York: Basic Books, 1960), p. 343.
6. Alfred Kazin, "The Language of Pundits," in his *Contemporaries* (New York: Knopf, 1961).
7. Throughout this book, *psychotherapy* will be used to denote any form of "talking" treatment given by a professional who has studied with those who have been influenced by Freud and his intellectual descendants, whether or not he later denounced or approved them. The professionals in this field are generally trained as psychoanalysts, psychiatrists, psychologists, social workers, or clergymen, all of whom may be called *psychotherapist* when operating within this framework.

The following is a brief summary of the various professions that practice psychotherapy:

Psychiatrists are physicians. As such, they have been graduated from medical school, completed an internship in a hospital, and have undertaken a residency in some psychiatric facility. Of the almost 14,000 physicians in the United States who say they are engaged in the full-time practice of psychiatry, about 40 per cent are certified by the American Board of Psychiatry and Neurology (U.S. Department of Health, Education, and Welfare, Public Health Service, *op. cit.*, p. 164).

Only a few psychiatrists are also *psychoanalysts*. A psychoanalyst has attended an institute which teaches psychoanalytic theory and technique to physicians who have completed a residency in psychiatry. Only 4 per cent of those physicians who say they practice full-time psychiatry also say they are members of the American Psychoanalytic Association, the only organization in the United States affiliated with the International Psychoanalytic Association, founded by Sigmund Freud. Some psychoanalysts belong to other societies, but none of these has more than 500 physicians as members (*Health Manpower Source Book*, p. 164). There is no legal bar, however, to any psychiatrist calling himself a psychoanalyst, whether he belongs to the American Psychoanalytic Association, to any other psychoanalytic association, or to none.

Although there are 20,000 members of the American Psychological Association, of whom about one-third are engaged in clinical service of one kind or another, only 3,000 are members of the Division of Clinical Psychology, the only group whose members have been specifically trained to deal with mental patients. *Psychologists* have at least a bachelor's degree, and 60 per cent also have a Ph.D. Just as a medical training emphasizes the general principles of medicine without necessarily delving very deeply into problems of the mentally disturbed, so a training in psychology emphasizes the general principles of both animal and human complex neurological functions (sometimes called mental functions), without necessarily dealing with "abnormal psychology." Many states now require a person to have a license if he wishes to call himself a psychologist, just as a person must have a license to call himself a doctor of medicine. Generally, a licensed psychologist must have a Ph.D., some supervised postdoctoral experience, and have passed an examination. Some psychologists have also attended a psychoanalytic institute (not one affiliated with the American Psychoanalytic Association, which does not allow psychologists to practice psychoanalysis) and call themselves psychoanalysts. Two-fifths of the clinical psychologists in private practice in New York City said they were graduated from a psychoanalytic or psychotherapeutic training institute or center (Report of the Subcommittee on Manpower of the New York City Regional Mental Health Planning Committee, October 1964, p. IV–22).

Of all the professionals dealing with mental outpatients, *social workers* are the only group whose majority are women. Because most social workers do not deal individually with the public but rather are employed by institutions and agencies, the field is not licensed. Although there were about 100,000 social workers in the United States in 1964, only about 7,200 worked in psychiatric settings (U.S. Department of Health, Education, and Welfare, Public Health Service, *Health Resources Statistics*, 1965, P.H.S. publication no. 1509, p. 142). Almost 20 per cent of New York City's 4,500 social workers work in a psychiatric setting, however (Subcommittee on Manpower, *op. cit.*, p. LV–35). Less than half of the social workers in the United States have had graduate training in social work, but almost all the psychiatric social workers hold at least a master's degree. An unknown number have had formal advanced training at a psychoanalytic or psychotherapeutic institute, and many have had a personal analysis.

Clergymen are the largest group of professionals in the United States, and the most frequently consulted about personal problems. Well over 6,000 ministers have been certified by the Council on Clinical Training as having completed a certified course of training and supervised practice in pastoral counseling. Several hundred of these are now primarily engaged in the private practice of psychotherapy (estimate by the staff of the Council on Clinical Training).

All these professions may practice psychotherapy or psychoanalysis, either in an institutional setting or in private practice, and regardless of background or training there are no legal barriers to any person's calling himself a psychotherapist or psychoanalyst. In fact, there are some famous "lay analysts" who have no advanced degree in medicine, psychology, or social work. A few even obtained training authorized by the International Psychoanalytic Association, although its American branch has always been opposed to the training of nonmedical personnel.

The difference between psychoanalysis and psychotherapy is a matter of considerable argument. Generally, psychoanalysis attempts to reconstruct a patient's personality, while psychotherapy goes into less depth and attempts to repair the damage without necessarily altering a person's basic personality. In traditional Freudian psychoanalysis, attention is mainly focused upon transference—the tendency of patients to attribute to the therapist the various characteristics of persons (especially parents) the patient has interacted with in the past. But since each school of psychoanalysis and psychotherapy defines "depth," "reconstruction," "transference," and "basic personality" in a somewhat different way, our definition is merely semantically correct. In any case, psychotherapy is the generic term with psychoanalysis as the special case.

Finally, it should be pointed out that many psychiatrists either do not practice psychotherapy as we have defined it or practice it quite infrequently. In fact, until after World War II, most training in psychiatry emphasized somatic therapies and patient management in institutional settings, rather than psychotherapy. British psychiatry, for example, has always had this emphasis, and many psychiatrists in the United States have been increasingly influenced by British methods as well as by other nonpsychotherapy developments of recent years.

8. Freud, "Further Recommendations in the Technique of Psychoanalysis," first published in *Zeitschrift*, Bd. 1, 1913: "Analytic therapy is almost unattainable for the poor, both for external and internal reasons."
9. Lawrence S. Kubie, "Social Forces and the Neurotic Process," in A. H. Leighton, J. A. Clausen, and R. N. Wilson (eds.), *Exploration in Social Psychiatry* (New York: Basic Books, 1957), pp. 83-84.
10. Gurin, *op. cit.*, Table 9.1.
11. Leo Srole, Thomas S. Langner, Stanley T. Michael, Marvin K. Opler, Thomas A. C. Rennie, *Mental Health in the Metropolis: The Midtown Manhattan Study* (New York: McGraw-Hill, 1962), p. 147. The over-all rate of going to psychotherapists in this sample was 13 per cent, over six times the rate of the national sample. This in part reflects the greater number of facilities in Manhattan as well as the greater psychiatric sophistication of its population. For all of New York City only a bit more than 4 per cent admit to ever seeing a psychiatrist or psychologist. (J. Elinson, E. Padilla, and M. E. Perkins, *The Public Image of Mental Health Services in New York City*, Columbia University School of Pub-

lic Health and The New York City Community Mental Health Board, 1965.)

12. Morton B. Cantor, "Karen Horney on the Psychoanalytic Technique: the Initial Interview," Part II, *American Journal of Psychoanalysis*, 17 (1957), 121-126.

13. For a review and critique of the literature on the use of health services in general, see Irwin M. Rosenstock, "Why People Use Health Services," *The Milbank Memorial Fund Quarterly*, 44 (July, 1966), Part 2, 94-124. For analyses of illness, symptoms, and medical care, see David Mechanic, "The Concept of Illness Behavior," *Journal of Chronic Disease*, 15 (1962), 189–194; J. D. Stoeckle et al., "On Going to See the Doctor, the Contributions of the Patient to the Decision to Seek Medical Aid," *Journal of Chronic Disease*, 16 (1963), 975–989; I. K. Zola, "Culture and Symptoms—An Analysis of Patients' Presenting Complaints," *American Sociological Review*, 31 (1966), 615–630; and the references in these works.

14. The first case is drawn from responses to one of our research questionnaires; the second represents responses to one of our research interviews. In both cases certain identifying facts have been changed.

15. Elinson, Padilla, and Perkins, *op. cit.*, Table 80.

16. *Ibid.*, Table 72.

17. For a discussion of stages in decision-making, see my "Reason Analysis," *Encyclopedia of the Social Sciences*, Second Edition (New York: Macmillan, 1968). A study of the process of seeking medical aid which uses reason analysis is Edward A. Suchman, "Stages of Illness and Medical Care," *Journal of Health and Human Behavior*, 6 (1965), 114–128.

18. *Action for Mental Health*, p. 291.

19. In a national sample only 42 of 2,450 persons had ever been to a psychiatrist. The New York City Midtown study uncovered 222 of 1,660, of whom only 40 were current patients. A study of all of New York City found 92 who had been to psychiatrists from a total sample of 2,118. Of these, only 16 said they were now seeing a psychiatrist.

20. See my "Reason Analysis," *op. cit.*, for bibliography and details of this method, which was first codified and developed by Paul F. Lazarsfeld.

21. Talcott Parsons and E. A. Shils, eds., *Toward a General Theory of Action* (Glencoe: The Free Press, 1951), esp. Chapter II.

22. Edmund G. Lowe, *Subways Are for Sleeping* (New York: Harcourt, Brace, 1957).

23. Part of this lack of discrimination may be traced to the fact that many of the metropolis' therapists have both read and absorbed the meaning of A. Hollingshead and F. C. Redlich, *Social Class and Mental Illness* (New York: Wiley, 1958), which showed the social class discrimination of clinics. For a complete analysis of acceptance and rejection of patients in our study, see Irma J. Lorenzen, *Acceptance or Rejection by Psychiatric Clinics*, unpublished Columbia University master's essay, 1967.

Data-Collection in a Psychiatric Setting

2

One lady to whom we sent a questionnaire wrote back:

Dear Doctors:
Thank you very much for sending me your questionnaire. I am returning it unanswered for the reason that I am not a member of the socioeconomic group for which it was apparently designed, . . .

The questionnaire presupposes a large degree of unsophistication on the part of the applicant: he must be able to think in terms of single causation, should feel that he belongs to a certain culture and so on. I am a 37-year-old intellectual of very complex experience and the language of this questionnaire suggests a kind of thinking too primitive to leave me anything but baffled and unable to find a relationship between it and me. . . .

Every study receives a few angry responses which, to protect their feelings, survey researchers call "crank" letters. This lady did, however, raise a host of issues about data-collection in such a sensitive area as psychiatry and psychotherapy. Though she could not be answered in the course of our study, she does deserve an answer in the form of this chapter on data-collection.

To begin with, there is only one good way of finding out why people go to psychiatrists, and that is by asking a fairly large number of persons why they did go. Records cannot be used for several reasons. Initial interviews conducted by psychiatrists and social workers are designed to yield information which aids diagnosis and prognosis. Motivation to go to a therapist is ascertained only to the extent that it is relevant to the goals of the initial or intake interview. Records of psychiatric screening interviews are quite variable and depend on the particular clinician as well as the style of a given clinic or hospital. Because of the purposes of the intake interview, the interviewer's opinion about a patient is entered in the records rather than the patient's own words describing why he came. A special inquiry must therefore be made about the patient's decision to enter therapy. To avoid contaminating the data by a patient's feelings, opinions and knowledge gained *after* beginning his therapy, the inquiry must be made at the time he first applies for treatment.

Who is to make this inquiry? Not clinicians, therapists, psychiatrists, psychologists or social workers—at least not in their clinical role. For the demands of the clinical role are different from the research role. Even should clinicians desire to gather sociological data, they owe their first responsibility to patients, not to impersonal research. Data collected to meet clinical needs are almost always incomplete sociology. The data must be gathered through special research techniques by persons playing a research role. These considerations also determine the research site. For if large numbers of patients must be queried, and neither records nor clinical intake interviews will do, and the questions must be asked at the very moment of application for therapy, then only clinic patients can serve as the source of data. Only in clinics is there a sufficiently steady stream of applicants coming to one place to make data-collection administratively feasible.

What questions should be asked? The general theoretical bases for the questions were covered in the first chapter. But there is quite a gap between the theory of reason analysis and actual questionnaires and interviews. The instruments of this study went through several stages of refinement. First, a questionnaire was developed in the spring of 1957 by Samuel Z. Klausner to study applicants to the Religion and Psychiatry Institute. This was completely revised by the present author, pretested in 30 interviews and administered as part-questionnaire, part-interview to 110 applicants during 1957-1958. After these data were analyzed, a new questionnaire was developed and administered to several clinics in 1958-1959. Some of these data are retained for the present study, which administered questionnaires and interviews in 1959-1960.

In what sort of clinics should inquiries be made? All sorts. The aim of this study is to discover, in a comparative way, why people go to clinics, and the reasons for going to one sort of clinic might be quite different from the reasons for going to another type of clinic. Fortunately, in New York City, the present world capital of psychotherapy, every imaginable type of clinic is represented. On the basis of records kept by the New York City Community Mental Health Board a list was made of all mental health clinics in Manhattan that have a large intake of patients.[1] They were divided into five types: nonhospital-connected clinics which included psychoanalytic clinics, psychotherapeutic clinics, and a religio-psychiatric clinic; and hospital-connected clinics which were separated into voluntary and municipal hospital affiliations. After much negotiation, the cooperation was obtained of almost every large nonhospital clinic in Manhattan (though one joined us too late for us to collect much data), and four voluntary hospitals—one Catholic, one Protestant Episcopal in affiliation, one connected with a large university medical center, and one large secular hospital (which also joined us too late). Because of a policy of excluding outsiders from doing research, the municipal hospitals could not join the research (though such prohibitions are no longer in force). As the chapter on clinics will show, the data collected do represent fairly the flow of patients in New York City as a whole to the four types of clinics we studied.

Should we use questionnaires or interviews? Clinic intake policies and limited financial resources dictated that both methods be used. Since most psychiatric clinics do some of their screening of applicants by mail, mailed questionnaires had to be used to study the entire population of applicants. Our basic procedure was developed in 1958-1959 in an experiment with 296 consecutive applications to the University Psychoanalytic Center.* After an applicant completed his application form, he was sent one of our research questionnaires with a cover letter from the clinic director explaining the purpose of the questionnaire and requesting his cooperation (see Appendix). Applicants who failed to return the questionnaire within three weeks were mailed another one. Eighty-three per cent eventually returned questionnaires in usable form. Moreover, the quality of response was high. The method worked so well that mailed questionnaires were also used for all psychoanalytic and psychotherapeutic clinics the next year, when we began data-collection in earnest (with the aid of an NIMH grant which we did not previously have). The psychoanalytic clinics which did their initial screening exclusively by mail gave us a response rate of 80 per cent to 90 cer cent,

---

* This name and all other clinic names in this book are pseudonyms.

as shown in Table 1. The psychotherapeutic clinics screened by telephone as well as mail, gave much more rapid decisions as to acceptance or rejection of the application, but their applicants returned only between 50 and 55 per cent of the written questionnaires. One of the clinics which screened by telephone immediately referred some applicants to other sources but questionnaires were sent to half of those referred and they too gave a response rate of about 50 per cent. Although there are other differences between clinics with high and low rates of return, the main difference must be caused by the more rapid decisions at clinics with low return rates, for despite the cover letter which states the research nature of the questionnaire and its voluntary character, applicants must have felt that their admission to a clinic was contingent upon their completion of the questionnaire.

But what about people like the angry lady whose letter began this chapter? Are respondents different from those not responding to the questionnaire? Surprisingly, there are no substantial differences.

TABLE 1 *Return Rate of Questionnaire*

Clinics	Usable Questionnaire Returned, %	Returned but not Processed, %	Total Number Sent
The University Psychoanalytic Center ('58-'59)	81	2	(296)
The University Psychoanalytic Center ('59-'60)	83	–	(179)
The Interpersonal Psychiatry Institute	92	2	(428)
The New Analytic Institute	*	*	*
The Center for Advanced Psychotherapy: referred	49	–	(126)
intake interview	55	–	(469)
Personal Psychology Institute	48	–	(112)

*Records of number sent lost. 11 returned.

First, official termination-of-treatment statistics do not differ substantially from our data. Second, demographic data, diagnosis, and disposition were collected on all cases who did not return questionnaires. An almost complete enumeration of such data was obtained only for the University Psychoanalytic Center. For other clinics, there was a significant number of nonrespondents for whom one or more characteristics were missing. There are no substantial differences on any item between those who responded and those who did not for the University Psychoanalytic Center. For other clinics there are also no significant differences between respondents and the nonrespondents on whom we have information, except that parents of children applying to the Personal Psychology Institute were less likely to return questionnaires.

Our "thirty-seven-year-old intellectual of very complex experience" does have a point, however. There is a tendency, although not a statistically significant one, for *less*-educated persons to be *more* likely to return the questionnaire, and for persons in the health professions to be less likely to return it. The unusual bias the lady remarked on was built into the questionnaire because, as she suspected, it was indeed designed to be answered even by the less-educated applicants. Some questions, therefore, were indeed too simple-minded. All in all, then, questionnaires filled out by applicants themselves were a remarkably successful data-collection device.

Questionnaires are far from the perfect data-gathering device for lower-class persons, however. Experiments in voluntary and municipal hospitals in 1958-1959 (before the latter were ruled off-limits) showed that on no account could satisfactory questionnaire data be obtained from the predominantly lower-class applicants to these clinics, except from St. Francis.* Interviews were necessary.† Though the purpose of the interviews was nonclinical, the setting might have induced respondents to believe that the interviewer was a doctor who could help them. On the other hand, a complete disassociation of research from service would probably have reduced patients' cooperation. The method used to bridge the two worlds of psychiatry and sociological research was worked out at the Religion and Psychiatry Institute in our earlier study of 110 applicants in 1957-1958 and was applied with minor variations to all the other clinics. All applicants were interviewed by the researchers for one hour at the time of their first intake interview with a psychiatrist or psychiatric social worker. Most interviews took place even before the clinicians saw the patients. A study of the interviews that took place after the clinical interview showed no differences from those given before it, provided that the research interview immediately followed the clinical interview. The clinic administrator in charge of scheduling intake arranged our interview so that it would appear to be a regular part of the clinic's procedures. Only at the time of the research interview were the patients told of the research. If they asked about the person they were seeing they were told he or she was a "sociologist."‡ (Most did not know what that was, but it sounded important and clearly was not a psychiatrist.)

Though the design was to interview consecutive applications, the unavailability of an interviewer (two interviewers had to cover four

* St. Francis Hospital did not allow data to be collected from patients referred within the hospital, who tended to be lower class.
† The interview guide was similar to the questionnaire in the Appendix but designed for oral delivery. Additional topics were included. Copies of the questionnaire may be obtained from the Bureau of Applied Social Research.
‡ The actual backgrounds of the interviewers included sociology, psychology, and the ministry.

clinics as much as ten miles apart) and occasional mix-ups in scheduling meant that an administrative factor entered between the design and the actual data-collection. The interviews do not, however, come from a statistically significantly different population from that reported by clinics to the State on termination of treatment forms. Hence the administrative factor is a random one.

Because data were collected through two different devices, the differences between the questionnaires and the interviews were studied to ascertain whether the results are comparable. Two devices facilitated this comparison. In the year previous to the main data-collection, 100 questionnaires were distributed to applicants to the Religion and Psychiatry Institute, as part of our experiments with data-collection. These questionnaires were filled out one hour prior to the intake interview. The next year 99 applicants were interviewed in the hour before intake with a similar instrument. Assuming the population of the clinic to be fairly constant, any differences in the responses to various questions could be attributed to differences between interviewing and filling out questionnaires. The differences were minor. In a second device for comparison, 48 applicants to the Interpersonal Psychiatry Institute who had already filled out a questionnaire were interviewed. An attempt was made to elicit further information and to clarify responses to the questionnaire. Any difference thus obtained between the interview and the questionnaire should be maximum because respondents were encouraged to add material or to change their minds. The interviews did elicit a better account of the incident which precipitated a person into therapy; they were also designed to cover some topics that had been omitted in the questionnaire because they were too complex for that medium. But in general, and within our coding categories, there were remarkably few differences between interviews and questonnaires. Without going into the details we can report that except where noted, differences between the questionnaire and the interview can be safely ignored in all our material.

Table 2 summarizes the number of questionnaires and interviews at each clinic that resulted from the data-collection methods we have described.

Now that the procedures for data-collection have been reviewed, we can come back to the reactions of the respondents to the questionnaires and the interviews. Not only did our "Dear Doctors" correspondents object to us, but the clinics themselves were most apprehensive about our procedures. Many strongly resisted our attempt to enlist their help with the study, although in the end, aside from the municipal hospitals (the decision about which was not made at the level of chief of psychiatric services), only two clinics refused outright to cooperate. What were their objections? First there was the administrative nuisance of interposing just one more step into an already complicated intake process. But more important, clinics felt that we wished to interpose a third party in the traditional doctor-patient relationship, and since we ourselves were not physicians nor in any way under clinic control, this might lead to possible damage to patients. Moreover, we might emotionally "drain" applicants before their intake interview, making psychiatric assessment difficult. In addition, all organizations are reluctant to open themselves to outsiders lest some special "secrets" of the organization be revealed—in much the same way that patients resist psychotherapy lest some of their dark secrets be exposed. Finally, even though most of the clinics we approached finally did agree to have us,[2] because of the way some clinics are organized the agreement had to be reaffirmed at each level of their hierarchy. Yet the process of agreement by and large served to improve questionnaire design. Some psychiatrists and other staff we consulted had excellent ideas for questions they wanted answered. On the other hand, some clinics insisted that we delete "sensitive" questions—some dealing with psychological matters and all concerned with social status. For example, one clinic did not allow race to be mentioned, another objected to questions about religion, a third to questions about psychiatrists, and a fourth objected to questions about Jewish psychiatrists.

Were the clinics right? Was the lady we quoted right? Did we really intrude on therapeutic process? By and large, we think not.

To begin with, we never encountered any gross disturbances. At the

TABLE 2 *Number of Questionnaires (Q) and Interviews (I) Collected from Ten Psychiatric Clinics in New York City**

Clinic	Instrument	Year	Number
Personal Psychology Institute	Q	1959-1960	54
University Psychoanalytic Center	Q	1958-1959	246
	Q	1959-1960	143
The New Analytic Institute	Q	1959-1960	11
Center for Advanced Psychotherapy	Q	1959-1960	313
Religion and Psychiatry Institute	Q	1958-1959	100
	I	1959-1960	99
St. Matthew's Hospital	I	1959-1960	61
Lincoln Hospital	I	1960	2
St. Francis Hospital	Q	1958-1959	17
	I	1959-1960	23
Center Hospital	I	1959-1960	32
Interpersonal Psychiatry Institute	Q	1959-1960	351
			1452

*158 experimental interviews are not included in the statistical analysis presented in this book.

time we appoached the clinics in our larger study, we were able to offer a year's experience with one clinic in interviewing psychiatric outpatients with no disasters and excellent patient cooperation, as well as a demonstrated ability on the part of all but two of the 140 applicants interviewed to answer our questions. No serious difficulties were encountered in any of the nine other clinics, despite the fact that clinicians were alerted to find fault with our intrusion. In one clinic, a social worker did find that patients were "talked out" after our interview, but no other clinic complained despite the fact that the same interviewer was used in several clinics. We did, however, agree to interview after intake in the one clinic where objections were raised.

Detailed responses to the questionnaire procedure were obtained in the course of the 48 interviews with those who had previously filled out a questionnaire. Of these 48, only 6 indicated clearly negative reactions. One person felt, "It was tiring. There were too many questions—too vague." Another said, "The questions tended to be classified in a certain group. I thought it should give you a chance to speak for yourself rather than [the research] ask questions." Some were ambivalent. "I guess I felt as though it was some sort of an imposition. Consciously I didn't mind it. I think I felt some hostility." And, "I didn't mind filling it out. Part of it annoyed me—drawing a picture and asking questions about other people." Most responses to our questionnaire, however, were more positive. "I found it a very interesting experience. I was forced to sit down. I was a little uncomfortable but I found it illuminating." "It was interesting and revealing. Asked me questions I hadn't thought about." "It was a little hard to write down what I felt on paper. But otherwise it was all right. Just by writing it down I felt better. The tension was relieved." In short, the questionnaire, just as an intake interview, put respondents through an emotional experience which for some amounted to a catharsis. Rather than reflecting poorly on the quality of our instrument, the emotional responses by applicants indicate that the questionnaire was meaningful to them. Perhaps this was the very problem of the "intellectual" quoted above. At the same time, we found no evidence that the questionnaire "damaged" anyone emotionally. The intake interviewers at the several clinics were indeed alerted to this possibility, but had only negative reports.

A few patients did have problems with our interview. The usual techniques of establishing rapport worked well with evasive respondents. For suspicious respondents, however, the scheduled format of questions may have been troublesome. One man, in response to each question said, "I don't understand what you mean." Our interviewer matter-of-factly replied, "I mean just what the question said." Talkative respondents, who threatened our tight schedule were told that we were not psychiatrists or, more bluntly, that we had quite a few questions to ask and not much time. Some respondents were not interested in the questions but rather wanted to tell a particular story of their own. Matter-of-fact statements as to the purpose of the research interview always overcame these problems without antagonizing respondents. Respondents who became hostile during the interview were reminded that the interview was entirely voluntary. All but one then wanted to go on. And the very structure of the interview helped those who were hostile at the beginning. When patients found the interview nonthreatening, they usually relaxed. Only four respondents were so upset or irrational that they could not be interviewed. When this happened they were returned to the waiting or reception room for a psychiatric interview. Most respondents who began the interview in an upset condition improved as the interview proceeded. When particular incidents recounted or questions asked evoked more affect than the interviewer felt capable of handling in the framework of our investigation, she shifted to other questions or issues, even at the cost of losing important material. The most important concern was getting the interview—not offering therapy.

Listing these problems may give the wrong impression, however. The overwhelming majority of respondents were cooperative. Most found our interview much less of a strain than the psychiatric one. And no psychiatrist ever complained that we upset patients or in any way interfered with the normal psychiatric interview. From our point of view, we feel that the general reliability and consistency of responses in our two types of instruments show that even disturbed respondents can be interviewed or given questionnaires similar to those given to normal respondents. The proof of our method, however, depends on the adequacy of the findings to be presented.

NOTES

1. We owe a great debt to Elena Padilla and the New York City Community Mental Health Board for their cooperation in this and every phase of our study.
2. The help of Dr. John Cotton in vouching for our competence and reliability and for insisting that there was little we could do to change patients is most gratefully acknowledged.

Therapists, Clinics, and Patients: The Organization of Outpatient Psychotherapy

❊

3

Interaction between patient and therapist begins long before they come face to face and is conditioned by the way psychiatry and psychotherapy are organized. To understand the process of applying for therapy at a clinic one must understand how clinics are organized and what types of clinic are available to different types of applicants. What we learn about clinics is also applicable to the private practice of psychotherapy. And since we intend in the last chapter to extrapolate from our findings implications for the general field of community mental health, we must know how clinics presently work.

There are four types of psychiatric clinic: psychoanalytic, psychotherapeutic, religio-psychiatric, and hospital. These four types differ in a number of crucial respects. Psychoanalytic clinics are chiefly oriented to training new psychoanalysts and to the perpetuation and development of psychoanalytic theory. Since they are more oriented to psychoanalytic associations than to the community at large, they receive less community support and are less subject to community control. Their patients are higher in social class and sophistication than those of any other type of clinic, and in this and many other respects psychoanalytic clinics come close to duplicating the conditions of private practice. In fact, to insure the adequate training of future psychoanalysts, such similarity is actually fostered by psychoanalytic clinics. In this study, psychoanalytic clinics are represented by the University Psychoanalytic Center, the New Analytic Institute, and the Interpersonal Psychiatry Institute.

Psychotherapeutic clinics differ from psychoanalytic clinics mainly in degree: their theory tends to be more eclectic, their patients of slightly lower social class and less sophistication, and their professional associations are less central to the conduct of the clinic. Psychotherapeutic clinics also tend to staff fewer medical personnel but more psychologists and social workers. Consequently, they are closer in pattern to the private practice of psychotherapy by nonmedical persons. The psychotherapeutic clinics in this study are the Center for Advanced Psychotherapy and the Personal Psychiatry Institute.

The religio-psychiatric clinics resemble psychotherapeutic clinics with one important difference: ministers do most of the therapy, and affiliation is not with a psychotherapeutic professional association but with associations of pastoral counselors.[1] Both religious and medical sources often tend to look askance at this new combination, and so this type receives the fewest referrals from professional sources. Yet religion-and-psychiatry is a growing movement in the United States; and any study which overlooks pastoral counseling either in a church, clinic, or a private setting is ignoring the most widely used form of counseling in the United States.[2] This type is here represented by the Religion and Psychiatry Institute.

Though they differ in many details, the organization of these three types of clinics is similar in that all tend to be governed by a consensus of colleagues rather than by a "bureaucracy"* system.

The last type, the hospital clinic, falls into the same patterns as other purely medical outpatient hospital clinics: it derives its patients from the urban lower class who tend to use the hospital as a polyclinic, so that it can barely cope with their large numbers. Hospitals, of course, are more bureaucratically organized than are independent psychiatric clinics. Representing hospital clinics in this study are Lincoln, St. Francis, St. Matthew's, and the Center Hospitals. These clinics are not at all typical of private practice and thus form an interesting foil to the others.

* *Bureaucracy* is a technical term used by sociologists to describe a system of hierarchical positions or offices, each with limited authority, in which each level reports to the one above it—the system which characterizes most executive functions of government and business.

✿ Clinic Organization

A bird's-eye view of clinic organization will help us understand how they work and who goes to them for treatment.[3]

Since it has little need for complex medical equipment, a psychiatric clinic, unlike most medical facilities, is chiefly an organization of people. A good place to start our story, then, is with the clinic leaders and the rest of its multifarious personnel. Each clinic in the study has a psychotherapist who is the nominal director—in every case serving on a part-time basis. In some clinics, a directorial committee composed of senior personnel helps to make policy. The executive committee of the psychoanalytic institutes themselves make major policy decisions, but the clinic director and his committee are always responsible to the larger organization of which the clinic is a part—a hospital, a training institute, or a voluntary organization. When training is an especially important aspect of the clinic, the director may be clearly subordinate to the persons or committee in charge of training. Serving under the director of the clinic are the various therapists: psychiatrists, psychologists, social workers, and ministers, as the case may be. In hospital clinics these professions are ranked in the order given, but in other clinics there is some attempt to level rank differences among these professions. State law, however, grants psychiatrists responsibility for the patients, and this tends to modify even the most egalitarian intentions.

In addition to the distinction among the professions which service the clinics, there are distinctions in rank among the various professional staff members. The major division is between the trainees on the one hand and the teachers and graduate staff on the other. Even within these strata there is a scale of ranks. A complex hospital clinic illustrates the range of positions. The chief of the Center Hospital clinic is also a member of the executive committee of the department of psychiatry of the medical school, and a faculty member of the University Psychoanalytic clinic. All this keeps him sufficiently busy so that much of the administration of the clinic must be turned over to an assistant chief, who is always a psychoanalyst. Other professional posts in the clinic include, roughly in order of rank, attending psychiatrists, a senior resident, and about 20 residents who supervise the 40 medical students each of whom gives a half-day a week for a three-month period. The only full-time personnel are three social workers. This gives the senior social worker more *de facto* power than her position might suggest, since she is the only one always on the spot when quick decisions must be made.

A typical psychoanalytic or psychotherapeutic institute clinic is somewhat less complex in structure: it is more often guided by committees than by a chief of service. The parent psychoanalytic institute usually provides a director or chairman responsible to an executive committee. Some institutes employ, in addition, a part-time director, but others administer the clinic through several standing committees of the institute as a whole. All committee members are of course graduate psychoanalysts who donate their executive leadership to the institute, though supervision of the 20 to 50 trainees or "candidates" is sometimes a paid activity. Attending graduate psychoanalysts supervise therapy, teach courses, and give training analyses to candidates. Other than membership in committees or chairmanship of them, rank is signified more by informal prestige than by formal authority. There are also paid social workers who have important functions in screening applicants for therapy, an administrative secretary, and a clerical staff. Again, since the social workers and especially the administrative secretary are likely to be on the spot full time, they tend to make more crucial decisions (such as who is an "emergency case") than their rank in the organization might indicate.

The personnel rosters are quite similar in both psychoanalytic and psychotherapeutic clinics. The religio-psychiatric type is also similar, except that they are faced with the problem, encountered in part even in psychotherapeutic clinics, of insuring adequate psychiatric supervision of therapy conducted by nonmedical personnel.

The clinic's process of screening patients who apply to it for treatment is of major concern to our study. Naturally, each clinic would like to get the best patients it can for its purposes. Psychoanalytic clinics generally accept few of those who apply to them, selecting only such as will make good training cases for their relatively small number of trainees. In the years we were doing our research, for example, the University Psychoanalytic Center received about 1500 inquiries a year, processed about 900 mailed application forms, and from these, attending psychoanalysts selected 260 applicants who were given a screening interview. Only about 15 per cent of applicants were accepted and about 170 patients were in treatment at any one time. The Interpersonal Psychiatry Institute took only 8 per cent of applicants though at the time it interviewed most of those who applied. These clinics variously have had social workers, attending psychiatrists and faculty members or even trainees, or some combination of these conduct the screening interview, and this mixture is characteristic of most types of clinics. The clinics occasionally change their policy about screening interviews, for the screening or intake interview has to fulfill many functions at once. In addition to insuring a supply of patients who will meet the needs of the clinic and deciding what might best help the patient, the screening interview must provide a diagnosis (a matter reserved to psychiatrists by law), a good sense of the patient's social history and financial standing, and must afford trainees an opportunity to learn how to conduct such an interview.

Psychotherapeutic clinics and the Religion and Psychiatry Institute generally take between 55 and 75 per cent of applicants, a much higher proportion than do psychoanalytic clinics, perhaps because they are more dependent on applicants to provide financial resources for the clinic. For example, the Center for Advanced Psychotherapy carried about 500 patients at the time of our research, most in one session a week given by about 40 trainees. On the other hand, in the Personal Psychiatry Institute, its 200 patients are treated exclusively by the 55 staff members. These clinics do not screen by mail and interview almost all applicants unless they are obviously too wealthy or too sick for the clinic to handle.

Most hospital clinics feel obligated to accept or place on a waiting list the very large majority of their applicants since the hospitals most clearly have a responsibility to the community at large. Even so, they can afford to offer only very short-term therapy to most applicants. Most applicants to hospital clinics walk in off the street, are referred by other clinics within the hospital, or are sent by the emergency service. The very large Center Hospital psychiatric clinic evaluates 800 patients a year, and since it cannot absorb anywhere near the number who apply, there is a high rate of referral to clinics and facilities outside its medical center. To handle this large number of applicants the Center Clinic has 3 social workers, 20 residents, 40 medical students, and 15 attending psychiatrists of various ranks. St. Francis Hospital clinic, however, except for patients referred by its other services, screens by mail.

In order to screen applicants and give them therapy, the staff of a clinic must relate not only to patients, but also to each other. Not surprisingly, the mode in which they are trained to relate to patients also spills over into their modes of relating to each other. Relations between clinic directors and their professional subordinates, even in hospital clinics, tend to be more collegial (an association of professional equals) than bureaucratic (an organization according to a hierarchical chain of command). The collegial form, which is characteristic of all organizations of professionals, is exaggerated in psychiatric clinics because of several factors. Norms engendered by psychoanalytic theory discourage "playing the role of papa" in an organization. A directorial committee, when present, helps to diffuse power and to make no one person responsible for being an "autocratic father." The system of supervision and case conference provides a second and much more powerful mode of reporting and control.

Each resident or trainee is assigned a senior therapist, often an attending psychiatrist, who supervises his work in weekly private conferences. Since ability in therapy is the main requirement of a graduate of a training program, the reports of the supervisor carry enormous weight. Hence his power over trainees is very great. Yet the supervisors often do not report to the clinic director but to the training director, and these are rarely the same person. When they are, the office of clinic director is quite powerful. Attending or staff psychotherapists are usually indirectly supervised through collegial case conferences. This procedure obviously reduces the power of an individual director. Moreover, the clinic is not the main place of work for the bulk of the staff (other than the trainees). Private practice is the major source of income for graduate psychotherapists. Hence, the sanctions available to a director are limited, and even the director himself is often committed to other activities. Lastly, and extremely important, the very role of therapist is a charismatic one, and therefore does not conveniently fit into a bureaucratic organization.

The strictly autonomous decisions made by the formal bureaucratic structure of a clinic tend therefore to be largely of a housekeeping nature: supplies, room assignments, arrangement of therapist hours, and so on. Since these matters are not likely to be of great interest to psychotherapists, they are usually delegated to the clerical, nonprofessional clinic or hospital staff. On the other hand, a number of these so-called housekeeping functions have significance to therapy, therapists, and patients. Included are the arrangement of appointments, especially for persons to be seen for the first time, record keeping, the collection of fees, and even assigning patients to specific therapists. Since these are semiprofessional activities, some of the clinics in our study assigned them to social workers, who are thus clearly noted as being less than full-fledged therapists. Nevertheless, the arrangement of appointments can be a genuine screening function, and thus of great importance to both patients and therapists.

The bald fact of the matter is that if one asks who "runs" a clinic, the answer is nobody and everybody. When we think of organizations, we tend to think of bureaucratically organized entities. Only the hospital clinics, however, and perhaps one of the psychotherapeutic clinics, even approach this model since they tend to have a more clearly defined system of ranks and authority. And as everyone knows who has been entertained by the world of medicine on TV, the charismatic authority of attending physicians can upset even the most bureaucratically organized hospital. The other clinics in our study, whatever their formal arrangements on organizational charts, tend to be collegially governed. Because much of the professional staff is part time and therefore cannot meet regularly in committee, collegial government under these circumstances may amount to almost no government. This is especially evident in the many and usually inefficient arrangements clinics make for running their intake services. Since bureaucracy is generally confined in a clinic to the clerical staff, and since bureaucracy can be a powerful tool, many things that patients think are carefully considered by the directorate of the clinic in a psychotherapeutic manner often turn out actually to have been clerical decisions. In one clinic, an efficient administrative secretary became so useful over the years, that when she left and her functions were reviewed, elaborate safeguards were introduced to insure that henceforth the professional staff would indeed make all decisions connected with therapy.

❁ Psychotherapists and Their Motivation to Serve

Clinics do a great deal for nothing or at least for very little money. That is how they work. Even the therapists or candidates who do get paid do not get what they might earn in private practice. Why do they do it, and how does their motivation affect the nature of clinics and the sort of patient they accept for treatment?

Psychiatric clinics in part resemble American hospitals: they are simultaneously the doctor's workshop, his postgraduate university, and the community's treatment center. These goals often conflict. Psychoanalytic influence on the practice of American psychiatry has somewhat altered the terms of conflict. In the practice of medicine and surgery, the most interesting cases are found in hospitals—namely, cases that can be helped through the application of complex medical and surgical procedures, possible only in hospitals; consequently, able doctors are drawn to hospital activities not only in order to be in a position to treat their own patients but also to improve their scientific knowledge and their practical skills.

But psychoanalytically influenced psychiatrists tend to find hospitalized cases less interesting than those they see in their private offices. They usually feel that psychotherapy, the preferred mode of treatment, cannot be effectively practiced on hospitalized patients. Consequently, the psychiatric outpatient clinic rather than the hospital is the focus of whatever is interesting to the psychiatrist outside of his own private practice. So, the more clinic patients tend to approximate the nature of cases seen in private practice, the "better" the clinic is. As a treatment center, which collects interesting cases, the outpatient clinic of a hospital is of limited value to psychotherapists. The director of one of the hospital clinics, however, suggested in a letter that attending psychiatrists on his staff had special interest in hospital cases:

Fortunately, for the sake of hospital inpatient services and hospital clinics, there are psychiatrists and psychoanalysts who like to vary their practice by working with a different type of patient. For them the response of a severely depressed patient, for example, with the properly chosen pharmacological agent can be just as rewarding in its own way as the elucidation of a subtle motivation in the analytic patient.

Yet it is also true that a hospital connection is very valuable to a psychiatrist working with private patients who are not classic psychoanalytic material and who might need sudden hospitalization. In any case, treatment of patients carries some weight in all clinics, if merely to assuage a therapist's medical or social conscience. Treatment as such seems more important to hospital clinics without direct university affiliations, to the Personal Psychology and the Religion and Psychiatry Institutes because of their ideologies, and to the Center for Advanced Psychotherapy for a variety of reasons. Conversely, the training function of a clinic rules the roost at University Psychoanalytic Center, Interpersonal Psychiatry Institute, and the Center Hospital clinic, and is becoming increasingly important at all other clinics for reasons soon to be explained.

Although now the dominant psychiatric persuasion in New York City, psychoanalytic psychiatry still resorts to the techniques of a revolutionary clique to gain social support and validation. Barred from the usual circles of academic medicine, the original circle of psychotherapists surrounding Freud found themselves meeting regularly at each other's homes to exchange ideas and innovations. This informal group grew into a formal society which developed a number of local psychoanalytic institutes. These institutes served to train new members and so became social and intellectual centers for alumni and faculty. Subsequent splits in the analytic movement multipled analytic societies and training institutes. Clinics, if present at all, were usually formed as an adjunct to the training center to insure a regular and suitable supply of training cases. This origin of clinics largely accounts for the primacy of training in the psychoanalytic clinics in our study. Because the psychoanalytic clinics are the direct heirs of the original psychoanalytic ideas that now in some form or other rule psychiatry in New York City, and they clearly have the "best" psychoanalytic patients, other clinics also began to conform to this pattern and to make training primary, relegating other clinic functions to a secondary role.

Now that "mental health" has become a popular slogan, there is a further reason for clinics to emphasize training functions. Almost everyone connected with the mental health professions feels that there is a shortage of trained psychiatrists and other therapists. As the rates of acceptance and rejection show, most persons who now apply to psychiatric clinics do not get full treatment. Any psychotherapist on the staffs of these clinics is personally exposed to the shortage of treatment facilities and hence is further motivated to promote the cause of training. In part, this is a self-fulfilling prophecy. For the more a clinic tends to become a training center, the fewer cases it can accept, and the greater the shortage of treatment facilities becomes.

The clinic therefore makes an important contribution to the analytic society or the training institute or to the residency program of a hospital by providing training cases, and the training program is a major motivation for the participation of therapists. The clinics in turn look to training centers for financial support, organizational leadership or coordination, and for treatment and advisory personnel. This relationship between clinic and training center may dominate the entire structure and operation of a clinic and is clearly true of the psychoanalytic clinics and Center Hospital which is part of a university medical center. A high rate of rejection of applicants—other things being equal— is an excellent indicator of the importance of training to a clinic. In any case, it is trainees (M.D.'s who have completed or almost completed their residency in psychiatry at the University Psychoanalytic Center; postresidency psychiatrists, psychologists, and social workers at other psychoanalytic and psychotherapeutic clinics; residents at hospital clinics and clergymen at the Religion and Psychiatry Institute) who do the bulk of clinic treatment (under supervision). Without trainees, therefore, none of these clinics could offer any but minimal service to the public.

Clinics also contribute directly to therapists. First, they sometimes pay them. Financial compensation is important to therapists at one of the psychotherapeutic clinics and at the Religion and Psychiatry Institute. Money is less important to hospital clinic residents and to therapists at psychoanalytic institutes who either now earn, or expect in the future to earn, fairly handsome fees from private practice. This source is not, however, as available to the clergymen at the Religion and Psychiatry Institute and to the psychologists or social workers who form at least half of the trainees at psychotherapeutic clinics.

The fact that the money received by clinic therapists is often nominal and that many attending psychiatrists in most of the clinics in our study are not paid at all points to the nonfinancial gains therapists receive from clinics. Psychiatry, which emphasizes two-person relationships, can be lonely as well as tedious. For training supervisors, the clinic affords an opportunity to escape from their therapist-patient routine. There are administrative meetings, clinic politics, and case conferences. Sociability seems to be an important factor in the success of minister-psychiatrist relationships in the Religion and Psychiatry Institute and is important to the success of virtually all the psychotherapeutic and psychoanalytic clinics.

In addition to good fellowship, however, a clinic gives psychotherapists a chance to exercise power and influence not only over patients, but over other psychotherapists, who in the context of clinics, always have a higher rank than their most exalted patients. Since it is a sociological law that persons tend to prefer interactions with those of similar or higher, rank, it follows that psychotherapists would prefer to interact with other psychotherapists or with training candidates rather than with the average clinic patient. And since rank tends to rub off through interaction, therapists who have active roles in institutes and clinics have higher prestige than other therapists who merely interact with patients. These tendencies give further impetus to training programs in those clinics, such as hospital clinics, which do not have a history of affiliation with a psychoanalytic institute. The opportunities for sociability, rank, and power vastly increase when a clinic devotes itself to training. Mere affiliation with the institute is thus an important motive for therapists who give their time to the psychoanalytic or psychotherapeutic clinics.

By encouraging interaction among therapists, clinics serve as social control devices and as value reinforcement centers for the psychotherapy movement. Tendencies of therapists in private practice to deviate from accepted standards and practices are corrected. Of course, the clinic not only controls but also educates. Every teacher learns far more than his pupils, and the same must be true of the relation between trainees and their supervisors.

For all these reasons, there is an overwhelming tendency for clinics which are not attached to hospitals to become training institutes. Although the typical history of psychoanalytic clinics shows that clinics follow upon institutes, the history of the psychotherapeutic clinics and the Religion and Psychiatry Institute—all of which began as clinics—suggests that there are strong forces which tend to produce institutes from clinics. The case of hospitals is different, for the psychiatric clinic is usually assimilated into existing patterns for training medical students, interns, and residents. Even here, the forces directed toward becoming chiefly a training center are almost irresistible.

One last function of a psychiatric clinic, generally unique to nonhospital clinics, is to provide therapists with patients for their private practice. This can come about in any one of several ways. Since psychotherapy involves so much of the personality of the practitioner, therapists prefer to make referrals to those whom they know fairly well in both their technical and human capacities. Regular interaction in a clinic setting gives therapists some opportunity to judge their associates and thus to establish informal referral networks. This seems characteristic of referrals made by most of the nonhospital clinics. Further, many applicants to a clinic may be directly referred to a private practitioner. Sometimes, patients specifically request this service because they know of no private practitioners and do not wish to trust to the phone book or a mental health association. In other cases, patients exceed the upper level of income acceptable for clinic treatment. When clinics are overcrowded and have long waiting lists, some otherwise suitable patients can be induced to pay fees, at least at the level demanded by trainees, in return for immediate private treatment. Occasionally, a patient is deemed "too sick," or not a good training case, and is privately referred. In all these cases, clinic administrators and admission therapists obviously prefer to make referrals to members of their own staff. Some clinics have even defined this procedure as part of their regular service, though it is quite costly to them.

Another channel for private patients is established by converting clinic patients into private patients. This can come about in several ways. First, patients who at first were earning little money may have been so helped by therapy as to be able to earn more and hence to pay private fees. Second, most clinics take on a patient for only a specified length of time, often geared to the training year, September through June, though analytic patients are guaranteed a longer time span of treatment. In practice, however, the limited time period available to a clinic patient is almost always insufficient. Yet, other patients are on the waiting list and must be seen. Even so, it is more difficult to resist treating a patient one knows than an applicant whom one does not know. Hence clinics often keep patients longer than the specified period. But not all patients can be kept and some are taken into a therapist's private practice or sent to other private therapists. This flow of patients from clinics to private practice does alleviate some pressure on the clinics and allows them to serve more applicants. The flow is limited, however, by the capacity of the patients to pay, and the number of private therapists' hours available. Hence, bringing patients into private practice is more common at nonhospital clinics which have both relatively affluent patients and some therapists who have open hours because they do not have the prestigeful medical degree. The practice of converting clinic into private patients obviously could lead to abuses, and some clinics ban the procedure. At the same time, this flow frees some treatment hours in overcrowded clinics.

❀ The Public and the Patients

Clinics may serve to support psychoanalytic institutes, provide for the training of future psychotherapists, and gratify the needs of psychiatrists and other psychotherapists in a variety of ways. Yet they would go out of business if they did not gain some measure of public support and did not recruit enough patients of the type they need. These last members of a clinic—the public and the patients—both receive from and give a great deal to psychiatric clinics.

Obviously, patients gain, or at least think they will gain, by applying to a psychiatric clinic. Whether they are truly helped is not the concern of this book. We do know, however, that 90 per cent of the applicants *thought* they would be "helped" in some way. Moreover, they hoped to receive treatment at lower cost than was otherwise available in the community. Between 80 and 90 per cent of applicants to all but the Religion and Psychiatry Institute said that the major advantage of a clinic over a private psychiatrist was its low cost. Applicants to the Religion and Psychiatry Institute, however, were more interested in the religious aspects of the clinic than in its low cost; and hospital clinic patients never really expected in any case to be able to be treated by private psychiatrists. With these exceptions, we found that the applicants' evaluations of the financial aspects of going to a clinic (as well as their estimate of the amount they could afford weekly for treatment) roughly matched the actual differences in fees charged by each clinic. The Center for Advanced Psychotherapy charges the highest fees, followed by the Religion and Psychiatry Institute and the Personal Psychology Institute, and then the University Psychoanalytic Center and the Interpersonal Psychiatry Institute. Hospital clinics are by far the lowest in cost.

Since the patients' fees do not fully compensate the clinics, they must find other sources for financial support, and it is usually the community at large, through taxes and voluntary contributions, which makes up a good deal of the difference. Naturally, the clinics which receive the most public funds generally charge the lowest fees.

The community, however, receives something in return for its support. By treating patients, the clinic offers the community a device for coping with persons who might otherwise be a serious drain on it. Even applicants who are merely "unhappy" are actual or potential deviants from their roles in society. By dealing with the unhappy, not to mention the overtly psychotic, the clinic acts as an agency of social control—a function no different in theory from that performed by the police, but with a greater emphasis on rehabilitation. The social welfare and job counseling aspects of clinics which attempt to integrate patients into the community are also not insignificant aspects of psychiatric service. Psychiatric clinics actually save the community a substantial amount of money by reducing time lost from work and helping to prevent crime. Moreover, merely keeping a person out of a mental hospital saves the state considerable expense. The hospital clinics, and the Religion and Psychiatry Institute to a lesser extent, are supported by the public because these clinics clearly recognize and attempt to exercise some social control functions. The psychotherapeutic and psychoanalytic clinics are less interested in such functions and in turn receive less community support, though in the long run their training operations may give the community traditional resources in terms of more therapists.

The money given by the community to clinics entitles it to moral and legal control over them. This is exercised, in a limited fashion, through granting clinics a license. The Community Mental Health Board also exerts some control, although less, probably, than it would like. The hospital clinics are most subject to community control; the psychoanalytic and psychotherapeutic clinics much less so.

On their part, patients also make important contributions to the clinic. First, they provide the basic human resources with which the clinic operates. Clinics are not unconcerned about the nature of the human material with which they work. Each clinic strives to get patients who are more likely to respond to the treatment offered, a procedure which has certain undesirable consequences for the clinic's social control functions, inasmuch as the patients most unlikely to respond are usually those whom the community needs most urgently to have brought under control. Second, patients, through their fees, provide financial support to the clinic. The sheer number of patients may also determine the extent of state support; a popular clinic might therefore claim a larger proportion of the state pie.

Third, patients contribute not only to the clinic as such, but both directly and indirectly to the therapists who practice there. Meeting the therapist's need to make people better is not a small matter. Indirectly, through their fees, patients also help to provide therapists with salaries in those clinics in which therapists are paid. In some "middle-income" clinics, this contribution is not so indirect, since the trainees are paid entirely from patient fees. In addition, in some clinics, patients provide trainees with a way of acquiring private patients.

Since the contributions of patients to both clinics and therapists are so clearly vital, clinics spend an enormous amount of effort in screening patients, for, as we have shown, many more apply than most clinics can treat.

There have been a large number of studies of the characteristics of patients selected by psychiatric clinics.[4] Almost all these studies show that clinics prefer young, nonpsychotic, highly motivated, better educated applicants. That is, patients are preferred who can communicate their feelings to middle-class therapists and whom the latter can judge to be likely to get better. This is also true over-all of New York State clinics.[5] Nevertheless, in a city like New York, with its multiple types of psychiatric services, there is no general rule for patient selection. Rather, each clinic selects those patients who best meet its current training and administrative needs and who best fit its ideology of psychotherapy or psychoanalysis. Since these needs and the ideology obviously vary, so does the model "good" patient, although it may be that most of the hospital clinics fit the pattern of previously reported findings. In general, each type of clinic tends to get only certain kinds of applicants to begin with, and the clinic's own selection process tends merely to exaggerate the effects of choices already made by the applicants themselves.[6]

One reason patients are so well preselected is that different clinics are tuned into quite different networks of referral. The notion of "referral" covers a multitude of processes which will be analyzed later. All we want to show here is the last source from which potential patients have heard about a clinic; this will give us some picture of a clinic's "watershed." (See Table 3.)

The psychoanalytic and psychotherapeutic clinics are closely linked to psychiatric sources. Almost 60 per cent of University's applicants had heard of the clinic through private psychiatrists or other psychiatric clinics. The Center for Advanced Psychotherapy is next in line with 50 per cent drawn from these sources, followed by Interpersonal with 40 per cent. The Personal Psychology Institute is far behind but does seem linked to community service and social work agencies. Among the hospital clinics, St. Francis resembles the psychotherapeutic clinics (because of its mail screening device), St. Matthew's gets some patients from psychiatric sources, but Center Hospital gets practically none. The Religion and Psychiatry Institute is also isolated from psychiatric referrals. Instead, it receives some referrals from ministers and, uniquely, a great proportion hear of the clinic through mass media, especially through books by its prominent leadership.

The institutional setting of some of the clinics also provides them with a large number of patients. The hospital clinics, with the exception of St. Francis, receive most of their patients through other clinics and services connected with their own hospitals.[7] Some applicants to the Religion and Psychiatry Institute come through contact with the church next door (noted in Table 3 as "Prior Contact with Institution"— which includes passing by and seeing a clinic's sign as well as being associated with an organization related to the clinic, and so on).

Aside from psychiatrists, the major sources of information for applicants to psychoanalytic and psychotherapeutic clinics are their families and friends. Interpersonal Institute applicants are very likely to have come through this source. Family and friends are also an important source for the Religion and Psychiatry Clinic.

Clinics themselves often make no referrals outward even though they do not keep all who apply. But when they do refer, they have sharply different practices, which further indicate the network into which they

TABLE 3 Latest Source of Information About the Clinic*

Source	University Psychoanalytic, %	Interpersonal Psychiatry, %	Advanced Psychotherapy, %	Personal Psychology, %	Religion and Psychiatry, %	St. Matthew's, %	St. Francis, %	Center Hospital, %
Mass Media	2	3	2	2	31	2	0	0
Prior contact with institution	3	1	1	2	10	57	13	53
Private psychotherapist	37	21	25	11	3	3	18	0
Psychiatric clinic	22	21	25	13	4	20	21	6
Social agency	5	11	6	23	2	2	3	3
Private doctor	2	2	7	6	2	3	8	9
Other medical	1	1	0	0	0	2	3	3
Other professional	0	1	1	0	15	2	13	0
Friends and family	27	40	33	43	34	10	21	25
Total	99	101	100	100	101	101	100	99
N	(386)	(350)	(310)	(53)	(192)	(61)	(38)	(32)

*New Analytic Institute and Lincoln Hospital excluded, since too few cases were collected to warrant tabulation.

are tied. The flow through the clinics seems to be as follows: University receives applicants from private psychiatrists, accepts very few, and sends the rest on to psychiatric clinics. The other psychoanalytic institute, Interpersonal, picks up applicants from private psychiatrists and from among the applicants' friends, keeps very few applicants, and sends those rejected to other clinics and psychiatrists. The Center for Advanced Psychotherapy also draws from psychiatrists and from friends of patients, but keeps a larger proportion for itself, and sends the rejected to private psychiatrists and psychologists. The Personal Psychology Institute draws far fewer from psychiatrists, keeps a high proportion, and sends the rest to private psychologists. The Religion and Psychiatry Institute gets applicants from rather unusual sources, and channels most of them to conventional psychiatric care. Limited data for the hospital clinics suggest a shuttle service from one low-cost treatment source to another. The flow in and out of clinics indicates that their watersheds are quite different and so they tend to have applicants of different social composition.

❀ Social Characteristics of Clinic Applicants

A review of the basic social characteristics of the applicants to various types of clinics shows that the applicants themselves are of different types. Table 4 summarizes the differences between clinics. Let us see what these differences mean.

Though a popular stereotype suggests that women are more concerned about emotional things and hence predominate among those applying for psychotherapy, this is actually true only of lower-class women.[8]

Sophistication generally erases the propensity of Western men to consider emotional matters as strictly women's business. Women do number between 65 and 70 per cent of applicants to hospital clinics, but these clinics attract a lower-class clientele. Even though women are 55 to 60 per cent of the applicants to other clinics, this figure is in proportion to their numbers among young adults in Manhattan, so that in fact only hospital clinics attract an undue proportion of women. The typical applicant to psychotherapeutic and psychoanalytic clinics, like patients in private therapy, is between twenty and thirty-five years old (25 per cent are under 25). By contrast, at least half of the applicants to hospital clinics (except St. Francis, with its screening by mail) are over thirty-five, and 60 per cent of applicants to the Religion and Psychiatry Institute are similarly over thirty-five.[9] Because of their youth, half of the applicants to psychoanalytic and psychotherapeutic clinics

TABLE 4 *Social Characteristics of Applicants*

Clinic	Women, %	Under 35 Years, %	Married, %	White, %	Native Born, %	Jewish, %	College* Graduate, %	"Insider," %	Student, %	Working Class, %	(N)
University Psychoanalytic	54	79	42	†	88	56	49	32	18	12	(383)
Interpersonal Psychiatry	59	82	25	96	93	59	39	22	28	16	(350)
Advanced Psychotherapy	57	68	36	94	89	58	32	22	12	14	(313)
Personal Psychology	57	64	33	98	87	57	19	14	10	17	(54)
Religion and Psychiatry	59	40	53	94	91	12	24	15	6	17	(195)
St. Matthew's	72	42	38	84	79	19	17	12	2	46	(60)
St. Francis	64	82	28	89	90	14	24	20	17	10	(39)
Center Hospital	69	46	72	73	52	†	0	4	0	59	(32)

*Excluding students.
†Not available.

are single. Other clinics receive a much larger proportion of married clientele.

It is often facetiously said that psychoanalysis is a "Jewish science," and in fact almost 60 per cent of all applicants to psychoanalytic and psychotherapeutic clinics are Jews.[10] But St. Francis Hospital, which is under Roman Catholic sponsorship, draws a group which is 60 per cent Catholic, and the Religion and Psychiatry Institute, headed by a Protestant clergyman, draws a group which is more than 70 per cent Protestant. Though Jews have been traditionally associated with the psychoanalytic movement, the attraction of members of other religions to psychotherapy obviously also depends on the religious organizational affiliation of the therapists.

In keeping with the psychoanalytic tradition, not only the religion applicants profess, but how much of it they practice is also related to clinic type. No matter what their religion, applicants to psychoanalytic and psychotherapeutic clinics are not very religious, and since the Jews in this sample are in any case less religious than the other groups, applicants to analytic clinics are, on the average, very much less religious than applicants to other clinics. Those applying to the Religion and Psychiatry Institute are, of course, the most religious, and hospital clinic applicants are about average. The Roman Catholic hospital, however, does *not* draw an especially religious group of Catholics.

Other ethnic factors are not quite as important in discriminating between one clinic and another. Negroes, despite their heavy concentration in Manhattan, simply do not apply to *any* of the clinics in this sample (less than 5 per cent of applicants) except to the Center Hospital where about 20 per cent are Negroes. And few foreign born apply to any but hospital clinics, where our English-speaking interviewers may have missed an additional number of Puerto Rican applicants.

Social class is the most important distinguishing trait among the applicants to clinics of various types. Generally, the more closely affiliated a clinic is with the orthodox psychoanalytic movement, the higher the social class of its applicants will be. In this study, class is indicated by an applicant's education and his type of occupation.[11] (Income is a fairly useless indicator of class in this study because income is closely related in the applicant's mind to acceptance by a clinic and the amount of fee he will have to pay—respondents told us intimate details of their sex lives but lied about their incomes.) Education in particular reflects the "psychoanalytic rank" of a clinic. Of the applicants to the only clinic in our study affiliated with the American Psychoanalytic Association, 50 per cent are college graduates; of the applicants to the Interpersonal Psychiatry Institute, 40 per cent are college graduates; but of the applicants to the psychotherapeutic clinic and the Religion and Psychiatry Institute, only between 20 and 35 per cent are college graduates.[12] The typical hospital clinic has between 5 and 15 per cent college graduates among its applicants, depending on neighborhood— and the Center Hospital Clinic had no such applicants at all in our sample.

Differences in the types of occupations of applicants attracted to the various clinics generally parallel the level of the applicants' education. For example, almost 40 per cent of the University Psychoanalytic Center applicants are managers or professionals, but two-thirds of Center Hospital applicants are workers. Yet the occupation of an individual indicates not only his opportunities in life's arena, but his general orientation to the world. Some occupations attract many "insiders" who are sophisticated about psychotherapy. The medical and mental health professions, teachers, persons in the arts, and even white-collar workers or executives in entertainment, communications, advertising, or education are good examples of "insiders." Among patients of some psychoanalysts in New York, 16 per cent are in some way occupied in the arts alone.[13] The clinics in our study definitely differ in their ability to attract these "specialists" in psychiatry and psychoanalysis. The University Psychoanalytic Center draws almost one-third of its applicants from this group, and the Interpersonal Psychiatry Institute and the Center for Advanced Psychotherapy find somewhat more than a fifth of their applicants in this category, but among hospital clinics only St. Francis approaches this proportion of "insiders." The Religion and Psychiatry clinic also draws relatively few "insiders" but attracts more executives and professionals who are not "insiders" than any other clinic, perhaps because the self-help writings of the president of the foundation operating the clinic often discuss the problems of businessmen and executives. It is important to observe that "insiders" and other professionals or executives do *not* differ in social rank. It is not social rank that brings the better educated to psychoanalysis but their greater sophistication and interest in psychotherapy.

Perhaps the unique feature of the psychoanalytic and psychotherapeutic clinics in our study, which differentiates them both from other clinics and from the private practice of psychoanalysis, is the relatively large number of college and postgraduate students attracted to these clinics. There are over 200 students in this study. Clearly, the students of today are the "insiders" of tomorrow. What attracts them to psychoanalytic clinics rather than to private practice is their current lack of funds. This is true even if their parents are well-to-do, since one of the key issues for this young group of applicants is the need to be independent of their parents.

In summary, the psychoanalytic clinics receive a young, single, well-educated, white, American born, and Jewish group who are characteristically "insiders" about psychotherapy. In this respect, these applicants are not typical of the New York Metropolitan area, but are quite like patients in private psychiatric practice. The psychotherapeutic clinics receive a similar set of applicants, although perhaps not of such high social standing. The Religion and Psychiatry Clinic attracts the backbone of America—middle-aged, married, white, Protestant businessmen, and especially their wives. The hospital clinics draw upon the urban working classes (and even a large proportion of relief clients); their applicants are also older and much more likely to be women. One hospital clinic, St. Francis, is an exception and appears much more like the psychoanalytic clinics, perhaps because of its location in Greenwich Village, but very likely, because its application procedure, which requires the writing of letters, makes it self-screening so that only those who would ordinarily apply to psychoanalytic clinics pass this literary barrier.

So we find that each type of clinic, even before screening, receives the type of patient in which it is most interested. Psychoanalytic and psychotherapeutic clinics get the best psychoanalytic patients, for youth, intelligence, sophistication, and cultural similarity to therapists are the social criteria which enable patients to meet the psychoanalytic model. The Religion and Psychiatry clinic gets patients most amenable to the ideology of its founder if not to that now practiced in the clinic, while the hospital clinics get patients who can usually be treated only with drugs and short-term therapy, although if a hospital is more interested in long-term therapy, this too can be accommodated.

✪ Conclusion

The psychiatric clinic system comprises three parts, each of which affects the others: the clinic organization, the staff and therapists, and the public and the patients. It all works as if by magic. The psychoanalytic and psychotherapeutic clinics are interested in training psychoanalysts and psychotherapists for private practice and in advancing the art and science of psychotherapy. They draw staff members who enjoy associating with each other and to whom the clinic goals are so important that they willingly give up some of their well-remunerated time in order to work with patients and supervise trainees. To further their training program, these clinics are dependent on getting patients who resemble, to a great extent, those that a psychoanalyst or psychotherapist might encounter in private practice. They also need the funds with which to operate the institute and the clinic. They in fact manage to get both. The psychoanalytic and psychotherapeutic clinics are tied into a referral system that sends them the "right" kind of patient so that even if they were to do random screening, they would be assured of relatively "good" cases. And their entire operation is seen as legitimate either by the state government, segments of the public, or patients —all of whom contribute to clinics in one degree or another. Psychoanalytic and psychotherapeutic clinics may differ somewhat in their organization, but they draw on such a similar pool of patients that henceforth we shall call both groups *analytic clinics.*

The religion and psychiatry movement has goals similar to those of the analytic clinics but in addition wishes to bring good pastoral counseling into religious institutions throughout the country. To do this it must have trained clergymen. Now most persons interested in psychoanalysis are not religious—in fact they may be antireligious. Nonetheless, the Religion and Psychiatry Institute manages to attract clients even in New York City who resemble the mass of American Protestant churchgoers with whom their pastoral counselors will eventually have to work.

Hospital clinics serve as treatment sources for the poorer and less sophisticated urban lower class. They are centers dedicated to treatment methods which include chemotherapy and other, not necessarily psychoanalytic, methods, along with some psychotherapy. Linked to medical practice, and heavily supported by the community at large, these clinics meet the training needs of general psychiatry and also manage to attract the sort of patient suitable for these needs.

No sociologist believes in magic, however, so how the system of patient recruitment does actually work will occupy our attention in the rest of the book. The fact that each type of clinic gets a certain type of patient needs to be explained. In the course of this explanation we will come to understand why people go to psychiatrists. Since analytic clinics draw on much the same group of patients as those who go to private psychiatrists and psychotherapists (in fact 65 per cent had already been to a private psychotherapist!), we can usually generalize the results of our analysis of analytic clinic applicants to the great bulk of private patients of psychotherapists and psychoanalysts. As a foil, we will have patients of very different sorts: "standard middle-class Americans" and the urban poor.

Lest anyone accuse a sociologist of seeing everything as rosy simply because a particular social system works at all, our last chapter will deal with community mental health, and we will return to some of the themes of this chapter. Community mental health, whatever it is, is not simply a collection of clinics satisfying their training needs or even attempting to cope with a mass of urban poor with very limited means of doing so. When the present system squarely attempts to satisfy the needs of the entire community it may face serious difficulties.

NOTES

1. For an analysis and history of the religion and psychiatry movement see Samuel Z. Klausner, *Psychiatry and Religion* (New York: The Free Press), 1964.
2. Gurin, Veroff, and Feld, *Americans View Their Mental Health*, p. 307.
3. All clinics are described as they were in 1960.
4. For a review of thirty-six such studies, see Irma J. Lorenzen, *Acceptance or Rejection by Psychiatric Clinics*, unpublished Columbia University Master's Essay, 1967.
5. Gerhart Saenger and John Cumming, "Study of Community Mental Health Clinics, Report I & II," Mental Health Research Unit, New York State Department of Mental Hygiene, Syracuse, New York, 1965 and 1966.
6. For a complete analysis, see Irma J. Lorenzen, *op. cit.*, *passim.* Lorenzen suggests that the unanimity shown in previous literature may be in part caused by the lack of heterogeneity in the clinics studied, or by the lumping together of statistics from different types of clinics.

   Neither her analysis nor that undertaken by others shows that clinic criteria are empirically well founded. The characteristics of patients which predict their selection by the clinics generally do not very well predict who will subsequently drop out of treatment.
7. An independent study of St. Francis in 1962 showed that 40 per cent were referred from units *within* the hospital. These applicants were excluded by the clinic from our study. They are probably lower in class origin than those screened by mail.
8. It is true that a national study of mental health (Gurin, *et al.*, *op. cit.*, p. 289) shows that women are more likely than men to say that they have used or could have used some professional help with their personal problems. But as I recalculate the data presented on pp. 278 and 33, women are barely, if at all, more likely than men to have seen a psychiatrist. And in the Midtown study in Manhattan (Srole, *et al.*, *Mental Health in the Metropolis: The Midtown Manhattan Study*, pp. 186-187), with age and marital status taken into account, the only difference between men and women is that young bachelors are *more* likely to go to psychiatrists. In fact, according to Srole, p. 174, most studies of hospital patients show higher hospitalization rates for men than for women. Only in an experiment offering limited psychiatric coverage for some Group Health Insurance subscribers in New York did women show higher rates of utilizing this new service (Helen Avnet, *Psychiatric Insurance*, New York: GHI, 1962). Even there, however, the differences disappear for the college graduates, who are the ones most prone to make use of the service. When our results differ from those characteristic of similar types of outpatient clinics in New York City, or from the official data reported to New York State, on all terminated cases by the clinics in our study, we shall indicate that a discrepancy exists. If not specifically indicated, however, our data do not differ, at the .05 level of significance (chi square test), from the figures reported in the *Statistical Report of Psychiatric Clinics in New York State for the Year Ended March 31, 1960* (State of New York Department of Mental Hygiene, January 1961). We wish to thank Dr. Elena Padilla, Director of Research, New York City Community Mental Health Board, for making special tabulations available to us. Our data for hospital clinics are generally similar to the data reported in Saenger and Cumming, *op. cit.*
9. Hospital clinics do have a slightly older group than the State figures show. Perhaps older applicants had more time available for our research interview (which was added to the regular clinic interview). Nevertheless, the relative differences between clinics remain even for the State data.

   The State figures for the Religion and Psychiatry Institute show 67 per cent women, a statistically significant difference from our finding. Their figure may be in error, however, since neither their own nor my data from the two previous years are substantially different from the 59 per cent we reported in Table 4.

10. In Midtown Manhattan, where the Interpersonal Psychiatry Institute and the Center for Advanced Psychotherapy are located, Srole finds that in proportion to their number in the population Jews are almost four times as likely to attend outpatient psychiatric clinics as Protestants or Catholics (p. 302). And among persons judged to be psychiatrically impaired, Jews in Midtown are 10 times as likely as Catholics and two and one half times as likely as Protestants to be current psychiatric outpatients (Srole, *op. cit.*, p. 302); Jews also constitute two-thirds of the patients of private New York psychoanalysts (Irving Bieber *et al.*, *Homosexuality* [New York: Basic Books, 1962], p. 27). Yet Jewish interest in psychiatry, despite the popular stereotype of Jewish concern with medicine, does not reflect a general hypochondriasis. A recent study of Washington Heights, the neighborhood in Manhattan where Center Hospital is located, shows that Jews are hardly more likely than any other ethnic group to consult physicians for physical illnesses (Edward A. Suchman, "Sociocultural Variations in Illness and Medical Care," *American Journal of Sociology*, 70, November, 1964, 319-331).

11. These indicators are *not* combined into a single index since, especially in the mental health field, occupational rank and educational level correlate somewhat differently with various dependent variables.

12. The psychoanalytic and psychotherapeutic clinics reflect the New York and national trend of better-educated persons to use psychiatric outpatient facilities. The better-educated or those of higher class on an index are from 6 to 20 times as likely as the least educated to have been to psychiatrists (Gurin, *op. cit.*, pp. 278, 333 [my calculation]; Srole, *op. cit.*, p. 241, 246; Avnet, *op. cit.*, p. 84). These rates refer to ambulatory patients. Hospital inpatients are more likely to come from lower-class groups. Indeed, the high rates for the better educated reflect their higher rate of consulting private psychiatrists, not their use of public clinics. In fact, 70 per cent of the patients of a group of New York analysts were at least college graduates (Bieber, *op. cit.*, p. 27). Conversely, in Midtown, New York, lower-class persons have three times the rate of higher-class persons in their use of psychiatric outpatient clinics. Thus, the psychoanalytic and psychotherapeutic clinics in our study are much more like private office practice, at least in the type of person attracted, than they are like most psychiatric clinics. The chief difference between a clinic like University Psychoanalytic Center and private psychoanalytic practice in New York lies in the higher proportion of clinic applicants who have started but not completed college. Lack of a complete higher education reduces earning power but not level of aspiration, thus forcing persons to apply to a clinic rather than to a private psychiatrist.

13. Bieber, *op. cit.*, p. 27.

The Theory of Our Friends

4

"No matter how much you all repel and avoid one another, you're all much more friends than you know. Allow me. I can explain it to you. We people are more personally engaged in what we do than the average folk, and therefore as we turn from one of our activities to another, we again find one another there. . . . Unlike the ordinary folk, if two of us have one acquaintance in common, we will prove to have three hundred in common, for we have these activities in common. We have gone to the same marginal schools; we have praised to the skies the dancer whom the rest of New York has not yet heard of; and if one of us steals off to a secluded coast that seems to us promising, he will meet another one of us walking naked toward him up King's Beach.

"Oh God, how true!" groaned Arthur, and without doubt they all glared at me with hatred for explaining to them the Theory of Our Friends.

"I'm not so overjoyed about it either, I assure you," I said, stung, "to come upon your faces everywhere! Nevertheless, I'll write it down, the history of our friends."[1]

In addition to the psychiatric clinics just described, these Friends are the heroes of this book. In their present guise they are called the Friends and Supporters of Psychotherapy and we are writing a chapter in their history. Although this society is not a real organization, the circle is real enough. Its existence makes it possible for an individual to select himself voluntarily for the painful experience of psychotherapy. Membership in the Friends has important consequences for the entire process of deciding to undertake psychotherapy. Over half of our sample of applicants for psychotherapy belong to the Friends.

Members of this circle have a number of distinguishing characteristics. Their "three hundred" friends are all likely to have similar problems and to have been to psychotherapists. Since these friends are knowledgeable and understanding about psychotherapy, applicants who are members of this circle are likely to have asked their friends for the name of a psychotherapist. And it follows that they have told their friends that they have applied to a psychiatric clinic.

Association with sophisticated cultural circles in New York City is an excellent way of becoming a member of the Friends. In our sample of clinic applicants, over 70 per cent of the culturally sophisticated—that is, those who were likely to go to concerts, cocktail parties, plays, and museums or art galleries at least several times a year—were also members of the Friends and Supporters of Psychotherapy. This means that while the better educated are more likely to be members of the Friends, many who have not even graduated from high school are also members. More important than social class is the type of circle in which one moves. Thus, persons in show business on Broadway, clericals on Madison Avenue, or window-dressers on Fifth Avenue are more likely to be members than Downtown businessmen or neighborhood salesmen. For there is a special "crowd" of *New Yorker* magazine fame that are the standard-bearers of the new "dynamic" psychology. Broadway, Madison, and Fifth Avenue are their nine-to-five locations. Single or divorced persons are especially likely to be members, largely because of their greater participation in New York City's sophisticated cultural life. They appear to belong to a particular generation, as well: those between forty and forty-four are most likely to be members; they came of age shortly after World War II, when Freud began to replace Marx as the prophet of the Friends.

Proof that we are dealing with a basic phenomenon of urban life, or especially of New York City, is that previous attendance at psychiatrists' offices is usually insufficient to bring any but working-class applicants into the fold of the Friends. In fact, there is little relationship between the number of previous visits to psychiatrists and membership in the Friends.

Our interest in the Friends is not occasioned by a desire to describe the Metropolis. This circle has direct and impressive consequences for the decision to undertake psychotherapy. Membership in the Friends affects the choice of psychiatric clinics, for the majority of applicants to analytic clinics are among the Friends, but very few applicants to other clinics are members. Since analytic clinics are the "right" kind of clinic, members of the Friends are more likely to have heard of the clinic to which they are applying through their acquaintances. Compared to the nonsophisticates, especially the less educated, the Friends are likely to know of more private psychiatrists as well as more about psychiatric clinics. They are also more likely to consult their friends about their problems and, indeed, are likely to have different problems from the nonsophisticates.

In short, membership in the Friends tells us more about the decision process than does any other single variable in this study. In this chapter we shall substantiate and expound the "Theory of Our Friends" which we have just briefly reviewed.

❁ *The New Urban Society*

The American city has been interpreted as a series of neighborhoods or ecologically determined communities. Especially prominent in explicating this view was the research done in the city of Chicago by sociologists of the University of Chicago.[2] They studied neighborhoods from the "Gold Coast" to the slums, and emphasized that the huge metropolis could be understood as a series of units, each with its own characteristics. This picture matched the reality of America up to the 1930's. Many persons lived and died without ever having left their own neighborhood. True, the neighborhoods were not static. A major Chicago research effort described the growth and change of American cities as a radial movement from the inner rings of a city outward to the suburbs. Within these rings, propinquity was a ruling force. The friends one made and the girl one married were chiefly determined by the pattern of neighborhood association. The circle of friends was a neighborhood circle.

An alternate view was suggested by Georg Simmel in his trenchant essay, "The Metropolis and Mental Life." To Simmel, a European, the modern city differs qualitatively from the subjective circle of the traditional small town. In the city, to protect himself from the potentially paralyzing onslaught of a myriad of human stimuli, man "outgrows all personal life" and transcends interpersonal intimacies. Imagine walking to work down the main street of a small American town. One nods and says hello to the people one meets on the route, whether one really knows them by sight or not. But the din that would be created in New York City if every person were similarly greeted on his way to work in the subway is inconceivable. The silences of the metropolitan apartment-house elevator, broken only by occasional comments about the weather, serve to symbolize this fear of intimacy which proximity breeds. The city man compensates for his blasé shell by seeking "individual independence and the elaboration of individuality itself." The metropolis not only allows man to follow his own interests and his own destiny but demands that he create them for himself. There is no neighborhood. There is only one's self and one's interests.

Neither of these views fully captures the spirit of the modern metropolis. The urban man is not fully a member of an ecologically defined neighborhood nor is he an island unto himself, elaborating his own individuality. The urban reality is in large measure an economic one. And so Raymond Vernon describes the metropolis as a region which specializes in "external economy" industries. Organizations which participate in external economy industries have a "compelling need to be close to other firms in order to make sales or hold down costs."[3] Similarly, at the level of the individual, the freedom that Simmel finds in the city is the freedom to seek out a community or circle of like-minded persons, such as the Friends and Supporters of Psychotherapy, who through their interaction meet the individual's special needs. These circles combine some of the characteristics of a neighborhood and some of the elaboration of individuality which a neighborhood cannot allow. The "three hundred" friends in common are typical of closeknit neighborhoods. The Friends do not necessarily live next door to each other, however. The privacy and freedom from observation that the metropolis grants allow each individual member of the Friends the illusion of having discovered his own King's Beach. Paradoxically, without this sense of isolation the group would cease to exist.

The Friends and Supporters of Psychotherapy are only one of many such circles, sets, or salons in the metropolis. The airplane has made possible a circle that transcends a single metropolis or even a nation. This circle has been appropriately labeled by journalists as the "Jet Set," and is said to be replacing "Cafe Society." The "Fight Crowd" is another such circle identified by newspaper writers. Although creative artists espouse the ideology of individualism noted by Simmel, there are in fact many subcommunities of artists, actors, writers, and musicians in the metropolis. Another more prosaic but no less important type of circle is the occupational community of typographical union members, which according to one study is a major factor in the International Typographical Union's two-party system.[4]

TYPES OF SOCIAL UNITS

To understand the basic characteristics of social circles we should examine three major dimensions of all social units: (1) degree of organization, especially as reflected in the organization of their leadership; (2) the density of the interaction among members; and (3) the degree to which units are instituted.[5] Some units, such as formal organizations —businesses, for example—are highly organized, have formal leadership, and the relation of each position in the organization to others is well known. Crowds, in contrast, are amorphous and have no clearly structured leadership. Density of interaction refers to the frequency and range of contacts one group member has with another.[6] In a free market, for example, there is frequent and wide-ranging interaction among members of the market. On the other hand, mass-media audience members are said to be isolated, each in front of his TV set. Finally, families are instituted because there is widespread agreement over a long span of time on a cluster of norms which define the sort of social relations expected between one family member and another as well as on the boundaries between families. Informal cliques and gangs studied by sociologists are not instituted in the same way. First, they do not have the most characteristic mark of an instituted group: a concept indigenous to the culture and used by members of the group to identify the sort of group they are; such concepts are family, community, neighborhood, business, shop, and nation. Second, and this follows upon the first mark of an instituted group, a person always knows when he is a member of an instituted unit. When units are not instituted it often takes sociological research to identify the group and its members.

If a unit is characterized by relatively dense interaction rates, then two additional dimensions become important: the basis for the interaction and the nature of the link between group members. Interaction may be based on propinquity, such as interaction within crowds, neighborhoods, or communities. Or interaction may be the result of a common set of interests, as in business and other formal organizations. But the distinction most important to our present discussion is between direct and indirect interaction. The former is "face-to-face" interaction typical of "primary groups." The latter is more typical of "secondary groups" in which interaction often takes place through a "chain of command" in which A interacts with B who in turn interacts with C. This pattern also characterizes markets and communities.

We can now define social sets, circles, and salons. Sets and circles exhibit the peculiar combination of indirect interaction based on common interest, together with a relatively low degree of institutionalization. Thus we match in our formal fashion the literary image provided by the exponent of the "Theory of Our Friends." The "friends" if they "have one acquaintance in common . . . have three hundred in common" (indirect dense interaction); they have "activities in common" (common interest), but they are not ordinarily aware of the nature of their relationships—"you're all much more friends than you know" (low institutionalization). They have no formal leadership, for "you all repel and avoid one another."

We cannot here comment in detail on Chart I, but it illustrates our typology and shows how circles and sets differ from other more commonly studied social units. Interaction within circles and sets is more indirect than within salons. Because relations between members are not highly instituted, circles, sets, and salons do have something in common with crowds, cliques, memberships of voluntary organizations, and with fans, mass society, and mass media audiences. All of these units are typical of mass societies, by the way, and the place of circles within such societies deserves careful attention. Note that while circles and sets are similar to memberships of voluntary organizations and to fans, such as Beatles or Yankee fans, they lack the focus provided by formal leadership—rational-legal in the case of organizations, and charismatic in the case of fans. Both formal contracts and equally binding extracontractual norms of markets distinguish markets from sets and circles. In their broad aspects—in formality of leadership and density of interaction—circles, sets, and salons are like communities and neighborhoods.[7] They have similar functions and are in many ways nongeographic communities. We can now see why Simmel proposed that in complex societies they may even take on some of the functions of geographical communities and even of families.

❀ Defining the Friends

With the formal definition of a circle—indirect interaction based on common interest and a low degree of institutionalization—we can locate the Friends and Supporters of Psychotherapy. They are defined through their contacts with others knowledgeable and understanding about psychotherapy. On the basis of a preliminary study, we predicted that comparing one's problems with others, checking with others who had been to therapists and asking them for referrals, and telling others that one is applying to a clinic should be more characteristics of the Friends than of other applicants.[8]

Participation in New York City's cultural life should also be associated with membership in the Friends, for circles are often cross cutting. Even casual observation of literary and artistic circles in New York seems to indicate a pronounced interest on their part in psychoanalysis—or at least this was so in the 1950's. Items asking respondents about the extent of their visits to theaters, concerts, museums and art galleries, and even cocktail parties were therefore placed in the final version of our questionnaires and interviews.

CHART 1 *Typology of Social Circles*

Formally Instituted Relations	Formality of Leadership	High Density of Interaction				Moderate Density of Interaction
		Indirect Chain of Interaction		Direct Chain of Interaction		
		Basis for Interaction				
		Propinquity	Interest	Propinquity	Interest	
Moderate	Informal		Social set or circle	Crowd	Salon	Mass Society
	Formal		Membership of voluntary organization, fans	Cliques, gang	Demonstrations, picket line, protest	Mass Media Audience
High	Informal	Community	Market	Neighborhood	Marketplace	Mass Society
	Formal	Tribe	Formal organization	Family	Live entertainment	Nation-State

Sophistication or membership in the Friends is not defined in terms of opinions or even knowledge about psychotherapy or cultural activities, for this would delineate our group in terms of their adherence to the norms of a subculture. In contradistinction to such a basis for definition, all the items selected by our theory refer to activities or interactions. The group of Friends is defined in terms of its social structure rather than according to the content of its ideas. The "Theory of Our Friends" is therefore a sociological not a cultural theory. It is a matter of separate concern to ascertain whether over and above the interests which bring it together this social group also has a set of common ideas or even an ideology.

How can we best test our theory? In addition to the model about to to be described, the final test of the Theory of Our Friends requires a sociometric test of those whom our model selects for membership in order to ascertain their degree of relatedness through acquaintance chains. Such a test is beyond our present means. By developing a model of how these items might be related we can, however, implicitly test the theory. If the Friends are a true social circle, then the attributes just suggested may not characterize each member of the group. Rather, they are attributes of the circle as a whole. In describing the national character of Americans or Russians, for example, one does not claim that every American or Russian has the traits ascribed to his country, or even that there exist "typical" Americans or Russians. The attempt is to capture an atmosphere, a climate of opinion, or a sense of the group.

This point of view implies a mathematical model.[9] Suppose one runs into one of the Friends, at random. One is likely to discover a person who is a theater-goer, a concert-goer, someone who knows others who have been in therapy, and so on. Non-Friends, when approached at random, are less likely to have these traits. Although these traits characterize the group as a whole, within each group the attributes are distributed at random among the members of that group. This is called "local independence" by Lazarsfeld and Anderson. The entire relationship between going to a concert and also going to a play, which is found in the population at large, is really accounted for by group membership. Thus, there are more visits to concerts and to plays among members of the Friends than among nonmembers; yet among the members, a person who goes to one event need not necessarily go to the other. For both of us to feel "in," it is entirely sufficient that I have been to the latest concert and you to the latest play. In fact, the random but frequent distribution of these traits is what makes for group conversation, mutual interest, and attraction, as every hostess knows. The structure of a circle allows these attributes to be traded, as it were, among the members, and the desire to trade helps the circle to develop. The indirect chain of interaction, the common interest, and the lack of instituted relations—all character-istic of social circles—are both the cause and the consequence of this arrangement. A social circle therefore means that many members of the circle have the group traits, but these traits are not related to one an-other among the members of the circle. The homogeneous quality of circles *yet without an instituted structure which specifies priorities or orders of items* (as in a Guttman scale) thus makes local independence within unordered classes the logical choice for a model.

While the principles which define a social circle may be reasonably straightforward, it actually takes a computer to work the whole thing out. Our knowledge of the circles with which we are dealing suggests that responses to eight items might indicate circle membership. The items suggested were: going to plays, concerts, cocktail parties, and museums or art galleries at least several times a year; and knowing others with similar problems, having friends who went to psychiatrists, telling a few people about coming to the clinic, and asking friends for a referral. Since each person could be classified as having said yes or no to each of the eight items, there are 2^8 or 256 possible combinations of answers. We need to know which combinations indicate membership in the Friends and Supporters of Psychotherapy and which do not. Further, we think there may actually be two *intersecting* circles—psychiatric sophisticates and cultural sophisticates. We want the computer to ar-range the responses so that members of the Friends are more likely to assent to these items, or at least to the items having to do with going to a psychiatrist, but we also want to follow the principle of local inde-pendence which states that *within* a given circle, merely knowing that a person has said yes to one item does not help us to know whether he said yes to any of the other items. We cannot expect a perfect fit to these requirements, but we should like to know how closely the actual data come to meeting them. If the data do not fit, then we shall have to come up with some other idea about social circles, or another set of items. Clearly the task is beyond the immediate application of com-mon sense, and we need a mathematical model—*latent class analysis*—and a big computer to do all the juggling.

Table 5 shows the result of this estimation by the computer.[10] The relative size of the four latent intersecting circles is indicated across the top of the table. In the body of the table are the theoretical propor-tions of the members of each circle who say yes to the eight items listed down the side of the table. Thus, 39 per cent of the applicants theo-retically belong to the circle we have called "cultural and psychiatric sophistication." Of them, 90 per cent go to plays, 72 per cent to concerts, and so on. Our social-circle theory which led to the latent class model does seem reasonable, for the 256 response patterns estimated by the

TABLE 5 *Theoretical Size of Circles and Proportion of Response to Eight Traits among Clinic Applicants, as Estimated by the Model*

Trait	Friends and Supporters of Psychotherapy		Others	
	Cultural and psychiatric sophistication (39%)	*Psychiatric sophistication only (17%)*	*Cultural sophistication only (15%)*	*No sophistication (29%)*
Cultural Sophistication	%	%	%	%
Go to plays several times a year or more	90	36	90	8
Go to concerts several times a year or more	72	8	62	8
Go to cocktail parties several times a year or more	45	33	31	8
Go to museums or art galleries several times a year or more	92	29	70	29
Psychiatric Sophistication				
Know others with similar problems	62	60	22	21
Know friends who went to a psychiatrist	92	88	46	36
Told "a few people" about coming to this clinic	77	75	29	28
Asked friends for a referral to a clinic or private psychiatrist	72	58	9	10

model (not shown in Table 5) match or fit the actual data very well ($\chi^2 = .87$ with 220 degrees of freedom left when the number of parameters necessary for the estimate are subtracted from the 256 response patterns).

THE MEANING OF THE MODEL

Now that we have a statistically satisfactory structure of items, what do they mean substantively? Are we correct in our labels for the four circles? What does the proportion of responses for the different circles tell about the Theory of Our Friends?[11]

Almost all who are culturally and psychiatrically sophisticated say they go to plays and museums or art galleries at least several times a year, whereas those who are only psychiatrically sophisticated go less often. The nonsophisticated hardly ever go to plays, but have a fair proportion of claimed museum attendance. The nonculturally sophisticated who are psychiatrically knowledgeable do attend plays more often than those with neither psychiatric nor cultural interests. Perhaps modern psychologically motivated drama attracts them.

Concert-going, a less frequent trait, stands in vivid contrast to these patterns. Not all who are culturally sophisticated make such a claim. Concerts, of course, are almost entirely nonverbal and thus have no special attraction for the psychiatrically sophisticated who are not also culturally sophisticated.

Cocktail-partygoing is even less frequent than concert attendance. But it is almost equally prevalent among all types of sophisticated circles —cultural or psychiatric. It is hardly found among the nonsophisticated. This lubricant of New York City sophistication, celebrated in New Yorker cartoons, is apparently to some extent functional for all sophisticated circles regardless of the content of their sophistication. The circles are instruments of social interaction, and cocktail parties both promote and are consequences of this social interaction.

The circle of our Friends consists of those in the first two latent classes. Almost everyone who belongs knows friends, other than family members, who have been to see psychiatrists. Less than one half of the others do, however. The norms also dictate that one must tell others outside the family circle that one is applying to a clinic. This presupposes that first, one is not especially ashamed of revealing this information, and second, that those to whom one speaks will be sympathetic and understanding. These conditions are obviously much more easily met among the Friends. As either a cause or consequence of revealing to others, or knowing about others who have been to psychiatrists, a member of the Friends is fairly likely to know of other persons who have problems similar to his own.

Asking friends for a referral is the one trait which most clearly discriminates between members of the Friends and others. Moreover, asking a friend for a referral to a psychiatrist is not a simple request. If one has a cold and is in a strange city or does not know a doctor, one does not hesitate to say, "I have a cold and fever. Do you know of a doctor to whom I might go?" But it is an altogether different matter to say, in effect, "I think I have a neurosis, do you know of a psychotherapist to whom I might go?" Only members of the Friends are likely both to have the courage to admit to such a need and to have friends who might actually know a good psychotherapist. Almost no one who is not a member of the Friends is in such a position. The importance of the way cultural circles crosscut the Friends and Supporters of Psychotherapy is shown by the fact that those who belong to the Friends and are also culturally sophisticated are somewhat more likely than those who are not culturally au courant to have this important but delicate relationship with their friends. Indeed, this trait, crucial to the process of seeking therapy, is the only noncultural feature which distinguishes between the two circles of Friends.

There are two circles of Friends because there are two ways of becoming a member of the Friends. One way is through active participation in New York City cultural circles. An interest in psychotherapy, it appears, is prevalent in such surroundings, although not all culturally active circles are also supporters of psychotherapy. Nevertheless, mingling with persons interested in the theater, concerts, and art will often bring one in contact with persons knowledgeable about psychotherapy. Another channel to the Friends is more direct. Since there is a large number of persons in New York interested in psychotherapy, one may drift into a "crowd" of Friends and Supporters of Psychotherapy who are not also interested in the arts. These two paths are characteristically taken by two quite different types of persons. In fact, a simple two-class structure does not fit the data quite as well as a four-class one.

❀ Characteristics of the Friends

A theory of the Friends and Supporters of Psychotherapy has been developed and tested by means of a mathematical model. The model fits our data and leads to reasonable substantive interpretations. In the pages to follow, we shall describe the characteristics of the members of the different circles. An applicant was assigned to the circle to which he most probably belongs on the basis of his responses to the eight items which define membership in the Friends.[12]

TYPE OF CLINIC

Membership in the Friends is highly associated with the type of clinic to which a person has applied, as Chart II shows. As might be expected, the analytic clinics draw heavily upon the Friends, while two of the hospital clinics, St. Matthew's and Center, draw very few members of the Friends. St. Francis, again because of its application policy, draws a sophisticated population that more resembles the analytic than the hospital clinics. Personal Psychology draws a less sophisticated group than any of the other analytic clinics, and the Religion and Psychiatry Institute lies roughly between Personal and the hospital clinics. The circle of Friends is thus a key variable in explaining why certain groups are drawn to different types of clinics. In part, people go to different types of clinics because others in their social circles go there.

The influence of membership in the Friends on the application process will be taken up in detail later on. At present, let us see whether an applicant's social position affects the likelihood of his being a mem-

CHART II *Proportion of Applicants to Eight Clinics Who Are Members of the Friends*

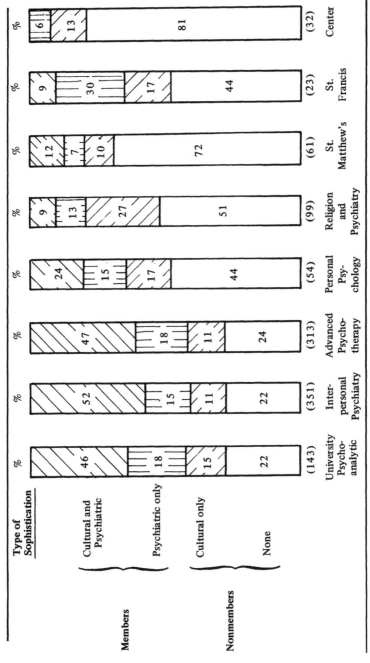

Note: Only clinics in the 1960 data-gathering are included.

ber of the Friends. In these analyses, we shall examine only applicants to analytic clinics—the stamping grounds of the Friends—unless there are noteworthy factors affecting the data at other clinics.

SOCIAL POSITION AND ETHNICITY

Cultural and psychiatric sophistication are both closely tied to the level of one's education, as Chart III shows. The details of Chart III are very revealing. First, it explains why those who have not even graduated from high school have applied to an analytic clinic; one normally thinks of psychoanalysis as suitable only for the well educated. About half of these poorly educated analytic clinic applicants are members of the Friends. A glance at the almost constant proportion of psychiatrically but not culturally sophisticated, at various levels of education, begins to explain how poorly educated persons become members of the Friends. Greater participation in New York cultural life comes with higher education; high culture is in turn associated with psychiatric sophistication. The route to membership in the Friends for the less educated, however, is in significant measure through pure psychiatric sophistication. The highest proportion of psychiatric sophistication unadulterated by participation in culture is found in the high-school graduate group. Twenty-one per cent of analytic clinic applicants who were high-school graduates but did not continue their education were psychiatrically but not culturally sophisticated. A high-school education gives a person the minimum ability to understand modern psychiatry but is not necessarily sufficient to guarantee cultural interests.

Membership in the Friends is, of course, associated with high social class, but this is not the most relevant way of explaining membership. Among analytic clinic applicants, for example, 54 per cent of those with the highest-ranking occupations were both culturally and psychiatrically sophisticated, as compared with 35 per cent of those with the lowest-ranking occupations.[13] This is a 19-percentage-point difference. The type rather than the social prestige of occupations held by applicants is more closely associated with membership in the Friends. Thus, in Chart IV we see that 60 per cent of men who are "insiders" but only 28 per cent of men who are blue-collar workers are culturally and psychiatrically sophisticated—a difference of 32 percentage points.

Insiders, it will be recalled, are those persons who work in occupations or industries sympathetic to psychiatry. Included are the health professions; teaching on both college and other levels; show business and the arts; and the communications, advertising and education industries, regardless of the particular job of the applicant. A secretary who works for an advertising agency is classified as an insider, along with a psychiatric resident, or an actor. Among the men, insiders are 17 percentage

CHART III *Proportion of Analytic-Clinic Applicants of Different Levels of Education Who Are Members of the Friends*

Education of Applicant*

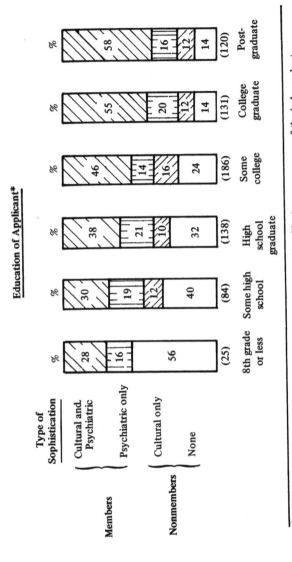

Type of Sophistication		
Members {	Cultural and Psychiatric	
	Psychiatric only	
Nonmembers {	Cultural only	
	None	

*Students excluded. In this and all following charts and tables, No Answers on any of the independent variables are excluded.

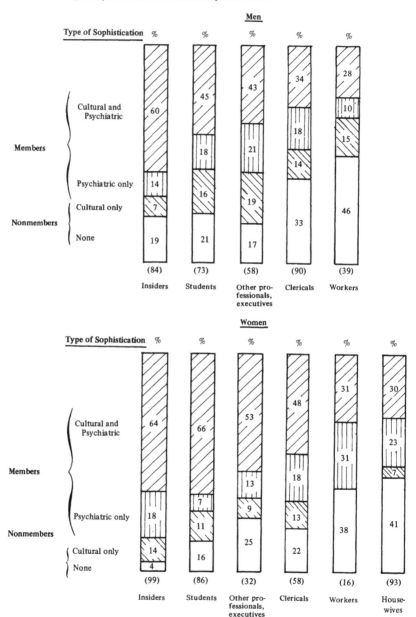

CHART IV *Proportion of Men and Women Analytic-Clinic Applicants of Different Types of Occupations Who Are Members of the Friends*

Men

Type of Sophistication

Members
- Cultural and Psychiatric
- Psychiatric only

Nonmembers
- Cultural only
- None

	Insiders	Students	Other professionals, executives	Clericals	Workers
	60	45	43	34	28
					10
		18	21	18	15
	14			14	
	7	16	19	33	46
	19	21	17		
	(84)	(73)	(58)	(90)	(39)

Women

Type of Sophistication

Members
- Cultural and Psychiatric

Nonmembers
- Psychiatric only
- Cultural only
- None

	Insiders	Students	Other professionals, executives	Clericals	Workers	Housewives
	64	66	53	48	31	30
					31	23
	18	7	13	18		7
		11	9	13		
	14	16	25	22	38	41
	4					
	(99)	(86)	(32)	(58)	(16)	(93)

points more likely than other professionals and executives of approximately the same social standing to be culturally and psychiatrically sophisticated. Certain types of occupation that have been associated with the public acceptance of modern psychodynamic theories thus remain the natural habitat of the Friends and Supporters of Psychotherapy. The "square" occupations—the businessmen, the lawyers, and the engineers—are perhaps too concerned with what can be directly apprehended through the senses to be caught up in a social movement that emphasizes the ineffable.[14]

The special climate of New York, generated by its sophisticated circles, is thus responsible for the development of the Friends, who constitute the majority of analytic clinic applicants. The Friends are also largely responsible for bringing a fair proportion of not especially well-educated persons into the psychoanalytic movement and thus attracting them to analytic clinics. The working-class applicants to analytic clinics tend, however, to be moving up the social ladder. Forty per cent of them would like professional or managerial jobs. And of the working-class men who do aspire to such high-level jobs, over 60 per cent ($n = 16$) are members of the Friends. Fewer than 25 per cent of the other working-class men ($n = 23$)—those without high aspirations—are members of the Friends. Further, of those who now have a high-level occupation, men who have moved up from a working-class background are more likely to be members of the Friends than men whose fathers were also executives, professionals, and businessmen—82 per cent ($n = 38$) as against 63 per cent ($n = 30$). Perhaps membership in the Friends actually facilitates upward social mobility; perhaps it is merely symbolic of this mobility along with other symbols, such as possession of modern oil paintings. In either case, it is conceivable that an application to an analytic clinic is indicative of upward social striving rather than a symptom of the psychic strains induced by the climb upward.

Class in New York City is intertwined with ethnicity. But ethnicity itself, when separated from social class, is extremely important in New York City life. Chart V distinguishes five major New York City ethnic groups: white Protestants, Catholics, Jews, Puerto Ricans, and non-whites. Class is represented by education.

Previously we saw that Jews are the majority of analytic clinic applicants, thus reinforcing the notion that psychoanalysis is a "Jewish science." On the other hand, with education controlled, white Protestant applicants to analytic clinics are more likely than any other ethnic group to be members of the Friends. In the cultural circles of New York, white Protestants are a minority group; perforce, they behave much like other minority groups who wish to be accepted by the majority; they outdo the majority at their own game. Where they are the majority, at the Religion and Psychiatry clinic, they evince less

CHART V *Proportion of Analytic-Clinic Applicants with Various Ethnic Backgrounds Who Are Members of the Friends*

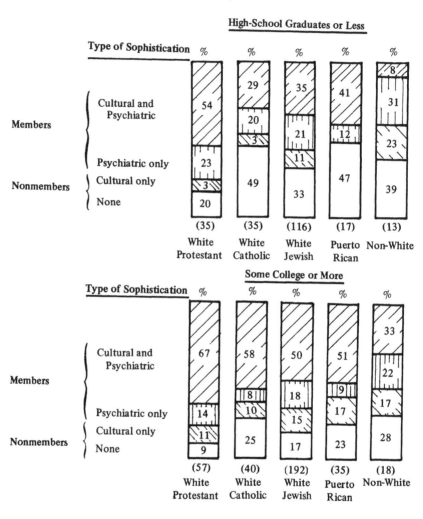

High-School Graduates or Less

| Type of Sophistication | | | % | % | % | % | % |

Members { Cultural and Psychiatric

Nonmembers { Psychiatric only / Cultural only / None

White Protestant (35), White Catholic (35), White Jewish (116), Puerto Rican (17), Non-White (13)

Some College or More

| Type of Sophistication | | | % | % | % | % | % |

Members { Cultural and Psychiatric

Nonmembers { Psychiatric only / Cultural only / None

White Protestant (57), White Catholic (40), White Jewish (192), Puerto Rican (35), Non-White (18)

Note: University excluded: no data on race.

interest in psychoanalysis, for only 19 per cent (n = 59) are members of the Friends. Protestants who are among the "in group" of the Friends are quite unlikely to apply to the Religion and Psychiatry clinic, for they are much less likely to be religious.* Catholic, Jewish, and

---

* 46 per cent of analytic clinic Protestant applicants are religious as compared to 65 per cent of the Protestants applying to the Religion and Psychiatry Institute. Only the nonreligious Protestants are especially likely to be members of the Friends.

Puerto Rican applicants to analytic clinics who are well educated have about the same proportion of members in the Friends. Among the less educated, however, Catholics (especially the more religious ones) and Puerto Ricans are less likely to be members of the Friends; Negroes are least likely to be members, regardless of level of education or type of clinic to which they have applied. Negroes generally seem less interested in psychoanalysis and psychiatry, at least in terms of the number who apply to the various clinics in New York. Perhaps they see their problems not in personal psychological terms but rather in terms of class and ethnic discrimination.

SEX, MARITAL STATUS, AND AGE

The effects of sex and age on membership in the Friends depend very much on an applicant's occupation and education. Especially important is the status of housewife, as shown in Chart IV. Housewives are 25 percentage points less likely than their sisters who have secretarial jobs to be culturally sophisticated. The majority of analytic clinic women applicants work, and they are even somewhat more likely than men to be members of the Friends; this is especially true of college students. Women students, but also women in other walks of life (except housewives), tend to become members of the Friends through their participation in cultural life. This participation is considerably greater than that of men, which accounts for the greater prevalence of women among the Friends.

The relative lack of sophistication of housewives calls attention to one of the major features of membership in the Friends. Single men and women, living alone or with roommates, are one of the important leavening agents of New York sophisticated living. They are culture heroes, of sorts, to the now somewhat more staid married persons who, through their nostalgia for a former status, help perpetuate the myth about gay bachelorhood. The simple structure of living within a family, on the other hand, creates certain obligations that cut down on the amount of time one can spend going to cultural events—unless, of course, one is unusually wealthy, a category absent from this sample of clinic applicants. For these reasons, single or divorced men and women who do not live with their parents are much more likely to be members of the Friends. For example, in the age range of twenty-five to thirty-four, the modal age for being a sophisticated single man or woman about town, well over 70 per cent of the men and over 80 per cent of the women applicants to analytic clinics who do not live with a spouse or with parents are members of the Friends. This compares to about 55 per cent membership for married men and women of these ages. The main difference is of course caused by the greater cultural sophistication of the single persons.

CHART VI   *Per Cent of Analytic-Clinic Applicants Who Are Members of the Friends, Adjusted for Education*

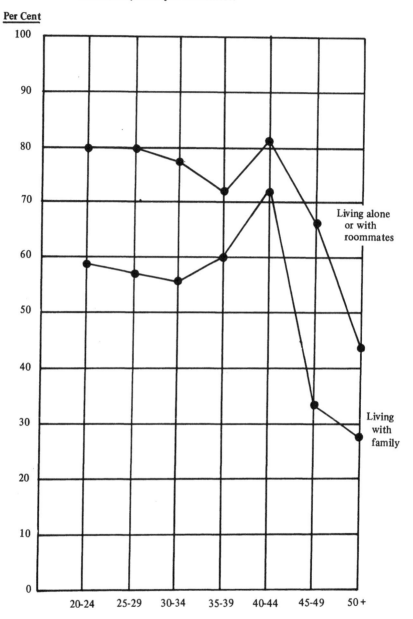

Per Cent

Age

Moreover, there is a generational effect here. Psychoanalytic thinking was never really popular in New York City until the many psycho-analysts expelled by Hitler from Germany and Austria found refuge in the United States and came to live in New York. The full flowering of the movement, and its replacement of Marxism as the dominant ideology of the young intellectuals, came after World War II. Persons who are now in their early forties came of age during this period. They thus remain the standard-bearers of the movement. Many of the Marxists turned to Freud, and they form a substantial proportion of older members of the Friends, as one can see, for example, by changes in the policy and inclinations of the *Partisan Review*. Many of the older Friends make enough money not to have to apply to clinics. Hence there are fewer of them in the sample. Nevertheless, relatively few persons over forty-five were exposed to the psychotherapy movement during their formative years. Consequently, there are few members of the Friends in the older group.

PREVIOUS PSYCHOTHERAPY

Thus far we have ignored the effect of psychotherapists themselves on membership in the Friends. Actually going to a psychotherapist might be thought to be one of the best ways of becoming a Friend and Supporter of Psychotherapy and far more effective than belonging to the right social circles. Yet previous psychotherapy leads to membership in the Friends only for some of the less educated applicants. For most, membership has largely to do with the innate character of one's social circle—something not easily altered by individual psychotherapy.

We cannot experimentally expose some persons to psychotherapy and not others, and then observe the results. Demonstrating the effect or lack of effect of previous psychotherapy on membership in the Friends is therefore a bit awkward. Let us begin, however, with the obvious. With the possible exception of hospital clinic applicants, there is al-most no relationship between previous psychotherapy and either cultural and psychiatric sophistication or psychiatric sophistication alone. Most hospital clinic applicants are poorly educated, however. When education is taken into account, analytic clinic applicants with less than a college education are, like the hospital applicants, somewhat more inclined to membership in the Friends if they have had extended psychiatric treat-ment. This is not true for the better educated who are the majority of applicants to analytic clinics and Religion and Psychiatry Institute applicants.

The complex way in which psychotherapy is associated with member-ship in the Friends is revealed by the difference between the better-educated and more poorly educated applicants. Going to a psychotherapist could produce membership in the Friends through direct or indirect influence. Therapy can bring a patient into direct contact with others who are in therapy, but since psychotherapy, as practiced, mainly consists of individual treatment, direct introduction to others in treatment is probably infrequent. Indirect effects are more likely. Therapy might make a patient more favorable to and knowledgeable about psychiatry. As a result of this change, he might then become more friendly with others who share his new ideas. In addition, psychotherapy may make a patient aware that others also go to psychiatrists by sensitizing him to the mere possibility of going to a therapist for treatment, just as when a person has a cold, he suddenly becomes aware of the "fact" that "everyone" else also has a cold. Whatever the route, contact with others who are in therapy can lead to assimilation into the circle of the Friends. Such "conversion" is likely to come about only if one has not previously had the chance to join the circle. Better-educated persons, through their normal social environment, are likely to have known others in treatment *and* to have been aware of the ideology of psychotherapy. For them, therefore, not joining the Friends is not a matter of lack of exposure but of lack of interest or the attractiveness of alternative circles.

Let us check the first assumption of this argument—that psychotherapy is related primarily to knowing others in treatment for less-educated applicants but not for the better-educated. First, in the population at large, the less-educated are less likely to know persons who have had psychotherapy. Fifty-one per cent of college graduates know a person in office treatment but only 11 per cent of those with less than a grammar-school education know such persons.[15] This difference is indeed partly caused by the nature of one's normal social surroundings. Persons tend to associate on a personal basis with others of the same social class, and lower-class persons are in fact less likely than higher-class persons to be in office or clinic psychotherapy.[16] Also, lower-class persons tend to have a narrower circle of friends of any kind. In our sample, the less-educated who have not had previous therapy are less likely to know of others in psychotherapy by almost 30 per cent. But the less-educated who have been to psychotherapists are almost as likely as the well-educated to know of others in treatment. Thus, the first part of our argument is demonstrated: Only among the less-educated is psychotherapy associated primarily with knowing others in treatment.

Membership in the Friends is partly defined through knowing others in treatment. Table 6, moreover, shows that knowledge of others is much more closely related to membership in the Friends than merely having previously attended a psychotherapist.

Among people with some college education, knowledge of others in treatment is the whole story; previous therapy does not count. Among

TABLE 6 *Per Cent of Applicants to Analytic Clinics Who Are Members of the Friends (by Education, Number of Previous Visits to Psychotherapists, and Knowledge of Others in Therapy)*

	High School Graduates or Less					
	Number of Previous Visits to Psychotherapists					
	None		1–20		21 or more	
Knowledge of Others in Therapy:						
Sophistication	No %	Yes %	No %	Yes %	No %	Yes %
Cultural and psychiatric	13	56	26	41	36	43
Psychiatric only	13	21	3	33	7	31
Cultural only	15	6	15	2	14	10
None	60	18	56	25	43	16
Total†	101%	101%	100%	101%	100%	100%
	(40)	(34)	(34)	(64)	(28)	(49)
	Some College or More*					
	Number of Previous Visits to Psychotherapists					
	None		1–20		21 or more	
Knowledge of Others in Therapy:						
Sophistication	No %	Yes %	No %	Yes %	No %	Yes %
Cultural and psychiatric	37	57	32	64	37	60
Psychiatric only	7	21	14	16	13	19
Cultural only	30	13	23	8	17	6
None	26	9	32	13	33	15
Total	100%	100%	101%	101%	100%	100%
	(27)	(70)	(44)	(103)	(52)	(121)

*Students excluded.
†In this and all subsequent tables, no answers, not applicable, or not collected in 1958–1959 are excluded.

the less-educated, however, both knowledge of others and previous therapy count in making one a member of the Friends. Both direct and indirect routes to membership seem operative. The likelihood that a less-educated analytic clinic applicant who does not know others in treatment belongs to the culturally sophisticated branch of the Friends depends directly on the amount of therapy he has had. Therapy plus knowledge of others, the indirect route, is associated among the less-educated with an increase in pure psychiatric sophistication.

But which causes which? Does therapy lead to knowledge of friends in therapy and thence to sophistication, or does sophistication lead to being able to stay in therapy or apply for more if the first time has failed? Staying in therapy must be the consequence of cultural and psychiatric sophistication, not a cause of it. It is absurd to think that psychotherapy alone can make one culturally sophisticated if one is not so to begin with. The indirect route, from therapy to knowing others in therapy to membership in the Friends, could however result in pure psychiatric sophistication, and psychiatric sophistication is indeed more frequent among the less-educated who have had some psychotherapy and now know others in therapy.

We conclude, therefore, that among the better-educated, psychotherapy does not affect imbedded personal patterns and relationships. The well-educated have already had their chance to join the Friends. If they have not yet done so, therapy is not going to make them more favorable to the Friends. But therapy is related to membership in the Friends among the less-educated in two ways: first, it helps them to stay in therapy, or at least to apply for more; second, a small proportion of less-educated applicants who have had therapy have been converted to membership in the Friends apparently through a two-step process: first they become aware of others in treatment and then through them become members of the Friends.

MEMBERSHIP IN THE FRIENDS: A SUMMARY PROFILE

The Friends and Supporters of Psychotherapy, as we have seen, tend to know others with similar problems, to have friends who have also gone to psychiatrists, to have asked their friends for a referral to a psychotherapist or psychiatric clinic, and to have told a few people about their application to the present clinic. Almost three-fourths of the circle of our Friends are also culturally sophisticated. This means that they are likely to have been to plays, concerts, museums or art galleries, and to cocktail parties at least several times a year. The Friends are found most often among the applicants to analytic clinics.

These traits do not come about by accident. Rather, location in certain social settings produces membership in the Friends. High education, high social class, but especially participation in an occupational milieu which emphasizes the artistic and the psychological—such as the health professions, teaching, communications and the arts—are all highly associated with membership in the Friends. Secularism, especially if one is Protestant or a poorly educated Catholic, is also important in creating appropriate conditions for membership. In a group predominantly Jewish, secular white Protestants are more likely than any other ethnic group to be members. Finally, bachelorhood, if lived apart from one's parents, facilitates cultural activity in New York and that in turn brings persons to the Friends. Applicants over forty-five years of age are just "out of it." Indeed, those who went "to the same marginal schools" and who "have praised to the skies the dancer whom the rest of New York has not yet heard of" are also the Friends and Supporters of Psychotherapy.

There are, however, other channels to the Friends than via New York City cultural sophistication. These channels tend to create members through psychiatric sophistication alone. Generally, those members of the Friends who come from positions in which members of the Friends are not prevalent—statuses such as housewives, workers, persons of low education, married persons, and the like—tend toward higher rates of psychiatric but not cultural sophistication. Thus, among housewives who are members of the Friends, over two-fifths are psychiatrically but not culturally sophisticated, whereas among "insiders" who are Friends, fewer than one-fifth are only psychiatrically sophisticated. These persons who are not naturally exposed to the Friends must be more directly recruited to membership through mass media favorable to psychiatry and through previous experience with psychotherapy.

✿ Consequences of Membership in the Friends

The moral of the History of Our Friends is contained in the rest of this book. Here, we shall briefly outline some of the consequences for deciding to enter psychotherapy that are attendant on membership in the Friends. As will become evident, membership in the Friends considerably eases the process of applying for therapy.[17]

First, although members do not necessarily identify more often than nonmembers with the status of psychiatric patient, they do tend to like such patients and to see more of them as having the same problems as their own. Their general opinions about psychiatry, however, do not differ radically from those of nonmembers, partially, we suspect, because we have not measured these opinions correctly. Members have also read somewhat more in psychiatry than nonmembers, although applicants to analytic clinics who are neither culturally nor psychiatrically sophisticated and who are poorly educated seem to excel in reading popular psychology such as is found in the *Ladies Home Journal* or other self-help material. Members also have general expectations of therapy that are more in line with those of psychotherapists themselves. They are less likely to expect advice and more likely to feel that they, not the therapist, will do most of the talking.

In each step of the decision to undertake psychotherapy, members of the Friends differ from others. Their problems tend to be different. There is a special syndrome of problems of the Friends which include sexual problems, difficulties in interpersonal relations, and dissatisfaction with oneself. It takes no special insight to see that each of these types

of problems corresponds to one of the major "causes" of emotional difficulties identified by the major schools of psychoanalysis. The matter
of presenting problems will be investigated in detail in the next chapters.

Since they have a knowledgeable social environment, members of the
Friends tend to report that a greater number of friends or relatives
noticed their problems; and they themselves are more likely voluntarily
to discuss their problems with friends and relatives. Yet in our assessment of reasons for coming to a clinic now, fewer of the Friends seem
to have come solely as a result of the pressure of others. Nevertheless, a
greater proportion of the Friends has heard of the clinic through their
friends or relatives; they are less likely to have been referred by nonpsychiatrist physicians or to have heard of the clinic through the mass
media. Finally, as might be expected, members of the Friends know of
more private psychotherapists and more clinics than do nonmembers,
thereby making their present choice a more rational one.

Our data in general show that membership in the Friends, whatever
the source of this membership, provides a potential applicant for psychotherapy with considerable social support in making what is, after all, a
much less lonely decision.

❦ Conclusion: How the Friends Contribute to the Psychotherapy System

The Friends and Supporters of Psychotherapy are a not-so-mythical
social circle, typical of the many such "crowds" fostered by a metropolitan environment. These circles are communities which are not neighborhoods but rather indirect chains of acquaintances linked by common
friends, interests, and values. Such nongeographical communities solve
implicit social problems for their members and for the metropolis at
large.

The circle of the Friends and Supporters of Psychotherapy solves a
problem of crucial importance to the psychotherapy movement and to
the individuals involved in the circle. Psychotherapy, of course, cannot
exist without clients. Most professions get clients through word of
mouth, professional referrals, and simply by existing in the usual social
environment of potential clients. Psychotherapists, too, receive clients
through these sources. But there is a difference. Although all professionals require a certain social distance from their clients to permit the
exercise of professional judgment and authority, psychotherapists require an even greater distance.[18] An important part of psychotherapy
consists of the client's playing out various values, modes of interaction
and feelings vis-à-vis the therapist. Since the therapist does not have

a clear place in the patient's life outside the therapy situation, the patient can engage in a full display of his own values, interactions, and emotions. The expression of these feelings is held to be crucial to effective therapy. In this type of therapy, then, the norms of the profession enjoin the therapist from interacting with the patient under any other circumstances than the therapy hour lest the patient's feelings be in some way obstructed. On the other hand, the social distance between therapists and patients makes both the recruitment of patients and the subsequent relationship with therapists more difficult. Potential patients do not know of any therapist to whom to go, and once they get there they do not know what to expect or how to act.

Contrast this with the situation of the minister, who is a part of the community of his "clients." Members of his congregation—and these comprise the majority of counselees with ministers—feel that it is possible just to "drop in" on the minister to chat. They also tend to know what to expect from the minister. In the course of their conversation they can reveal some of their personal problems. Easy access to ministers means, however, that ministers can counsel with their parishioners only at certain levels. Data show that when problems become more involved or too "deep" both minister and parishioner feel that they "know each other too well." The counseling relationship is then terminated, whether with or without a referral to a more distant professional.

General practitioners are a profession more closely related to psychotherapists. Indeed the psychotherapist models himself on the medical profession. General practitioners are socially closer to their patients than are psychotherapists, however. Most persons have a family physician. Almost no one has a family psychiatrist. Patients have been to doctors from an early age and know what to expect. The physician manages to maintain his emotional distance from patients and thereby preserves much of his authority by focusing on the specific issue of physical disability and illness. As both our study and others show, even emotional illness is treated by most general practitioners as a physical matter. They prescribe pills. Specificity is helpful to most tasks of the physician, but does not appear to be what most applicants to psychiatric clinics need, since their problems are of such a general nature.

Barred from the usual social contact with patients, yet needing a close relationship both to recruit patients and to work with them successfully, psychotherapists early in their history began to develop circles of friends and supporters. Freud formed the Vienna Psycho-Analytical Society in 1908 from a group which, beginning in 1902, met every Wednesday evening in Freud's waiting room.[19] In the beginning the group was informal and admitted laymen. Later, the group became a formal organization complete with bitter internecine feuds and restricted itself to psychoanalysts whose ideas were compatible with

Freud's. Freud and others, both enemies and friends, addressed groups of laymen and nonmedical academics not connected with the formal association. An entire chapter of Jones's biography is devoted to "Non-Medical Application of Psychoanalysis."[20] The result was that

> with the reviews just mentioned, the growing psychoanalytical literature, and the constant polemical discussion and diatribes conducted by his opponents at every meeting of psychiatrists and of the many general medical meetings, no educated person in German could have failed to know of the existence of Freud's work in the period before the World War and have perhaps some rough idea of its nature.[21]

At this time, jocularly sensitive to the future growth of the Friends, Freud said, "The best sign of the acceptance of psychoanalysis would be when the Viennese shops advertised 'gifts for all stages of the transference.' "[22] Jones adds, "That has not happened in Vienna, but I am told it has in New York."[23] I have been unable to find such advertisements in New York, but the indicators of the Friends found in this chapter serve the same function. In many ways, the modern circle of our Friends has made the psychoanalytic movement possible. For they provide a bridge between therapist and patient which shortens the social distance between them. How the Friends accomplish this function will be apparent in the following chapters.

NOTES

Portions of this chapter appeared in the *American Sociological Review*, 31 (1966). I am indebted to Neil Henry for adapting a method and supervising the construction of a 7094 program to solve the basic problem of this chapter, as well as his helpful comments on my explication of latent structure. David Elesh also contributed helpful comments.
1. Paul Goodman, *The Empire City* (New York: Bobbs-Merrill, 1959), p. 67. The passage came to my attention through an article by Marcus Cunliffe, "The History of Our Friends, on Paul Goodman," *Encounter* (June 1962), 28. Professor Cunliffe comments further about the setting of our friends, drawing from a character in a Delmore Schwartz story. In Schwartz's middle-class Jewish setting of the 1930's when Marx, not Freud, was the god, the girl complains that for years she has never been allowed to finish a sentence. In Cunliffe's paraphrase, "Everyone thinks that he has a subtle understanding of everyone else, but that he himself is misunderstood." This is still true of the same circles today. But now, as Goodman himself farcically describes it in Part II of the *Empire City*, psychotherapy is the cure for a lack of social conscience, as well as for feelings of lack of communication with others. Many of those who were once Marxists are now supporters of psychotherapy.
2. Representative is R. E. Park, E. W. Burgess, and R. D. McKenzie, *The City* (Chicago: The University of Chicago Press, 1925). For a more extensive bibliography of previous work on social circles, see my article in the *American Sociological Review, op. cit.*

3. Raymond Vernon, *Metropolis 1985* (New York: Anchor Books, 1963), pp. 27-28.
4. Seymour M. Lipset, Martin Trow, and James Coleman, *Union Democracy* (New York: The Free Press, 1956).
5. We regret joining a long tradition of finding dimensions for groups, yet because of a lack of interest on the part of sociologists in social circles, existing sets of dimensions do not seem quite adequate to separating social circles from other units. For references to other attempts at dimensions of groups and for a comprehensive list of group attributes, see Merton, *Social Theory and Social Structure*, 2nd ed. (New York: The Free Press, 1957), pp. 308-326.
6. This is probably Durkheim's meaning of density as used in *The Division of Labor* (New York: The Free Press, 1947), p. 257.
7. Some of the cells in our chart are empty. They represent structurally unstable situations. The combination of propinquity, indirect but dense interaction, together with low institutionalization is unstable, since such interaction cannot be sustained without turning into interaction not on the basis of propinquity but of interest. Or, such interaction may result in a community characterized by relatively high institutionalization. This combination is especially unstable should formal leadership develop. Finally, whether mass society, characterized by low rates of interaction and lack of leadership, can also have instituted relations appropriate to these conditions is a moot point. Certainly the relationships between strangers in a metropolitan area are well instituted, as Simmel has pointed out. Alarmist social critiques, on the other hand, find this situation charged with anomic elements.
8. For details of the previous study and the preliminary theory of the Friends, see Charles Kadushin, "Social Distance between Client and Professional," *American Journal of Sociology*, 68 (1962), 517-531, esp. 528ff.
9. Paul F. Lazarsfeld developed the theory of latent structure—the model we are using. In his "Latent Structure Analysis," in Sigmond Koch, ed., *Psychology: A Study of a Science* (New York: McGraw-Hill, 1959), he assigns probabilities of response to individuals rather than to a group. An individual who "really" belongs to a class has a certain probability of responding to the item when it is repeatedly administered to him. Thus, a "true" *New York Times* reader does not necessarily read it every day, but reads the newspaper with a fixed probability. Our interpretation emphasizes group data and interprets probabilities as the relative frequency of a trait within a given class. The responses are independent not from one administration to the next but between the various members of a class. The mathematical expression of these interpretations is, of course, the same. James C. Coleman, *Introduction to Mathematical Sociology* (New York: The Free Press, 1964), pp. 382ff. also notes that the concept of a latent factor underlying manifest response patterns implies that in a given set of responses of a number of persons, variability of response (either over time or between items supposed to indicate the same thing) can be located either *within* individuals or *between* individuals. He offers a model which separates "social variability from the psychological variability." Our analysis was developed before we read his model which does not seem conveniently applicable to a situation of four social groups and eight items. His notion that attitude distributions may be used, through a mathematical model, to indicate the existence of social as well as individual types is similar to ours and an exceedingly important idea. In our interpretation we allow for random individual variation within a group, assume the *group* to be the "cause" of the over-all configuration of items, but have no way of distinguishing the two sorts of variation. Further work along these lines is much needed.
10. Raymond Boudon and Neil Henry, with the assistance of David Elesh and Harry Milholland, developed estimation procedures for our data. A National Science Foundation grant to Lazarsfeld and Henry developed the IBM 7094 program used for the maximum likelihood estimate used here. The procedure itself and the maximum likelihood method of assigning respondents to classes are described fully in R. B. McHugh, "Efficient Estimation and Local Identifi-

cation in Latent Class Analysis," *Psychometrika*, 21 (1956), 331-347; 23 (1958), 273; T. W. Anderson, "Some Scaling Models and Estimation Procedures in the Latent Class Model," in U. Grenander (ed.), *Probability and Statistics* (New York: Wiley, 1959); P. Lazarsfeld and N. Henry, *Latent Structure Analysis* (Boston: Houghton Mifflin, 1968) explains our procedures in greater detail.

11. We are limited in our interpretations by the fact that we have a select aggregation of clinic applicants. However, a recent study of a random sample of New Yorkers, 75 per cent of whom were high-school graduates or less, which used very similar items, reports *manifest* marginals for the entire sample much like those for our nonsophisticated *latent* group: 11 per cent were to a play last month, 5 per cent to a concert, and 16 per cent know someone who goes to a psychiatrist regularly (Elinson, *et al., The Public Image of Mental Health Services*, Tables 48, 67). Our procedure really does seem to pull out the special "members of the Friends" even in a select population.

12. The assignment was made by examining each response pattern and assigning it to the circle to which it most probably belonged. The Latent Structure determines this assignment. See Paul F. Lazarsfeld, "A Conceptual Introduction to Latent Structure Analysis," in his *Mathematical Thinking in the Social Sciences* (Glencoe: The Free Press, 1954), pp. 378-379. This classification leads to "empirical" classes that are not exactly the same sizes as the "theoretical" classes of Table No. 5. The proportion within each empirical class which has a positive response to any item is also not exactly the same.

13. Rank determined by Hollingshead's modification of Edwards' scale. His first two categories are combined to yield the high group, the next-to-highest group is his category 3, the third category is his category 4, and the lowest consists of his 5th through 7th ranks. See Hollingshead and Redlich, *Social Class and Mental Illness*, pp. 390-391.

14. This point was suggested by Vernon Dibble. See his "Occupations and Ideologies," *American Journal of Sociology*, 68 (1962), 229-242, for an analysis of the way occupational ideologies come to have broader cultural and social influence.

15. NORC Survey Number 367.

16. Srole *et al., Mental Health in the Metropolis: The Midtown Manhattan Study*, pp. 241-243.

17. All the findings to be reviewed here hold true even when education is taken into account.

18. A more detailed analysis of this issue is found in my "Social Distance Between Client and Professional," *op. cit.*

19. Ernest Jones, *The Life and Work of Sigmund Freud* (New York: Basic Books, 1955), v. 2, p. 8.

20. *Ibid.*, Chapter 14.

21. *Ibid.*, p. 120.

22. *Ibid.*, p. 163.

23. *Ibid.*

THE REALIZATION OF
A PROBLEM
II

The Sociology of Presenting Problems

5

Many human relationships just happen. They need no special reason for them to occur. That is, there are expressive rather than instrumental reasons for many acts. For example, friends may telephone or ring the doorbell and say, "I was just wondering how you are," or "I was just dropping by." In modern business or professional relationships, however, one does not just drop by. There has to be a specific reason for action. The shoemaker is seen because there are shoes to repair; the doctor because a broken leg must be set; and the psychiatrist because people have problems. Some professionals such as ministers do receive casual visits, but that is because they are an integral part of a community called a church or parish. The psychiatrist has no flock, however. No one just drops by his neighborhood psychiatrist to say hello. A special reason, called a "problem," is required. In fact, an applicant's "ticket of admission" to psychotherapy is his problem, and these problems are very important to applicants. They give considerable thought to the way they present themselves in interviews. Most of the applicants who answered questionnaires were even more diligent: the typical applicant wrote over a hundred words in description of his problems, despite the rather narrow space allotted to his answer. Even the less educated, who, it will be remembered, were somewhat *more* prone to return the questionnaire, wrote at length. Almost 60 per cent of those who were not high-school graduates wrote at least 65 words.

To be clear about anything one must name the phenomena under discussion. All the great system-makers in psychiatry, in the interest of clarity, developed their own terminology for describing psychiatric problems. This multiplicity of classifications has, of course, led to more obfuscation than understanding. Even a partial amalgamation of various previous classification schemes, the *Diagnostic Manual* of the American Psychiatric Association, is for reasons to be examined in detail in the next chapter totally unsuitable for describing the way applicants present themselves to psychiatric clinics.

With considerable reluctance we must therefore add to the confusion by proposing still another classification of presenting problems. Ours, however, is devoid of any diagnostic intent. It is useful for understanding why people come to psychiatrists. After the scheme has been illustrated from actual case material, we shall show how its elements empirically cluster into four types of presenting problems, and how these in turn are related to the decision to seek therapy at three types of clinics.

We classified as "presenting problems" the problems applicants mentioned when asked for a general description of their problems, as well as the main things that are now bothering them. Responses to the question asking how they first noticed their problems and answers to the checklist of problems which followed the spontaneous replies are not included as presenting problems, though they are similarly classified.* Most applicants presented more than one problem. Reducing an applicant's response to that of a single problem would be extremely misleading, for it would imply an unspecified theory as to which problems are "really" the most important. Unless we specifically note that we are considering the applicant's own opinion as to which problem he himself considers the most important, all data on problems refer to *all* of his presenting problems.

Second, in classifying problems, every attempt was made to stay as close as possible to an applicant's original intent. The young social worker quoted in Chapter 1 was classified as having among her problems anxiety and lack of confidence (exactly what she said), categories

---

* The items on the checklist and the exact wording of the questions on the various forms administered are found in the Appendix.

that were in turn grouped with "general anxiety" and "self-values" in a manner to be explained shortly. The airplane mechanic said, "I don't worry about anything." This response appears to indicate a mechanism of "denial" since the rest of the interview reveals to a psychologically sophisticated observer that the man is "really" very anxious. But he himself did not say so. Therefore he was *not* coded as having said he was anxious, or as having indicated even a synonym of anxiety. By following this rule of literal coding, we were able to maintain fairly high reliability.[1] Any interpretation of the meaning of responses can then be ascertained through the process of objective statistical analysis and not confounded with the clinical judgment of a coder.[2]

❂ *The Classification Scheme*

Lack of a clinical interpretation of the data does not mean that no theory was invoked in the scheme of categories. Any classification of psychiatric problems constitutes a miniature theory of human behavior and ours is no exception. Derived from Talcott Parsons' theory of action, the major divisions are (1) biosocial problems, (2) inner emotional problems, and (3) social problems, for these refer to the basic analytic systems which describe individual action.[3]

Biosocial problems were further subdivided into physical and sexual difficulties. The inner emotional category was divided into the modes of motivational orientation—cognitive, cathectic, and evaluative.[4] The social category was separated into ever widening spheres—the primary group, the economic activity or major role, and the total social system. Within each of the areas mentioned, further divisions are apparent. An explanation of these categories and some examples now follow.

❂ *Biosocial Problems*

Biosocial problems are so called because, in order for an individual to consult a professional therapist, all purely biological difficulties must be expressed in terms of a social disturbance. For example, the common cold is not a "problem" or an occasion for professional advice until it interferes with a person's fulfillment of his social duties.[5] All of us who have brought notes from our mothers or doctors to school to explain our absences are familiar with this phenomenon. Included in our category of the biosocial are physical symptoms, drug and alcohol addiction, and heterosexual or homosexual difficulties.

PHYSICAL PROBLEMS

Somatic Problems. Somatic complaints include such things as headaches, fatigue (and insomnia), faintness, stomach disorders, appetite disturbances, heart palpitations, tremors, seizures (and paralysis), and "bad health" in general.[6] Both the social worker and the airplane mechanic were classified as having somatic complaints. About one-fourth of analytic clinic applicants, less than one-fifth of religio-psychiatric clinic applicants, but one-half of hospital clinic applicants presented one or more somatic complaints.

Alcoholism. Alcoholism (almost no drug addicts applied for psychiatric treatment) is presented by only 1 per cent of analytic-clinic applicants but by proportionately five and seven times as many religio-psychiatric and hospital clinic applicants.

SEXUAL PROBLEMS

Without gainsaying that complaints of interpersonal difficulties usually accompany and are a part of sexual problems, we classified all sexual problems separately as biosocial. Included under heterosexual complaints are such problems as frigidity, impotence, masturbation, over/or underactivity, feelings of general sexual inadequacy, and inability to relate properly or regularly to the opposite sex. To be coded as homosexual, however, an applicant had to specifically state that as his problem. Unless he himself said that he was a "latent homosexual" (in which case he was classed as having a problem with homosexuality), no inferences on the part of a coder were allowed. In view of the traditional emphases of analytic clinics, it is not surprising that Table 7 shows that these clinics attract over twice as many applicants with sexual problems as any other type of clinic. One-fourth of analytic-clinic applicants had such complaints. Typical of these persons is the forty-year-old single male applicant to the Interpersonal Psychiatry Institute who wrote, "I have never been able to maintain a serious relationship with someone of the opposite sex. I live a good deal in my imagination and masturbate every day for sexual satisfaction."

❊ *Inner Emotional Problems*

The next division of presenting complaints in Table 7 deals with problems of inner emotional adjustment. These difficulties can be located in three major motivational areas: cognitive orientations—those

TABLE 7 *Proportion of Different Problems Presented to Three Types of Clinics*

	Analytic Clinics	Religio-Psychiatric Clinic	Hospital Clinics
Biosocial Problems	49%*	30%	65%
Physical	24	17	55
Somatic	23	15	51
Drug and alcohol	1	5	7
Sexual	31	14	13
Heterosexual	25	11	10
Homosexual	8	4	2
Inner Emotional Problems	83	63	63
Cognitive	24	9	17
Thought processes	21	7	14
Orientation	5	3	6
Cathectic	55	38	47
Depression and Immobility	25	9	19
Loss of control	9	9	9
Specific fears	12	10	11
General anxiety	33	21	24
Evaluative	54	41	13
Social and cultural values	11	13	2
Self-values	49	33	12
Social Problems	77	74	58
Specific	61	66	54
Primary groups	33	46	27
Spouse	15	34	12
Other love object	3	3	4
Other relatives, friends	18	15	14
Major occupational role	35	21	25
Performance	28	15	21
Future	11	4	7
Interpersonal conflict	3	4	2
Entire social situation	9	8	14
General Interpersonal	43	18	14
Movement toward people	6	3	1
Movement against people	11	3	1
Movement away from people	42	14	13
No Problem, Others Have Problems	5	10	4
Average number of problems per applicant	4.0	2.7	2.8
Total number of applicants*	1111	195	134

*Neither the indented nor the totals add directly, since each applicant may have indicated more than one problem in any category.

aspects of motivational structure with which an individual sees and apprehends the world; cathectic orientations—those orientations which provide one's feelings and emotional energy; and evaluative orientations —those in which a person compares, weighs, and evaluates objects which were selected by means of his cognitions and cathexes. All these processes actually take place simultaneously, and therefore any complaint about one's inner emotions actually deals with all three orientations at once. Nonetheless, any given presenting complaint or statement can be classified according to the orientation which seems to be most problematic.

Problems of an inner emotional nature form the overwhelming majority of problems presented to analytic clinics (83 per cent), but vie for primacy with social adjustment problems among religio-psychiatric-clinic applicants (63 per cent inner emotional but 74 per cent social adjustment) and with biological adjustment problems among hospital-clinic applicants (63 per cent inner emotional but 65 per cent biosocial).

COGNITIVE PROBLEMS

Thought Processes. Cognitive, cathectic, and evaluative problems are further differentiated in Table 7. Cognitive problems include thought processes and orientation problems. Thought-process problems are manifested by complaints of poor concentration—the lower-class man who said, "I notice that I don't have self-concentration"; an inability to come to decisions—the coed who wrote, "I generally freeze when it comes to making decisions"; and obsessions, confusions, and the like, typified by the white-collar worker who wrote, "I find myself usually preoccupied with things that are not at hand . . . inability to retain directions, the syntax of a story, etc. . . ." A religio-psychiatric clinic is least likely to be presented with these problems. Unexpectedly, the analytic clinics seem to draw proportionately more thought problems. This will be explained in Chapter 7 in terms of the social mobility aspirations of analytic-clinic applicants.

Orientation. Problems of more general cognitive disorientation are presented by only 5 per cent of the sample. Included in this category are a respondent's own complaints that he suffers from a lack of orientation ("I don't know where I am"), unreality ("My life does not seem real"), or other sensations of floating or distortions of reality such as visions and voices. Note that there are no substantial differences between types of clinics in the proportion of applicants that are willing to admit or are themselves aware of these traditionally "psychotic" symptoms.

CATHECTIC PROBLEMS

Applicants who complained of difficulties associated with the level of their emotional energy were classed as having cathectic problems. This is one of the largest single categories of presenting problems. Over half the analytic-clinic applicants, a bit under half the hospital-clinic patients, and two-fifths of religio-psychiatric-clinic applicants manifested at least one problem in this area. Cathectic problems may be of several types.

Depression and Immobility. These persons felt that they had a low level of emotional energy. A male graduate student says, "I have had periodic severe depressions." An applicant who is occasionally employed in the theater complained of immobility. "Laziness—no jobs to speak of—quitting things I start. . . . Sleeping all day and staying up all night drinking coffee . . . not doing *anything!*" For both these persons, the cause of their lassitude or depression may be the blocking of large amounts of emotional energy. But that is not what they feel. They know that they are emotionally depleted. In keeping with its "positive" orientation, the Religion and Psychiatry Institute is least likely to draw complaints of depression or immobility.

Loss of Control. In reporting loss of control such as, "uncontrollable crying and screaming and choking and shaking fits," or other such tantrums and hysteria, an applicant is stating, in effect, that he has too high a level of emotional energy. His feelings are bursting out all over and cannot be contained. "Losing my mind," a type of loss of control, was also classed here. Nine per cent of the applicants to each type of clinic felt they had such problems.

Specific Fears. An applicant may also cathect certain objects or situations so that he feels his transfer of emotional energy to these objects to be unreasonable, interfering with his normal level of emotional activity. Fears "of dark and and closed" places, "cancer," death or suicide —"I fear that something tells me to throw myself out of the window" (actual attempts or desires to commit suicide are classed under depression)—"bad dreams," and so on are all classed here. These fears also seem equally distributed among the several types of clinics.

General Anxiety. In contrast to the above symptoms which are fairly specific, many persons such as the young social worker quoted earlier also mentioned feelings of general uneasiness, anxiety, tension or nervousness. Diffuse feelings of unhappiness were also classified here if they could not be noted as outright depression. One-third of analytic-clinic applicants, one-fifth of Religion and Psychiatry Institute applicants, and one-fourth of hospital-clinic applicants expressed feelings of general anxiety.

EVALUATIVE PROBLEMS

Through cognitive and cathectic orientations a person perceives the world and himself and invests these perceptions with emotional energy. The world so apprehended is given significance through the processes of valuation and evaluation. The significance of the objects, channels, and possibilities that one apprehends determines how one's resources are to be allocated. Problems of significance concern over half the analytic-clinic applicants, two-fifths of the Religion and Psychiatry Institute applicants, but little over 10 per cent of hospital-clinic applicants. Merely achieving health and emotional energy are sufficient problems to these persons. Worrying about evaluation is perhaps a luxury to them.

Social and Cultural Values. Two aspects of the matter of significance concern us: the standards and values by which significance is judged, and the outcome of this judgment or evaluation—an outcome which inevitably reflects upon oneself. The category of social and cultural values includes statements that show a concern with or a reaction to the standards of evaluation set by one's society or culture. For example, an artist applying to an analytic clinic directly attacked her values: "I have ambivalent feelings about the way I live. I am in conflict with my values." Others presented feelings of guilt, shame, or sin, and issues of right and wrong. Mentioned by 11 and 13 per cent of analytic and Religion and Psychiatry Institute patients, respectively, these social and cultural problems seem of less interest to hospital-clinic applicants. Only 2 per cent of them raised such issues.

Self-Values. An applicant may state that he cannot meet his *own* demands, whatever they are. The most common complaint in the area of self-values is "a lack of self-esteem and confidence which has . . . prevented me from utilizing my education and abilities to the fullest." Others are dissatisfied with themselves because they haven't accomplished anything ("I have an ever-present sense of a wasted life"), or because they do not know where they are going ("I lack direction and the ability to stand by whatever values I profess and work for them").

Low self-evaluation is a symptom most typical of applicants to analytic clinics. Table 7 shows that half are affected. One-third of the Religion and Psychiatry Institute but less than 10 per cent of hospital-clinic applicants present problems of self-values.

⚙ *Social Problems*

We now turn to a different level of problems: man's adjustment not to his body or his inner feelings but his adjustment to his social surroundings. Impairment in one's ability to cope effectively with society is a major determinant in the decision to seek psychotherapy. Table 7 shows that about 75 per cent of applicants to analytic clinics or to the Religion and Psychiatry Institute and 60 per cent of hospital-clinic applicants indicated at least one problem of social adjustment.

SPECIFIC SOCIAL PROBLEMS

Almost all who complained of their social adjustment spoke of problems in relating to specific persons, sets of persons, or to institutional areas. Social interaction in modern American society can be divided into three major areas of increasingly wider scope: primary relationships—family and friendship networks; economic relationships—one's job or other major social role such as housewife or student; and political relationships—one's relationship to the total system. Problems in each of these areas were separately noted.

Primary Group. Included here are persons who experienced difficulties with their spouses, such as the forty-four-year-old housewife applying to the Religion and Psychiatry Institute who said, "My husband has told me that he doesn't care for me and would like to break up our marriage." One-third of the applicants to this clinic mentioned marital problems. This was the most frequent complaint presented to the Religion and Psychiatry Institute.

To include similar complaints about persons to whom applicants were not married, the category of "love object" was added. About 5 per cent of the total sample reported problems in this area. There is little difference between clinics in the frequency of this complaint.

Finally, a person may experience conflict with his children, in-laws, parents, other relatives, or friends. The most frequent complaint stems from women who have difficulties with their children: A thirty-four-year-old Negro woman on relief said, "I want to care for my children but they get on my nerves. Sometimes I just want to scream." About 17 per cent of the total sample reported these problems, whose prevalence does not seem to vary appreciably from one type of clinic to another.

Major Occupational Role. A role may constitute a person's full-time occupation whether or not it provides a cash reward. Such roles or occupations, like those of student or housewife, are a considerable source of difficulty in modern society. Persons may have problems with the way they *perform* their roles ("I have run away from scholastic endeavors. . . . When I had to work and support myself I did not keep the jobs I had . . ."). They may worry about their occupational future, or be unable to get along with people on the job they hold (". . . a somewhat pugnacious, aggressive personality that leads to conflicts with people. Primarily college instructors. Because of these clashes I have been denied the opportunity to obtain my degree.").

Major social role problems, when grouped together, account for over one-third of applicants to the analytic clinics, one-quarter of hospital-clinic applicants, and one-fifth of the Religion and Psychiatry Institute applicants.

Total Social Situation. Last, in the realm of specific social adjustment are those who feel they have a problem because they have difficulties with their entire social situation, such as the artist who said his problems stemmed from "the state of arbitrariness and insecurity in the fine arts," or those with financial problems and those who have directly clashed with society, such as the man who said that his major problem is "compulsive sexual behavior which may lead to imprisonment and physical harm. . . . Problem was not too severe up until . . . arrested for loitering in the subway. . . ." Less than 10 per cent of all applicants have such problems, which are more frequently presented to hospital clinics.

GENERAL INTERPERSONAL PROBLEMS

Instead of complaining about specific relationships, an applicant may express problems with his social environment in terms of his general mode of relating to other persons. Karen Horney suggests that individuals tend to adopt one or several of the following three general strategies of coping with others: they may move *toward* other persons, *against* them, or *away from* them.[7] We shall interpret these categories in the order in which she developed them.

Movement toward People. In movement toward people, "one accepts his own helplessness, and in spite of his estrangement and fears tries to win the affection of others and to lean upon them."[8] This pattern is commonly called dependency. For example, a twenty-two-year-old girl wrote, "Up to now I've been terribly dependent on my parents and have hated it."

Movement against People. In this case, one "accepts and takes for granted the hostility around him, and determines, consciously or unconsciously, to fight. He implicitly distrusts the feelings and intentions of others toward himself."[9] We included in this category persons who expressed hostility and aggressiveness as a problem, who felt that losing their tempers or being angry with others was inappropriate. Those who felt feelings of persecution or felt they were not liked or accepted by others were interpreted to mean they felt they themselves did not like other persons. This interpretation represents our only explicit use of psychoanalytic theory in the coding scheme. Thus, a thirty-year-old secretary who wrote that she has "uncontrollable temper tantrums— inability to adjust to other people, I insist on my own way regardless of whom it inconveniences or hurts . . ." was classified as moving *against* people.

As Table 7 shows, both movement toward and movement against people were infrequently mentioned categories. Apparently, one does not usually recognize or admit to these traits in oneself. It is interesting to note that they are most common among analytic-clinic applicants.

Movement away from People. In moving away from people, a person moves neither toward nor against. Rather, he "keeps apart. He feels he has not much in common with them [people] and they do not understand him anyhow."[10] Horney often refers to this mode of coping with persons as detachment or isolation. In our coding, persons who said they felt withdrawn, afraid to meet and talk with people, who could not communicate with others, who felt passive or unable to form a relationship with others were placed in this category. For example, a forty-year-old housewife said that her main problem is "people. I still feel that although my husband and children love me very much I'm lonesome. The fact that if I know I'm going to be where there are more than two or three people makes me uneasy about going."

Perhaps Karen Horney sensed the importance of this problem to persons undertaking analytic psychotherapy, for she devoted more space to a description of the character neurosis associated with this mode of adaptation than to any other type. Over 40 per cent of applicants to analytic clinics mention this problem, almost four times as many as present it to any other type of clinic. After self-value problems, this is the most frequent analytic-clinic presenting problem.

❀ No Problem, Others Have Problems

The final category consists of all those persons who think that they do not have problems or that someone else has problems. This type of "problem" constitutes a relatively small proportion of those brought to any clinic, although 10 per cent of the applicants to the Religion and Psychiatry Institute are willing to place the problem on someone else's shoulders. Many of those who come without a "problem" think they ought to have one. For example, a young student applying to an analytic clinic wrote, "My problem is that I have no problem (in my opinion) and yet am doing badly in school. My main problem is that I'm not bothered. . . ."

Table 7 summarizes both the classification scheme and the statistical findings on the relationship between presenting problems and psychiatric clinics. The relationships are strong and consistent. But the table is too complex to be discussed in detail. Instead, we shall reduce this large set of problems to a smaller set more ideally suited to show how different types of clinics receive different types of presenting problems.

✿ How Problems Group

Some of the problems just reviewed "go together"; the person who presents one particular problem is also likely to present certain others. One could think of many possible common-sense groupings of presenting problems. For example, persons with marital problems might also be likely to complain of sexual difficulties. There are many forces operating on the applicants, however, not all of them obvious. But logic is not a substitute for data. Our classification scheme merely checks on whether we have allotted room for all possible problems. The clustering shown below represents the results of an empirical cluster analysis of the major problem headings. Four not so obvious types of presenting problems then emerge: psychiatric, performance, psychoanalytic, and projected problems.

The psychiatric problems include cognitive, cathectic, and physical problems. These are the types of problems often associated with classical psychiatric symptoms. They are also somewhat related to the performance and psychoanalytic clusters.

Performance problems are those described above as major social role problems. The difficulties in getting things done seem to be related to both the psychiatric and the psychoanalytic clusters. Psychoanalytic problems are those believed by the psychoanalytically oriented Friends and Supporters of Psychotherapy to be the "right" problems. Included are sexual, evaluative, and interpersonal problems. This cluster has the strongest set of internal relationships. It is strongly negatively associated with projected problems.

The last cluster of problems—the projected problems—are so called because persons who have them tend to blame other people for their problems, that is, they project their difficulties. Primary-group problems, situational difficulties, and having no problem at all obviously belong to this group, which is distinguished largely by its set of negative relationships with all other problems.

There are several reasons why the problem areas cluster as they do. For example, there is a high association between cathectic and physical complaints. It is a well-known principle of psychiatry that psychological states, especially anxiety and other symptoms in the cathectic group, may result in physical symptoms. On the other hand, especially among lower-class applicants, serious physical symptoms cause worry and anxiety. This is directly expressed by some applicants. Cathectic symptoms are the only inner emotional problem respondents are likely to identify as being physically "caused."

The relationship between cathectic and physical presenting problems is not only one of direct cause and effect. For some groups, especially lower-class applicants to hospital clinics, a high-rate of physical symptoms is associated with a low rate of presenting cathectic problems. Psychoanalytic theory tells us that cathectic problems may be unwittingly converted into physical symptoms. This conversion seems to depend in part on the social acceptability of physical as against cathectic symptoms. Hysteria was at one time a middle-class illness; now that the middle class has become more sophisticated psychologically, hysteria has become more characteristically a lower-class illness. Despite this kind of mutual exclusivity between the two types of symptoms, they remain bound in the same cluster. For the "R_2" below the main diagonal of Table 8 indicates the degree to which physical and cathectic symptoms have the same profile of relationships with the other problem areas. If they are substitutable for one another, then even though the same person may not have both symptoms, he will have other symptoms or problems compatible with the physical-cathectic entity. An "R_2" of .31 shows this to be true.

Each of the problem areas in the prescribed cluster has been identified with one of the major schools or trends in modern psychoanalysis. Sexual problems are, of course, Freud's patent discovery. Evaluative problems are emphasized by some of the Neo-Freudians, such as Horney and Fromm. They and Sullivan have also been concerned with interpersonal relationships as the genesis of psychiatric problems. Apparently our applicants find some truth in all schools, for he who presents one of these problems is likely to present the others.

There is also a substantive theoretical link among the three problem areas of the psychoanalytic cluster. Interpersonal problems are the psychological counterpart to problems of evaluation. For he who says I do not like myself or even my larger self—society—is also likely to feel that he cannot get along with other people. Sexual problems are, of course, a limited aspect of interpersonal problems. Finally, there is a strong relationship between the presentation of sexual problems and feelings of guilt, which in turn are manifested by having problems with one's value system.

Traditional psychiatric problems and the newer psychoanalytic problems are not, however, mutually exclusive clusters. Table 8 shows that if a person presents one type of problem he may also present the other. Yet by and large their "profile" of relationship with other problem areas is quite different, as shown by the largely negative "R_2." The two biosocial problems—sexual and physical—are the keys to the difference between the psychiatric and the psychoanalytic clusters. Sexual prob-

TABLE 8 *Problem Cluster for Applicants to New York City Psychiatric Clinics*

	Psychiatric			Performance	Psychoanalytic			Projected		
	Physical	Cognitive	Cathectic	Major Role	Evaluative	Interpersonal	Sexual	Primary Group	Situation	No Problem
Physical		00	17	−03	−13	−05	−12	−11	−02	−11
Cognitive	−02		10	09	04	05	−08	−09	−07	−08
Cathectic	31	16		03	02	06	−12	−16	−03	−13
Major Role	−11	11	00		06	12	−01	−12	05	−11
Evaluative	−31	01	−04	07		20	08	−07	−02	−15
Interpersonal	−18	03	03	16	34		09	−06	−06	−16
Sexual	−30	−23	−32	−09	13	12		05	−05	−02
Primary Group	−24	−26	−38	−30	−18	−20	10		05	−06
Situation	−08	−23	−15	00	−14	−23	−15	08		05
No Problem	−18	−18	−26	−25	−15	−36	−22	−05	−05	

(Phi Coefficients above the main diagonal; Pearson R_2 are below)

Note: Phi is equal to $\sqrt{\frac{X^2}{N}}$ and is the same as Pearsonian product movement correlation for the case of a true dichotomy. For 1452 cases a phi of .021 is significant at the .01 level of confidence. Pearson R_2 is the correlation between the phi coefficients for any pair of problems. Thus the profile of phi coefficients for physical problems has a −.02 Pearsonian product moment correlation with the profile of phi coefficients for cognitive problems. The profile refers, of course, to the phi contingency of one problem with all the other problems in the matrix. See Tryon, "Domain sampling formulation of cluster and factor analysis," *Psychometrika*, 24 (1959), 113-134. We are indebted to Irving Silverman for his version of cluster analysis and his IBM 650 program for accomplishing it.

lems are strongly related to the other psychoanalytic problems; physical symptoms are strongly related to the other psychiatric problems. But sexual problems are negatively related to psychiatric problems and, similarly, physical symptoms are negatively related to psychoanalytic problems. Sexual and physical problems are therefore keys to the entire process of decision from the realization of one's problems to the application to a clinic.

Physical symptoms send applicants to hospital clinics and sexual problems bring them to analytic clinics. The physical symptoms are symbolic of the institution of modern medicine and of concern with the body rather than the soul. Sexual problems have been transformed to mean problems with emotional life. Freud's early key to psychiatry, the physical and the sexual, thus remains of great consequence in the decision to seek therapy.

Most emotional problems, whether psychiatric or psychoanalytic, are related to difficulties in performance. Which is cause and which is effect is often difficult to determine. But there is no question of the pervasive nature of performance problems. They are negatively related to the two specific problems of the psychiatric and psychoanalytic clusters—physical and sexual problems—but somewhat related to cognitive, cathectic, and evaluative problems, and strongly related to interpersonal problems.

The essential characteristic of problems in the projected cluster is that, like automobile accidents, they are usually "the other fellow's fault." Hence these problems are generally negatively related to any problem that implies personal responsibility. The negative relationship between interpersonal and primary-group problems is a case in point. One might expect that he who has specific complaints about individual relationships would also say that he cannot get along with people in general. But this is not so. If one has the "insight" to "know" that specific interpersonal conflicts are caused by a more generic factor, then there is no point in presenting the less insightful detailed battles. There are two exceptions to the general rule, however. Situational problems are related to major role problems. After all, if one has difficulties in performing, it is convenient to blame the situation. Second, sexual problems are associated with marital problems. Whether marital problems cause sexual problems or the reverse is true is a moot point and certainly one not demonstrable from our data.

In this section we have developed a logical classification of presenting problems. The scheme rests on the notion that there are three basic types of problems for any individual: his biosocial problems, his inner emotional problems, and his problems with society. The most important biosocial problems are the over-all physical symptoms and specific sexual problems. Inner emotional problems can be cognitive—what is seen; cathectic—what is felt; and evaluative—what is weighed and rated. Social system problems can be specific primary group, occupational role, or total situation problems, or they can be more diffuse inabilities to cope with human relationships. It is our feeling that this scheme is logically coherent, easy to use, and related to the process of deciding to enter psychotherapy.

The empirically derived clustering here presented covers a wide range of problems indeed; it is one way of grouping all of life. Such attempts at the universal produce strange bedfellows and eliminate many fine distinctions. Life is too complicated to be summed up in four categories. That is why even the "strong" relationships in the clusters are, in comparison with other types of clusters in social science, fairly modest. Nevertheless, the value of this four-way grouping of problems will become immediately apparent when in the next section we analyze the relationship between presenting problems and types of clinics.

❀ Relation of Type of Clinic to Types of Problems

In this section we shall show that the classification of problems just attempted leads to a sociology of presenting problems. There is a matching between type of clinic and the type of problem presented to it. As Table 7 showed, different types of clinic receive drastically different types of presenting problems.

The degree to which persons with different types of problems are filtered into different types of clinic is shown most dramatically when the empirical clustering of problems is tabulated against clinic type, as shown in Table 9.

TABLE 9 *Type of Problem and Type of Clinic*

Type of Problem	Analytic Clinics, %	Religio-Psychiatric Clinic, %	Hospital Clinics, %
Psychiatric	69	49	84
Performance	35	25	26
Psychoanalytic	78	53	31
Projected	41	60	39
Total N	(1118)	(199)	(135)

Psychoanalytic problems are most popular among analytic-clinic applicants; psychiatric problems are exhibited by almost all the applicants to hospital clinics; religio-psychiatric applicants most frequently present projected problems. Since performance problems are often a manifestation of other problems or, in turn, cause them, they are almost equally presented in all types of clinics.

The general scheme seems reasonable. Let us see how it works out in detail by referring back to Table 7, which lists the specific presenting problems. Here we see that analytic clinics receive a higher proportion of sexual and homosexual complaints, thought problems, and cathectic problems, especially those involving depression and general anxiety. Problems of self-values and interpersonal problems seem to be specialties of the house, as it were. Analytic clinics are *unlikely* to receive problems of alcoholism or drug addiction. It should also be noted that in terms of our classification scheme, analytic clinics receive *more* problems per applicant than does any other type of clinic.[11]

Moreover, the psychoanalytic clinics receive the emotional problems stressed by their leading theorists. If Freud emphasized sexual problems, then so do applicants to analytic clinics. And if Fromm, Horney, Sullivan, and others have stressed the importance of feelings of self-inadequacy and poor interpersonal relationships in the genesis of mental disturbance, so do the applicants to analytic clinics. Even the high intellectual achievement of psychoanalytic theory has its parallel in reports of thought difficulties among applicants. The fine lines that divide one analytic thinker and his supporting institute from other thinkers and their institutes, however, are not perceived by applicants. All the clinics we have called "analytic" receive roughly the same proportion of each type of problems.

The Religion and Psychiatry Institute receives proportionately more marital problems than any other clinic. In fact, 75 per cent of married women under 35 applying to this clinic present some primary-group problem. Otherwise, the types of problem presented are similar to those of the analytic clinics, except that role performance, interpersonal, and sexual problems are less frequently reported here and, in conformity with the founder of the clinic's "positive" orientation, it receives few reports of depression. In short, the Religion and Psychiatry Institute receives the problems characteristically presented to ministers in their pastoral roles.[12]

Hospital clinics specialize in reports of physical symptoms. They demonstrate their integration with medical facilities by receiving a large proportion of patients with physical symptoms. Relative to analytic-clinic applicants, those going to a hospital clinic are quite unlikely to present any other than physical symptoms, cognitive problems, and cathectic disturbances.

Whatever the reason for these differences, they do exist. Even a casual observer must be struck by the close match between the problems presented by applicants for treatment and the ideological or institutional position of the various types of clinics.

There is, therefore, a sociology of the process of applying to a psychiatric clinic, for the matching between patient and clinic cannot be magically accidental. That even the leading psychoanalytic theories appear to be partly reflections of the nature of the patients drawn to psychoanalysis means that we must go beyond psychoanalytic theory in search of explanations for the harmony between "supply" and "demand" in the psychiatric outpatient marketplace.

The five reasons developed in the first chapter for differences among individual applicants also apply to the differences among clinics. (See pp. 6–7.) Different types of clinics do receive applicants from quite different social positions, as we saw in Chapter 3. Hence their applicants may have different sets of problems simply because of the different pressures to which their different social positions expose them. Since applicants of different positions also have different ways of reacting to or expressing their problems, the problems received by clinics may merely reflect that difference in social position. Then too, applicants to analytic clinics are much more likely to be members of the Friends and Supporters of Psychotherapy or to have previously undertaken extensive psychotherapy. Controlling for social position or psychiatric sophistication does reduce some of the differences among clinics in the types of problems presented to them. Nevertheless, all the differences noted remain and are of considerable magnitude. We must therefore conclude that the dynamics of referral and the expectations of the nature of the psychiatric treatment (reasons four and five) must be heavy contributors to the observed differences in the types of problems presented to the various clinics.

Indeed, a detailed statistical examination of changes in the way a person first conceived of his problem and the way he finally presents it to a clinic shows that applicants tend to increase their proportion of "suitable" problems, and drop their proportion of "wrong" problems. For example, applicants to analytic clinics are more likely to add sexual problems to their original set of problems and drop physical symptoms. Hospital applicants do the reverse.

The following case illustrates the complex matching and decision-making process which may bring a person to an analytic clinic while at the same time changing that person's notion of what the problem really is.

Margaret is a twenty-nine-year-old single woman. Her parents, with whom she lives, are Orthodox Jewish immigrants from Central Europe. Her father is a businessman in the garment industry. She herself is a schoolteacher. She is both culturally and psychiatrically sophisticated although, as we shall see, the degree of sophistication is a fairly recent acquisition. She enjoys outdoor sports such as skiing and horseback-riding. She feels that *Families with problems* (the italicized words were given to respondents as the beginning of a sentence which they were to complete in any way they wished) "need help." But *Keeping trouble to yourself* "is the best policy." *Most friends* "are not really friends," and *Most people I know* "are false."

She first noticed her problem in the following way. "The weight problem has been with me since I'm a teenager. It was discussed with my family physician. He felt or suggested at the time that I seek guidance but I guess I never would admit that something was wrong, that I couldn't control myself. I've now come to the realization that I am in great need of someone else's guidance."

From her answers to the questionnaire, we learn that the process of realization of the need for guidance seems to have come about in this manner:

Although her family physician had been consulted "for overweight on and off for the past twelve years," she "only began to think of these things [Inner Emotions, an item on our checklist] this past year."

In the last year or so, both "a fellow" and a close "girl friend" had commented about her problems without being specifically asked to do so. "They all felt my mother was involved." She found these comments helpful "in that it made me think about it."

Following her friend's comments, they discussed the difficulties. They "only spoke about or around the problem since it was brought up by her and now that we have a close relationship I value very much having someone to talk to." Her friend appears to have a similar problem: "Her problem is relating with men." She was advised to take a vacation and to see a psychiatrist or psychologist.

It appears that the (girl) friend is also a patient at the clinic. In January, a month before the date of her reply to the questionnaire, she asked this friend if she knew of any psychiatric clinics. "I have never felt so discouraged about things. Also, I have this depressed, unhappy feeling that has come into particular focus this past year." Although she specifically asked her friend about applying to the clinic, her friend had previously mentioned the clinic without knowing that she was interested in applying to it. Indeed, in the "last couple of years I know friends and acquaintances" who are seeing psychotherapists. Now that she herself has applied, she has told a few friends about it, but not her family.

Finally, in answer to the question, "Please write a general description of your problem," she writes: "I have only recently realized that I am not the happy secure person that I thought myself to be. I have been overweight for some time now and have never been able to bring myself to do something about it. Here I am 28 [sic] and have gone out with many men but find that I can't seem to get interested in any one." She feels that the main things about her problem that are bothering her now are first, "weight," and second, "relationships with men."

This girl has changed her notion of what constitutes her problem, indeed, her self-concept. She does not drop the idea that she has a weight problem, but through contact with a friend who is attending the clinic and others, she comes to realize that interpersonal problems are also involved in her difficulties. She thus comes to match the theoretical orientation of this particular clinic. Notice that by virtue of her type of occupation and cultural sophistication she has, in the last few years, fallen in with a group that are members of the Friends and Supporters of Psychotherapy. She too is now a "member." In "joining" she has changed her ideas about her problems and has also been guided to a psychiatric clinic.

Conversions are not easy, however. The girl still feels her major problem is weight. She has not fully accepted an image of herself as a psychoanalytic patient since a good patient should feel that her basic problem is an emotional one. In responding to the question, "What kinds of people do you think come here for help?" she further indicated her limited perspective: "People whose problems can be helped within a limited time." She also indicated that it was relatively easy for her to come to the clinic, thus showing an apparent lack of strong emotional involvement in the decision. Indeed, she did not show up for her first interview at the clinic.

From this case it is apparent that the entire channel which leads a person to a particular clinic, the very subject of our study, influences an applicant's recognition and formulation of certain types of problems. It is evident that not only does the type of problem a person has determine his choice of clinic, but his choice of clinic in turn determines the type of problem he presents. The close matching between a clinic's institutional affiliation or ideological orientation and the type of problems it receives is therefore a product of the total process of client decision-making.

NOTES

1. A staff of about 10 coders under the direction of two coding supervisors (Mrs. Jan Eckert Azumi and Mrs. Vivian Biasotti Vallier) performed this operation. Considerable group discussion developed common norms of classification. Independent checks showed that the author would have made the same classification as the coders on any of the 23 indented categories in Table 7 about 85 per cent of the time. No claim is made that persons who did not participate in this group would have classified the material in exactly the same way as this group of coders. We do claim, however, that if our training procedures and instructions were followed, other persons would also agree with our classification about 85 per cent of the time. Interestingly, a study of older psychiatric patients which uses a very similar but independently derived method of classifying presenting problems but which did *not* use a training program for coding (K. Warner Schaie, Lois R. Chatham, James M. A. Weiss, "The Multiprofessional Intake Assessment of Older Psychiatric Patients," *Journal of Psychiatric Research*, Vol. I [1962], pp. 92-100) concluded "that when the same units of description were used, raters with different professional background did not show any significant differences in their complaint assessment. In fact there was marked agreement among panel members and the principal differences found were related to the distinct complaint pattern ascribed to different patients." (p. 99.)
2. For the differences between clinical assessment of an individual case and statistical ascertainment, see Paul F. Lazarsfeld and Morris Rosenberg, *The Language of Social Research* (New York: The Free Press, 1955), Introduction to Section V.
3. Talcott Parsons, *et al.*, *Towards a General Theory of Action*; we have added the biological, and collapsed the social and cultural into one category, since for prac-

tical if not analytic purposes, problems originating in one rather than the other are not easily distinguished.

4. *Ibid.*, p. 59.
5. See Parsons, *The Social System* (New York: The Free Press, 1951), Chapter X, for a discussion of illness as nonfulfillment of social roles.
6. Each of the 23 indented categories, such as somatic symptoms, was coded into a number of subcategories. Over 100 subcategories were recorded.
7. Karen Horney, *Our Inner Conflicts: A Constructive Theory of Neurosis* (New York: W. W. Norton, 1945), pp. 42-45, and chapters II-V. We are not following the details of her theory of neurotic character, however, in this classification.
8. *Ibid.*, p. 42.
9. *Ibid.*, p. 43.
10. *Ibid.*, p. 43.
11. This is *not* caused by the different instruments in use in different types of clinics. In research conducted at the Religion and Psychiatric Institute 100 applicants received a questionnaire, and 99 were interviewed. All applicants completed this procedure at the time of their first visit to the Clinic. Questionnaire completion or interview took about one hour. The average number of problems elicited from the questionnaires is identical with that obtained in the interviews. Lest the place in which the research was administered be construed to be a possible factor (persons who fill out questionnaires at home have more time to think of different problems), we remind the reader that the 48 persons interviewed at the Interpersonal Psychiatry Institute did not, on the average, present more or fewer problems than they had previously written up in completing the questionnaire at home.
12. See Kadushin, "Social Distance Between Client and Professional," *American Journal of Sociology*, 68 (1962), and E. Cumming and C. Harrington, "Clergyman as Counselor," *American Journal of Sociology*, LXIX (1963), 234-243.

Presenting Problems and
Psychiatric Diagnoses

✹

6

The problems which are presented to different types of psychiatric clinics are filtered through the process of application. Because the nature of one's friends and one's social position affect this presentation, there is a sociology of presenting problems.

Is there not, however, also a psychiatry of presenting problems? Are we not trying to stage *Hamlet* without the confused Dane? Thus far, nothing has been said about the true emotional illnesses of applicants. Rather, only their own and necessarily distorted opinions of their conditions have been recorded. In this chapter, we shall discuss the traditional, objective way of dealing with presenting problems—psychiatric diagnosis.

Unfortunately, psychiatric diagnosis is not uniform and therefore not useful. Almost all psychiatrists and social scientists who have dealt with psychiatric diagnosis in a statistical fashion have reported high variability among clinics, administrative units, hospitals, and individual clinicians in their use of diagnostic categories. Some clinicians call almost every patient schizophrenic; others rarely use the term. When the same individual or the same protocol is reviewed by different psychiatrists, or even by the same psychiatrist at different times, there is far from perfect agreement as to diagnostic classification. And as one might suspect, psychiatrists do not agree on the meaning of the diagnostic categories.[1]

Our data agree with these negative findings. Unlike other studies, however, we can pinpoint two factors which psychiatry believes to be most relevant to a patient's diagnosis: his presenting problems and his social situation. Yet even these cornerstones do not illumine diagnosis because (1) despite a similarity in problems presented to different types of clinics, there is wide variation in the distribution of diagnoses even within one type of clinic; (2) there is little relationship between the way we coded presenting problems and psychiatric diagnosis; (3) diagnostic categories are only minimally related to social factors; (4) when both presenting problems and the social situation of applicants are taken into account, there is disagreement among clinics in the interpretation of the same type of problem presented by persons of similar background.

There are several explanations for these facts. Because psychiatric theory and concepts are not well agreed upon, the rules by which diagnosticians move from the manifest responses of patients to their underlying psychiatric diagnoses are incoherent or poorly specified. Therefore, the social situation of clinics becomes more important in determining diagnosis than the characteristics of applicants. The divergent theories of the various clinics also account for much of the difference among them in diagnosis. Each clinic's position is fixed in the process of routinizing the complex scientific vocabulary of diagnosis. Through social interaction, each clinic develops its own set of norms for the application of diagnostic terminology, for each seems to have a favorite diagnostic category. Finally, administrative reasons force many clinicians who would not otherwise do so to make diagnoses. Consequently, the diagnoses themselves seem to follow a clinic's administrative exigencies.

Let us try to demonstrate these facts and support these explanations.

❁ *The Recording of Diagnoses*

As part of our follow-up of patients, the clinic's diagnosis of the applicant was recorded verbatim on a special form. The diagnoses were then coded according to the instructions in the *Diagnostic and Statistical Manual, Mental Disorders* of the American Psychiatric Association.[2]

In most cases, it was easy to fit the clinic's diagnosis to the categories of this standard manual. All clinics receiving financial help from the Community Mental Health Board are in fact required to make diagnoses in conformity with the *Diagnostic Manual*. Not all clinics in our study receive this aid, however. University Psychoanalytic Institute, the Center for Advanced Psychotherapy, and Interpersonal Psychiatry Institute are therefore free to make use of whatever diagnostic categories they choose. Interpersonal solves the diagnostic problem by making a formal diagnosis only for those cases which are being considered for treatment. The other two clinics hold by and large to the accepted nomenclature, although fitting their categories to those of the Manual occasionally posed some problems.

Not all clinics are included in our analysis. Interpersonal is excluded because of the few formal diagnoses recorded. The New Analytic Institute and Lincoln Hospital are omitted because they had too few cases in our study to make statistical analysis worthwhile, and Center Hospital is not listed because of our difficulties in locating records.

A large number of diagnoses in University Psychoanalytic Institute and in other psychoanalytically oriented clinics were made in combinations not permitted by the *Diagnostic Manual*. The favorite tactic was the assignment of both a neurotic diagnosis or a personality disorder diagnosis together with a diagnosis of underlying schizophrenia. Since this fits modern psychoanalytic theory, the diagnosis was recorded as given. That diagnosis which the clinician felt to be more important or "basic" was recorded as the first diagnosis. Three diagnoses were allowed for in our coding scheme. This chapter uses only the *first*, or most important diagnosis.

☼ Variation in Diagnostic Patterns

About one-third of the applicants to the University Psychoanalytic Center, the Religion and Psychiatry Institute, and St. Matthew's and St. Francis Hospital outpatient clinics are identified as schizophrenic as shown in Table 10. The Center for Advanced Psychotherapy, however, uses the category of schizophrenia only half as often as this group of clinics, and the Personal Psychology Institute almost never diagnoses an applicant as schizophrenic.

Religion and Psychiatry and University Center are similar in their relatively sparing use of diagnoses of neurosis and their heavy reliance on personality trait or pattern diagnoses. Advanced Psychotherapy calls over half of its applicants personality trait problems. Personal Psychology feels that two-fifths of the applicants are neurotic.

Not only do these clinics differ among themselves, but they also differ from the average diagnoses reported by other comparable clinics and

TABLE 10 *Psychiatric Diagnoses Made by Six Psychiatric Clinics*

Major Diagnosis	Personal Psychology %	University Psychoanalytic %	Advanced Psychotherapy %	Religion and Psychiatry %	St. Matthew's %	St. Francis %
Acute and chronic brain disorders	0	0	0	0	0	0
Involutional psychotic reaction	0	1	0	5	13	0
Affective reactions	2	0	0	1	3	0
Schizophrenic reactions	2	35	17	31	37	32
Paranoid reactions	0	2	0	1	3	0
Other psychotic reactions	0	3	0	0	0	0
Psychophysiologic autonomic and visceral disorders	0	1	1	0	0	0
Psychoneurotic disorders	41	9	17	5	23	16
Personality pattern disturbance	16	26	3	42	7	11
Personality trait disturbance	27	16	57	7	7	26
Sociopathic personality disturbance	2	5	5	3	7	16
Special symptom reaction	0	1	0	0	0	0
Transient situational personality disorders	10	2	0	5	0	0
Mental deficiencies	0	0	0	0	0	0
Total	100%	101%	100%	100%	100%	101%
N	(49)	(312)	(160)	(112)	(30)	(19)

practitioners. Table 11 shows the diagnoses made by "our" clinics, all licensed voluntary-hospital clinics in New York City in 1960, all licensed nongovernmental nonhospital clinics in New York in 1960, all the private psychiatrists participating in Group Health Insurance's (GHI) trial of insuring mental disorders in 1959–1961, and a collection of cases reported by members of the Society of Medical Psychoanalysts in the 1950's. Since all the data come from the same time period, any differences in diagnostic patterns in this table cannot be caused by differing fashions of diagnosis at different times. Four of the clinics in our sample have much higher rates of diagnosis of psychosis than have any of the comparison groups. St. Francis comes closest in its rate of psychoses to the comparable nongovernmental hospital clinics. The psychiatrists in private practice—the GHI group and the Medical Psychoanalysts—are similar to each other and to Personal Psychology in the relatively heavy use of "neurosis." Other clinics in our study as well as the comparable New York City clinics do not find such a high proportion of neurosis among their patients. In the nonpsychosis category, the GHI psychiatrists find the fewest personality disorders. Next come the New York City voluntary-hospital clinics, and in our own group, St. Matthew. Otherwise, our clinics show higher rates of personality disorders than do even the cases reported by the Medical Psychoanalysts.

These trends are not a statistical artifact caused by omission of nondiagnosed cases. Differing rates of nondiagnosis in different clinics bear no relationship to the distributions of recorded diagnosis.

❁ Diagnosis and Presenting Problem

A potential cause for varying patterns of diagnosis among the different clinics is the fact that patients with different problems are recruited to different types of clinics. For example, clinics whose patients present more cognitive problems might report more schizophrenia. Nevertheless, differences in the type of problems presented by patients cannot be the basic cause for the observed pattern of diagnosis, for grouping clinics by presenting problems produces the now familiar distinction between analytic, religio-psychiatric, and hospital clinics. Yet this grouping is in no way similar to the one suggested by the patterns of diagnosis. On the contrary, University Psychoanalytic and the Religion and Psychiatry Institute are similar in their high rates of schizophrenia and personality disorder diagnoses. The two hospital clinics also are loosely linked to this group because of their high proportion of schizophrenia diagnosis. On the other hand, the hospital clinics infrequently diagnose applicants as having personality disorders. Personal Psychology and Ad-

TABLE 11 *Summary of Psychiatric Diagnoses Made by Six Psychiatric Clinics, New York City Clinics, GHI Psychiatrists, and Selected Psychoanalysts*

Diagnosis	Personal Psychology %	University Psycho-analytic %	Advanced Psycho-therapy %	Religion and Psychiatry %	St. Matthew's %	St. Francis %	NYC[1] Nongovernment Hospitals %	NYC[1] Other %	GHI[2] %	Psycho-analysts[3] %
Chronic brain	0	0	0	0	0	0	6	3	1	0
Psychosis	4	41	17	38	56	32	27	15	22	20
Neurosis	41	9	17	5	23	16	28	19	46	42
Personality	45	46	65	52	21	53	22	37	16	36
Transient situation	10	2	0	5	0	0	10	19	12	–
Mental deficiency	0	0	0	0	0	0	2	1	–	0
Other	0	2	1	0	0	0	4	1	2	2
No deviation	0	0	0	0	0	0	1	5	1	–
N	(49)	(312)	(160)	(112)	(30)	(19)	(2878)	(6187)	(843)	(100)

[1] *Statistical Report of Psychiatric Clinics in New York State* for the year ended March 31, 1960, Table 9, p. 34 (with undiagnosed removed).
[2] Avnet, *Psychiatric Insurance*, Table 73, p. 148 (with multiple diagnoses removed).
[3] Bieber, et al., *Homosexuality*, Table II – 3, p. 28, comparison heterosexual cases.

vanced Psychotherapy, the two psychotherapeutic clinics, each have very different ways of diagnosing patients.

The idiosyncrasies of the clinics are more clearly indicated by their use of detailed diagnoses. Of the more than 70 diagnoses available in the *Diagnostic Manual*, each clinic uses but a few. All except Personal Psychology agree that "schizophrenic" is a term that need not be further specified (contrary to the *Manual's* instructions), or else that it means so-called latent, chronic or ambulatory or borderline schizophrenia, or the equivalent term, pseudoneurotic. This view of schizophrenia stems from an analytic orientation, supported by the findings of projective tests, that regards ego disintegration as important in defining schizophrenia. If this position is taken, clinically observed bizarre or "out of contact" behavior is not a necessary condition for a diagnosis of schizophrenia.[3] Moreover, many applicants who were diagnosed as borderline schizophrenics, pseudoneurotic, or latent schizophrenics were also said to have neurotic symptoms or disorders. That is, to the casual eye, they might appear to be neurotic, rather than psychotic. If one does not accept this view of schizophrenia, and Personal Psychology apparently does not, then few outpatients could be called schizophrenics, since they are sufficiently "in contact" to be able to apply to a clinic by themselves.[4]

There are patterns within other diagnostic groups as well. The proportion diagnosed as anxiety reactions among the psychoneurotic disorders ranges in different clinics from 14 to 65 per cent. Schizoid-personality diagnoses range from zero to 62 per cent of all personality-pattern disturbances. "Passive-aggressive" is the favorite personality-trait-disturbances diagnosis for two clinics, but it is used for only 10 per cent of such diagnoses at University Psychoanalytic. Here, "compulsive" is the favored category. Further, the distribution of diagnoses does not correspond to the distribution of presenting problems. Clinics thus vary widely in respect to their "favorite" diagnosis.

Since the pattern of problems presented to a clinic does not account for the distribution of diagnoses, it is not surprising that the presenting problems of an individual patient afford an uncertain basis for predicting his diagnosis. Each presenting problem was compared to the primary diagnosis given by each of the four clinics for whom we have sufficient cases. This procedure produced 124 tables, summarized in Table 12, which may be read in the following way. In the upper left-hand corner under *Personal Psychology* and opposite the presenting problem "somatic" is the diagnosis "neurotic." This means that there was a high degree of association between the presenting problem—physical symptoms—and the clinic's diagnosis—neurotic. But there was no relationship between physical symptoms and the diagnosis "neurotic" for applicants to the other clinics. The rest of the chart may be similarly read.

The few areas of uniform agreement between what patients say and what a clinic diagnoses are confined to the areas of traditional concern to psychiatry: inner emotional problems of a cognitive or cathectic nature, and primary-group problems. None of the topics of basic interest to psychoanalytic theory—sexual, interpersonal, and evaluative problems—show any uniformity of diagnosis.

In an area of traditional psychiatry it is apparent that applicants who present a cognitive problem are indeed likely to be diagnosed schizophrenic, if a clinic uses this category frequently. Our category of cognitive problems in fact has an almost direct counterpart in the *Diagnostic Manual's* definition of schizophrenic reactions: "a group of psychotic reactions characterized by fundamental disturbances in reality relationships and concept formations," as well as by other symptoms.[5] Nonetheless, only at University Psychoanalytic does the relationship with schizophrenia hold true for all categories of cognitive presenting problems. Even there, the association, while fairly large, is not overwhelming. Forty-nine per cent of University applicants who presented a cognitive problem (N = 71) were diagnosed schizophrenic, as against 31 per cent who did not present this problem (N = 241) and were diagnosed schizophrenic.

Except for the Religion and Psychiatry Institute there is fair agreement that persons who present cathectic problems are neurotic, although the diagnosis of specific cathectic complaints varies from clinic to clinic. Typical of the modest relationships in this area is the association between the presentation of general anxiety and University Psychoanalytic's diagnosis of neurosis. Fourteen per cent of those who said they felt anxious (N = 119) were diagnosed neurotic as against 6 per cent of the others (N = 193).

The most impressive agreement among clinics is the assignment of primary-group problems to the passive-aggressive category. There is also general agreement that applicants with these problems are not schizophrenic.

The only other area of general agreement is in the classification of homosexuals as sociopathic. This agreement is in part the result of one of our coding rules which said that if a clinic merely noted that an applicant was a homosexual, without specifying any other diagnosis, then he was to be classed "sociopathic," according to the instructions in the *Diagnostic Manual.*[6]

Relationships between what a patient considers his most important problem and a clinic's diagnosis are even weaker than the ones just reported which take into account all of a patient's problems. Further,

TABLE 12 *Summary of Associations between Diagnoses and Presenting Problem for Four Psychiatric Clinics*

| | Clinic's Typical Diagnosis | | | |
Presenting Problem	Personal Psychology	University Psychoanalytic	Advanced Psychotherapy	Religion and Psychiatry
Biosocial				
Physical				
Somatic	Neurotic	Schizophrenic	Not Schizophrenic	*
Alcoholism	*		*	*
Sexual				
Heterosexual	*	Personality Pattern	*	Schizophrenic, Schizoid
Homosexual	Sociopathic	Sociopathic	Sociopathic	Schizophrenic
Inner Emotion				
Cognitive	*	Schizophrenic	*	Schizophrenic
Thought problems	*	Schizophrenic	Schizophrenic, Neurotic	*
Cognitive orientation	*	Schizophrenic	Schizophrenic	*
Cathectic	Neurotic	Neurotic	Neurotic	Schizophrenic
Depression and immobility	Neurotic	Schizoid	Neurotic	Schizophrenic
Loss of control	Neurotic	Schizophrenic	*	Schizophrenic
Specific fears	Personality pattern	Phobic	Phobic	Schizophrenic
Anxiety	Neurotic	Neurotic	Neurotic	*
Evaluative	*	Schizophrenic	*	Schizoid
Social values	*	*	*	*
Self values	Personality pattern	*	*	*

Social			
Major role	*	*	*
Performance	*	*	*
Future	*	*	*
Interpersonal conflict	*	*	*
Primary group			
Spouse	⎱ Passive Aggressive	⎱ Passive Aggressive / Not Schizophrenic	⎱ Passive Aggressive / Not Schizophrenic
Love object	⎰	⎰	⎰
Other relatives			
Friends			
Total Situation	*	*	*
General interpersonal	Personality pattern	*	*
Away from people	*	*	Schizoid
Against people	*	*	*
Toward people	*	*	*
No Problem, Others Have Problems	Transient situational	*	*

*No association

the patient's location of his problem—that is, whether the applicant feels his problem is caused by physical conditions, his situation, his childhood, his friends, or what have you—is a still poorer way of predicting diagnosis.

In short, no matter how the data are manipulated, patients' problems are simply not consistently related to their clinical diagnosis.

❊ Social Factors and Diagnosis

Thus far we have analyzed a traditional facet of diagnosis: the patient as he presents himself. Recent research in psychiatry has called attention to the importance of latent factors such as social class, age, and sex in the determination of diagnosis. Since the various clinics in our study differ with respect to the class and age of their applicants, some of the confusion over diagnosis may simply be the result of social differences among their applicants. Moreover, if presenting problems cannot predict diagnosis, perhaps the applicant's social background can account for a large proportion of the variation in diagnosis.

Age and sex are social factors that should be most directly related to diagnostic categories. Schizophrenia is supposed to be a disease of young adults, for example. Yet there are only a few consistent differences between older and younger applicants, and between men and women in the frequency of schizophrenia diagnosed. If heavy use of the term "schizoid" for younger applicants to the Religion and Psychiatry Institute counts as a diagnosis of schizophrenia[7] (the clinic may be unwilling to label young persons with an "incurable" disease), then indeed all clinics which use this diagnosis use it more frequently for younger applicants. All clinics also follow the Manual's definition of involutional psychosis, applying it only to older applicants. Transient situational disorders are also more likely to be ascribed to older applicants.

Both University Psychoanalytic and Advanced Psychotherapy, but not the others, agree that older women applicants are more likely to be neurotic. Both also agree that men applicants are more likely than women to be schizophrenic, but disagree as to which age group is so affected. All clinics, however, find more homosexuals among the men, and hence men are more likely to be diagnosed sociopathic. There are no other trends which are true for more than one clinic.[8]

Controls for age and sex also do not affect the differences reported among clinics in diagnosis.[9] Moreover, in view of the oft-noted relationship between schizophrenia and social class, we also compared separately an applicant's sophistication, education, his own occupation and his breadwinner's occupation* with the diagnoses made by the same four clinics with which we have been working. Again, regardless of whatever factor is controlled, the differences among clinics remain. What is more, social class is not consistently related to diagnosis in our sample.

Sophistication is also not consistently related to diagnosis. Nor is formal education strongly related to any specific diagnosis. Those with very little education, however, are *not* more likely to be termed schizophrenic, as previous reports might have led us to believe, although University tends to call the less educated psychotic. Persons with postgraduate education, however, are uniformly less likely than others, even with sex and age controlled, to be diagnosed schizophrenic. But this is not really a matter of social class. Rather, it is more akin to not giving a "bad" diagnosis to an applicant who is very much like the examining psychotherapist. Perhaps the evident accomplishments of a person with postgraduate training also serve to reduce the likelihood of his being called schizophrenic. Again, University Psychoanalytic applicants who have the special intellectual training of a postgraduate education are more likely to be diagnosed as compulsive.

Workers are *not* more likely to be diagnosed schizophrenic, or anything else, for that matter. The group with the highest rate of schizophrenia is students. Control for age largely erases this difference, however. Yet with age and sex taken into account, the very highest occupational group (executives and professionals) does receive a more favorable diagnosis in all clinics. This may be the result of the same factors that influenced clinicians in their judgment of persons with postgraduate training. Housewives, by the way, are more likely to be diagnosed neurotic by both University and Advanced Psychotherapy, even when compared to women of the same age group who are working.

The last indicator of social class considered, the breadwinner's occupation, exhibits about the same patterns as education and one's own occupation.

We must therefore conclude that social factors are *not* strongly or consistently related to diagnosis, nor do they account for differences in diagnosis among different clinics. The lack of relationship between social class and diagnosis is especially surprising, in view of the published literature to the contrary.[10] Perhaps as a result of this literature clinicians are becoming aware of what they may feel is a class bias. Data we collected from the Religion and Psychiatry Institute in 1957, before the

* "Breadwinner" here and following is taken to mean the occupation of the respondent if he is living alone and is supporting himself, or is living with a spouse and the spouse either is not working or is employed at a less prestigeful job; it means the occupation of the husband if he has the better or only job; it means the occupation of the father for students and other such dependents.

wide circulation of the evidence relating social class to diagnosis, showed a strong relationship between schizophrenia and low social class. In 1960 there were no such relationships.

❖ Social Factors, Presenting Problems, and Diagnosis

Neither the presenting problems nor the social situations of applicants are uniformly related to the diagnosis of their illnesses by psychiatrists. Perhaps clinicians react differently to the same problem if it is presented by persons of different background. *Who* says it, may count for as much as *what* is said. Certainly part of diagnosis consists in evaluating the social functioning of an applicant. If a housewife says that she cannot think or concentrate properly, this may have a different consequence for her than if a student presents this problem. Hence she might receive a different diagnosis. Any over-all relationship between presenting problems and diagnosis would thus be obscured.

To test the effects of social position upon the evaluation of presenting problems, we selected the effect of an applicant's social class on the diagnosis of cognitive presenting problems. Cognitive problems have been shown to be related to diagnoses of schizophrenia, and social class is supposed to be related to schizophrenia, although it has not been shown to be so in our data. Some of the literature hints that diagnosticians are "tougher" on lower-class than on middle-class patients. Should a middle-class and a lower-class person present the same problem the latter may be more likely to be called "psychotic." A crucial test is provided by using cases from University Psychoanalytic Institute and from Advanced Psychotherapy, for despite the similarity of their applicants in both social class and presenting problems, University makes twice as many diagnoses of schizophrenia as does Advanced Psychotherapy (Table 13).

The response of diagnosticians from both clinics to cognitive presenting problems is indeed affected by the social position of applicants. As expected, applicants of low education and less prestigeful occupations are more likely to be called schizophrenic when they present cognitive problems. But this is also true of insiders.

The two clinics differ in their reactions in a number of important areas, however. University Psychoanalytic is equally severe with students, insiders, clericals, and workers; the Center for Advanced Psychotherapy responds to cognitive problems with a more frequent diagnosis of schizophrenia only if the applicant is an insider or a worker. University is somewhat harsher on members of the Friends; Advanced is indifferent. Nor do the two clinics react uniformly to persons of the same educational level and the same presenting problem. University

TABLE 13 *Proportion of Applicants to University Psychoanalytic Center and the Center for Advanced Psychotherapy Who Were Diagnosed Schizophrenic, According to Whether They Presented Cognitive Problems or Not, and Their Social Class Background*

Social Background	University Psychoanalytic Clinic				Center for Advanced Psychotherapy			
	Presenting Problem				Presenting Problem			
	Cognitive		Not Cognitive		Cognitive		Not Cognitive	
	%	N	%	N	%	N	%	N
Sophistication								
Member of the Friends	53	(15)	28	(60)	15	(29)	21	(78)
Not a member	44	(9)	32	(38)	16	(15)	20	(38)
Own Education (excluding students)								
Some high school	50	(4)	35	(17)	20	(5)	17	(12)
High school graduate	25	(8)	37	(27)	29	(7)	13	(30)
Some college	71	(17)	33	(55)	14	(14)	20	(30)
College graduate	57	(14)	31	(48)	14	(7)	15	(13)
Postgraduate	17	(12)	19	(52)	25	(4)	5	(19)
Own Occupation								
Insider	50	(20)	26	(73)	22	(9)	7	(26)
Student	56	(16)	36	(39)	29	(7)	20	(10)
Executive and professional	14	(7)	23	(30)	0	(3)	0	(14)
Clerical	57	(14)	35	(52)	13	(15)	26	(42)
Worker	67	(3)	20	(5)	57	(3)	13	(8)
Housewife	44	(9)	31	(26)	0	(5)	0	(13)

Psychoanalytic clinic applicants who went to college but no further, and who present cognitive problems, are much more likely to be called schizophrenic than applicants with a similar background who do not present cognitive problems. This is not true of applicants to the Center for Advanced Psychotherapy. There, persons with cognitive problems are likely to be diagnosed schizophrenic only if they are high-school graduates or graduate-school level in educational achievement.

An analysis of these apparently jumbled findings casts some light on the general problem of this chapter: the relationship between presenting problems and diagnosis. According to one view, difficulties in thinking and concentration are "normal" to those who engage in artistic and intellectual activities. Cognitive problems, when presented by such persons, should not be taken as indicating severe ego damage and hence schizophrenia. On the other hand, should working-class men complain of cognitive malfunction, they may be seriously ill, since workers are not ordinarily concerned with these processes. A second view holds that inability to think is a serious problem precisely because an individual is an intellectual and hence dependent on his wits. An applicant's handicap in performing his usual social functions is indicative of the seriousness of his ego split.

University Psychoanalytic Clinic must subscribe to both these views. If the working-class applicant says he has cognitive problems, then he is schizophrenic, but then so is the intellectual or member of the Friends with cognitive presenting problems unless he has distinguished himself by being able to perform postgraduate work. The Center for Advanced Psychotherapy is more conservative in its use of schizophrenia as a diagnosis. Should lower-class persons present cognitive problems, then they are likely to be diagnosed schizophrenic. At the other end of the social scale, only very high-level intellectual functions such as those required by insider occupations or professions are felt to be affected by complaints of poor cognitive abilities.

☼ Accounting for Confusion

We have discovered that neither the differences in the nature of patients' problems nor their social background systematically explains the wide variability of diagnosis. We must therefore examine the very nature and theory of diagnosis. Diagnosis is a form of classification, and classification is a particular type of measurement. Measurement, in science, depends on scientific theory; it is not an automatic or natural property of things. The measurement of weight depends on theory relating mass, force, and acceleration. These concepts themselves have a history and have been the source of controversy. Similarly, diagnosis in psychiatry depends on theories of the nature, etiology, and course of psychiatric disorders. Physicists now by and large agree as to the underlying theory of weight. The same cannot be said about psychiatrists and mental illness. Some even deny that illness is an appropriate concept for psychiatry. Since the concepts of psychiatry are cloudy, each clinic strives to impose as much order as it can.[11] The clinic as a social unit becomes the most important determinant of diagnosis. The theoretical orientation of a clinic, the interaction between therapists, and even the administrative problems of operating a clinic come to have as much influence over diagnosis as the actual condition of patients.

Before suggesting that social factors within a clinic are crucial to an understanding of diagnosis, we must discuss a few technical problems of classification. Some of the causes for the poor agreement we observed between presenting problems and diagnosis must surely be assigned to differences between the purpose of our classification system and that implied by the *Diagnostic Manual*. The multitude of stimuli which clinicians take into account in making diagnoses and the poorly defined set of rules for linking what is observed to what is inferred are also responsible for the low associations between problems and diagnoses. These issues are all interrelated.

Psychiatric diagnosis uses a conceptual scheme far different from the one we employed to classify an applicant's problems. We took every statement at its face value and attempted to classify it according to a frame of reference which has relevance for the decision to seek therapy. The psychiatrist, however, rarely treats patient statements as *prima facie* evidence. Rather, he assumes that every statement must reflect something else, something of which the patient may not even be aware. His classification scheme is partly descriptive of symptoms, partly etiological, and partly predictive of the future course of the illness.

Clinicians do not, in their diagnosis, note each presenting problem as we do. Rather, they attempt to make some global assessment of the meaning of the combination of symptoms. It is a statistically unreasonable task to relate all combinations of the 23 basic presenting problems to the diagnostic categories. (There are 2^{23} such patterns.) Yet this is what psychiatrists do when they arrive at a diagnosis. Moreover, the actual words of the patient, all that we have to go on, form only one of many fragments of evidence used in the diagnostic process. Posture, voice, mode of speech, facial expression, and many other factors bear on the clinical evaluation.

Nevertheless, the patient himself is, or should be, the stimulus for the diagnosis. However complex, there must be some rules for getting from what a patient says (or looks like) to the actual diagnosis. After all, if a patient says he is Napoleon, this is usually taken to mean that he is a paranoid schizophrenic. This patient statement is not taken literally, but there is a clear rule for getting from the statement to a diagnosis. As long as there are clear rules for this procedure, there must be some relationship between patient statements and psychiatric diagnosis, even if the association is not an obvious one.

Our evidence suggests that if these rules do exist, they are not consistently applied. A candid discussion by the two psychiatrists who evaluated 1600 protocols from a population sample in New York City revealed "that almost every one of these pathogenic responses (in the protocols) was subject to exception."[12]

In addition to the sheer difficulty of clinically evaluating a multitude of factors, there are special historical reasons in psychiatry for the present confusion. Our data have shown a fair association between cognitive, cathectic, and primary-group problems and diagnosis, but poor and inconsistent associations between role performance, physical symptoms, and other problems on the one hand and diagnosis on the other. Those presenting problems with higher relationships to diagnosis are the ones associated with traditional nosological categories. The set of problems usually associated with psychoanalytic theory—sexual, self-evaluative and interpersonal problems—show the poorest relationship to diagnosis. Moreover, it is not clear on even a priori grounds how they should be related. One of the consequences, therefore, of the psycho-analytic influence on all of our clinics is the break-up of traditional diagnosis. Psychiatrists are now even less certain about the rules which guide the journey from the manifest to the latent.

Social certainty comes to replace theoretical or conceptual clarity. Just as patients' problems are socially validated, so too are our profes-sional diagnoses. The grouping of diagnoses in our collection of clinics closely reflects the line of influence of psychiatric theory in New York City. University Psychoanalytic Center influences the theories of Center Hospital through the latter's association with the department of psychi-atry at the University Medical Center. The Religion and Psychiatry's diagnostic team was trained at Center Hospital. The chief of service at St. Matthew is a graduate of University Psychoanalytic Center. No wonder these four clinics, despite their remarkably different types of patients, all have similar distributions of diagnoses.

This consensus within clinics does not come about automatically. Rather, it is the result of the very process of diagnosis and is inherent in the fact that medicine is an applied science. For the translation of a multitude of abstract ideas into language suitable to a confined and repetitive situation is characteristic of applied science. Medical diagnosis is thus a prime instance of the routinization of scientific vocabulary. De-spite the over 70 psychiatric diagnoses available, each clinic makes use of only a few. No one can remember and properly apply such a large set of concepts, so the selection of a limited number makes life easier. The guidelines for this routinization are largely social. Many small-group experiments have shown that in the absence of clear cognitive standards, persons whose actions are visible to one another tend to develop common cognitive standards.[13] We have already seen that the patient does indeed present an ambiguous stimulus, especially in the light of the uncertain state of psychiatric concepts and theories. Con-tinued therapist interaction, coupled with similar prior training and similar administrative needs, thus encourages each group of diagnosti-cians to define ambiguous clinical cases in some consistent way. Yet the definitions of one group of therapists need not necessarily coincide with those developed by another group.

Lack of certainty does not absolve psychiatrists from the social re-sponsibility of making diagnoses, even though many prefer not to make them for the very reasons suggested by our analysis. Administrative requirements of the state as well as the internal requirement of a clinic as opposed to private practice—other clinicians must have some idea as to what one's patients are like—force most clinics to attach diagnostic labels to most patients. Since the forces which make for the necessity of a diagnosis are administrative, the diagnosis itself is often used as an administrative device, although clinicians themselves may not be conscious of this fact.

Many clinics in our sample can select only a small proportion of their applicants for treatment. It is easier to justify turning away an applicant if he is said to be "too sick" to be treated through outpatient psychotherapy or analysis. Therefore, the clinics with the least room are likely to make the most "bad" diagnoses. Despite protestations to the contrary by some clinicians of these clinics, psychosis and especially schizophrenia are felt to be difficult to treat. On the other hand, neuroses, the type of disorder made famous by Freud, are held to be more amenable to orthodox psychotherapy. Personality disorders respond slowly to psychotherapy but on the other hand usually constitute less of an emergency than other cases and therefore appear to be less "sick."

The relationship between the proportion of cases accepted, waiting time, and number of hours allotted for treatment on the one hand, and diagnostic patterns on the other hand, is completely consistent with the interpretation of diagnosis as an administrative device. In fact, diagnosis is one of the very few facts about a patient related to his acceptance or rejection. In general, all clinics tend to reject patients who were diagnosed psychotic. Further, Personal and Advanced clinics which take a higher proportion of applicants than the others (see Chapter 3), in fact do have the fewest diagnoses of schizophrenia. Personal Psychology takes the highest proportion of applicants and makes the most frequent diagnoses of neurosis. Its average treatment time is less than that offered by the Center for Advanced Psychotherapy. The latter, therefore, has many more diagnoses of personality disorder, since these take longer to treat! Significantly, the psychiatrists participating in GHI's experiment were limited to no more than 15 individual psychotherapy sessions. They showed the fewest diagnoses of personality disorder and the highest proportion of neurosis. In reporting about cases in treatment for a median of 225 hours, the Medical Psychoanalysts reported high rates of both neurosis and personality disorder. University takes very few patients (most of whom are diagnosed "compulsive"). St. Matthew's, St. Francis, and the Religion and Psychiatry Institute all have long waiting lists. They are also the clinics with the highest rates of diagnosed psychosis.

No one of the three social factors we have discussed—theoretical orientation, routinization of vocabulary, and administrative need—is probably sufficient in itself to account for the differences among clinics in diagnostic usage. These factors do tend to cluster, however, thus providing for a powerful force in an otherwise pliant situation.

We have found wide variation in typical psychiatric diagnoses used by various clinics in our study, few relationships between presenting problems and diagnosis, minimal associations between social factors and diagnosis, and inconsistent usage of diagnosis when both social factors and presenting problems are taken into account. Because the rules of procedure from evidence presented by the patient to the diagnosis inferred by the psychiatrist are unclear, and are being further upset by psychoanalytic theory, differences in psychiatric theory and administrative practice are paramount in accounting for the discrepancies among clinics in their diagnostic patterns. Pressure to arrive at some coherent scheme forces each clinic to stereotype patients into a few diagnostic categories. Some clinics, such as Interpersonal Psychiatry, avoid the whole problem by making very few diagnoses.

Little in this discussion is new to the psychiatrists in our clinics who are attempting to make diagnoses. The consequence to our study of this weakness in the validity and reliability of diagnosis is less obvious. If what we have said is true, then there is no "objective" truth about our applicants and their problems. If they do not know what is "really" wrong with them, neither does anyone else, or at least it is not possible to agree as to what is "really" wrong. In this sample of applicants, there are only individuals who present psychiatrists with problems which they feel are troublesome. They hope that something can be done about these problems.

We shall therefore deal with these felt difficulties as serious data and attempt to understand why applicants with certain kinds of backgrounds and certain previous experiences feel that the problems they represent are adequate reasons for seeking psychotherapy. We shall no longer refer to a patient's diagnosis.

NOTES

1. A recent review of this field is Richard H. Blum, "Case Identification in Psychiatric Epidemiology: Methods and Problems," *The Milbank Memorial Fund Quarterly*, 40 (1962), 253-288. For further references, see the Bibliography.
2. Committee on Nomenclature and Statistics of the American Psychiatric Association (Washington, D.C.: American Psychiatric Association Mental Hospital Service, 1952). Special thanks are due to Ellen Coser, who did the coding.
3. Otto Fenichel, *The Psychoanalytic Theory of Neurosis* (New York: W. W. Norton, 1945), pp. 415-417, 443-446.
4. For a systematic statement of the orthodox clinical view of schizophrenia, see J. K. Wing, "A Simple and Reliable Subclassification of Chronic Schizophrenia," *Journal of Mental Science*, 107 (1961), 862-875.
5. *Op. cit.*, p. 26.
6. *Ibid.*, p. 39.
7. Data not shown.

8. Detailed tabulations of these and other findings about diagnoses are available from the author.

9. Our findings are replicated by the *Statistical Report of Psychiatric Clinics in New York State,* Table 10, p. 35, except that they tend to diagnose children as having transient situational disorders.

10. An exception which agrees with our data is the more recent study in Jerusalem by R. Moses and J. Shanan, "Psychiatric Outpatient Clinic," *Archives of General Psychiatry,* 4 (1961), 60-73.

11. For a discussion of some of the consequences of uncertainty in medicine see R. C. Fox, "Training for Uncertainty," in R. K. Merton *et al.* (eds.), *The Student Physician* (Cambridge: Harvard University Press, 1957), pp. 207-241.

12. Srole, *et al., Mental Health in the Metropolis* (New York: McGraw Hill, 1962), p. 396.

13. See H. L. Zetterberg, "Compliant Actions," *Acta Sociologica,* 2 (1957), 179-201.

The Effect of Sophistication, Training, and Social Reality on the Presentation of Self

❂

7

To psychotherapists, presenting problems are "defenses." Though the definition of the concept "defense" varies from one psychotherapeutic system to another, we shall take "defense" to mean a psychological device or mechanism which a person uses to protect himself from feelings he cannot accept.[1] In this view, when a person applies to a psychotherapist, he presents those problems which best accord with his self-concept. In fact, if he feels himself to be bad and worthless he will probably present himself in the worst possible light.

By regarding presenting problems as defenses, psychotherapists serve notice that the manifest content of the problem conceals as much as it reveals. Since the problems brought by patients are held to be reflections of deeper and more fundamental psychological processes and states, psychotherapists feel that they can make much better predictions about individual behavior if they know the underlying "psychodynamics." As surface manifestations, presenting problems are regarded as unreliable. Hence the inferred psychological states become the psychotherapists' "reality" while the presenting problems recede into a secondary status. Some psychoanalysts even feel that treating a patient for his symptoms alone is an inferior form of treatment. This tendency to regard presenting problems as "mere" defenses is a strategic error, however, for several reasons.

First, the basic assumption of psychoanalysis is that what patients have to say is valuable information. Presenting problems clearly serve as indicators of the deeper unobservable states, provided, of course, one knows how to interpret the problems. At present, however, the rules for interpreting them are not as clear or as well developed as we might like them to be, but that is quite another matter. What is more important is that the problems warn the patient himself that he needs professional help. A patient seeks help for the pain which he feels, and arguments as to what his "real" illness may be or even whether he is "really" sick tend to obscure the very important function of psychic pain. Problems are also strongly related to the type of place to which a patient goes for help. In Chapter 3 we saw that different types of clinics receive patients with very different types of problems. Moreover, and most important for our purposes, presenting problems as reasons for seeking therapy point to the vital social processes which underlie the decision to seek therapy. These forces are by no means obvious. Just as the psychological processes underlying a person's manifest problems are largely hidden from him, so the social forces which cause his motivation are also concealed from his view. He is too enmeshed in his social situation to see the larger forces to which he responds. That is why the reasons an applicant gives us for seeking therapy do not directly reveal these forces. Yet by aggregating many cases and analyzing them statistically, the sociologist places himself beyond the specific case and by virtue of this distance can see the larger social processes which underlie individual reasons.

Five social forces were earlier outlined which impinge upon presenting problems. First, different social structures create different problems for their participants. Second, given the same feeling or problem there are different socially and culturally structured ways of reacting to it. Third, persons in various social positions may have different ways of verbally expressing their feelings or problems.* These first three factors operate in all situations. Factors four and five apply especially to applicants for psychotherapy. People who go to psychotherapists are influenced by the opinions of others as they thread their way through the referral network, and these opinions affect the types of problems they

---

* Forces two and three locate the main opportunities for the operation of defense mechanisms. The same feeling generated by a given pressure may be acceptable to persons of one culture but not to those of another. Hence, even under the same pressure, one group will utilize a defense mechanism whereas another will not.

eventually present. The final force which affects the formulation of presenting problems derives from a person's anticipation of the reaction of a therapist. Applicants may report to a therapist those things which they expect will interest him. So applicants to a psychoanalytic therapist report sexual problems in accord with a stereotyped conception of psychoanalysis, while applicants to a clinic located in a hospital may respond to the therapist's white coat by emphasizing the medical aspects of their emotional problems. We have already dealt with this matter by showing that different problems are brought to different clinics, and in the next chapter we shall show the effect of personal influence on the realization that one has a problem. Here we wish to take up the first three forces mentioned above. In essence, they constitute a tension between verbal facility and social reality, a tension between social sophistication and social pressures.

The more a person knows about therapy, the more likely he is to feel that certain tensions within himself signal his need for professional psychiatric attention. And the more his symptoms prevent him from meeting the needs of his life situation, the more likely he is to feel the need for psychiatric consultation. The question here is, which counts for more—sophistication or reality? The several cases we presented all manifested physical symptoms of one sort or another. The social worker and the airplane mechanic presented in Chapter 1 had "stomach pains" and "trouble with my heart," respectively. The schoolteacher presented in Chapter 5 complained of being "overweight." The first question, then, is how sophisticated must one be to "know" that physical symptoms often portend psychiatric difficulties? On the other hand, do not the less sophisticated and less knowledgeable about psychotherapy find it much easier to express their emotional stresses in physical terms? And is it not true that certain segments of the population, such as lower-class persons, are much more apt to be more physically sick than other persons? Does not the reality of some people's lives make it probable that they will have somatic symptoms which may not be indicative of psychiatric disorders? And do not some jobs require greater physical health than others? This sort of argument can be extended to other presenting problems. One of Freud's major influences upon Western civilization was his revelation that all sorts of emotional problems may in fact be related to sexual problems. Those who know more about psychoanalysis or who have been influenced by others who know about this subject therefore might decide that they ought to see a psychiatrist because they have sexual problems. On the other hand, assuming that sexual problems *do* indicate psychiatric difficulties, certain people just because of their social position may be more likely to encounter sexual problems, or at least to be placed in situations in which their innate sexual inadequacy becomes more visible. Traditionally, men are supposed to be more adventurous sexually and to place more stock in their own sexual adequacy than do women. So it is entirely possible that regardless of their early sexual traumas, men are on the average more likely than women to become aware of their emotional problems through some failure in a sexual situation. Both social sophistication and social reality, then, are factors making for the realization that one has a psychiatric problem.

Which is more important in what kinds of situations? Is sophistication or reality the determining factor in bringing problems to people's attention? These are the basic questions we hope to answer in this chapter.

❊ Ways of Becoming Sophisticated

One meaning of "sophistication" is the quality of being worldly wise and cultivated, as opposed to being natural, or natively simple.[2] Those who are sophisticated may have a cultivated set of problems rather than those they might naturally possess. Obviously there are many kinds of sophistication as well as many ways of acquiring it. A person's degree of sophistication can be measured in terms of the way he has acquired it, that is, a graduate of the Cordon Bleu cooking school will be sophisticated about food. Or sophistication can be ascertained in terms of the resulting cultivated taste one has acquired, such as preferring *pâté de canard en croûte* to chicken pie. The sociologist, of course, prefers to measure sophistication in terms of social situations that might lead to a sophisticated outlook, and then independently to ascertain whether or not that outlook has in fact been acquired. The most general social situation which can serve as an indicator of having acquired sophistication is having gone to school. The more education one has acquired, the greater one's general sophistication. This indicator is better than none at all and it is easily ascertained in surveys. For our purposes, however, we need a measure much more closely related to psychological or psychiatric sophistication. In this area, there are three basic ways of acquiring sophistication: reading books about psychology and psychiatry, belonging to a social circle interested in psychology and psychiatry, and actually going to a psychotherapist. In our sample of clinic applicants, level of education is related to all three specific indicators of psychiatric sophistication, and reading books is related to membership in the Friends and Supporters of Psychotherapy, but not much related to going to a psychotherapist. And the number of visits to a psychotherapist is fairly unrelated to membership in the Friends. So these four indicators do measure somewhat separate things.

Reading has not yet entered our discussion, so a brief account of the data we collected might be helpful.[3] First we asked respondents to "check below those writings which you have seen or read in search of help with your problems."[4] Included among other sources were newspaper and magazine articles and books. We then asked for the title and author of materials read. Finally, toward the end of the questionnaire we asked, "Which of the following is a regular part of your life?" Reading books was included in a long list of leisure-time and religious activities. Almost all of the applicants to clinics (93 per cent) claimed that reading was a regular part of their lives. Almost 75 per cent claimed they read about mental health, and 53 per cent of the total number of applicants could actually back up this claim with a title. Though the phrasing of questions about reading affects the proportion who say they read, our sample leads the general population in general reading and especially in reading about mental health no matter how questions were asked.[5] One reason people who apply to psychiatric clinics read more about mental health is that they are better educated than average, and education is strongly related to the likelihood of reading anything, including mental health literature. In addition, the applicants' personal interest in psychology has a great deal to do with increasing their reading in general and their reading about mental health in particular, even among those with less education. Seventy per cent of persons with only an eighth-grade education who applied to analytic clinics ($N = 27$) could actually name the title of a book or article in the mental health field, and almost 70 per cent of applicants to the Religion and Psychiatry Institute who had not graduated from high school ($N = 17$) could name a title. Only about 20 per cent of hospital-clinic applicants with similar education actually named titles, but another 30 per cent did claim to have read something. In short, the need to discover more about one's problems induces applicants to read. A number of persons who said they did *not* read regularly as a general part of their life's activities did name the title of a piece they had read *in search of help with their problems*. About 15 per cent of grammar-school-educated applicants to analytic clinics read *only* in search of help—almost three times as many as those with more education. The impact of one's needs on the likelihood of reading mental health literature is further illustrated by the difference between those who became members of the Friends and Supporters of Psychotherapy through their general cultural sophistication and those who were members but were not culturally sophisticated. Twenty-five per cent of the latter named a mental health title ($N = 71$) but *did not read as a regular part of their lives*. Only 7 per cent of culturally sophisticated members of the Friends who named mental health titles ($N = 241$) failed to check off the fact that they read regularly anyway. The unsophisticated members of the Friends come to this circle because of their special interest in psychiatric problems. This interest boosted their reading in the mental health field (and in general) far beyond that which might normally be expected from persons with their modest interest in culture.

Readers of mental health literature cited two types of material: "serious" and "popular." Eighty per cent of the "serious" items were by either Freud or his students; the other 20 per cent were texts. In the popular category, journalistic accounts of modern psychology and psychoanalysis accounted for almost 40 per cent of the items; self-help books, 20 per cent; and books about sex, almost 10 per cent. Religious works, philosophy, medicine, and fiction each accounted for between 5 and 10 per cent of the remaining popular works. Not surprisingly, the chief determinant of *serious* psychology reading is level of education and cultural sophistication—except among applicants to the Religion and Psychiatry Institute, many of whom were attracted to the clinic by the books of authors associated with it.

To return to the measurement of psychiatric sophistication: we shall use four measures. Each measures slightly different things. Previous visits to a psychiatrist or other psychotherapists obviouly measure the direct impact of treatment itself. Somewhat less specific but still rather pointed avenues to sophistication are books and articles read. Membership in the Friends and Supporters of Psychotherapy is a measure of exposure to a social milieu interested in psychotherapy. Finally, level of education to some extent indicates general social class and to a certain extent indicates an applicant's over-all level of sophistication. To see how sophistication and social position interact in bringing problems to a patient's attention, let us begin with our previous example of physical symptoms.

☸ *Physical Symptoms: A Working-Class Burden or the Defense of the Unsophisticated?*

One of the best-known "facts" in modern studies of society and medicine is the relationship between social class and illness. Since Malthus' *Essay on Population*, written at the end of the eighteenth century, social scientists have assumed that the poor are sicker than the rich and die sooner. This fact, if true, is crucial in assessing the relationship between social class and the presentation of physical symptoms to psychiatrists. Our data, and those collected by others who have worked in this field,[6] show that working-class persons are much more likely than others to present physical symptoms as psychiatric problems. The institution most closely connected with the lower class, the outpatient psychiatry department of hospitals, specializes in receiving complaints of a physical nature. Does this mean that these working-class applicants merely reflect the facts of their social surroundings? If one collects a set of lower-class individuals at random, is one then likely to find more persons with physical symptoms?

A thorough search of the literature on social class and physical illness fails to support the well-known "fact" that lower-class persons in contemporary United States have more conditions, diseases, or symptoms of ill health than higher-class persons.[7] In other countries, with less advanced systems of sanitation, public health, medicine, and nutrition, lower-class persons do continue to be sicker. But in the United States, all recent household sample surveys show that among persons in the population at large, those of lower income or less occupational prestige report about the same number of illnesses or conditions as those of other social classes. This is especially true of New York City,[8] where social class differentials in the number of reported illnesses or conditions are very small. Moreover, the only satisfactory long-term study of these matters shows that persons in Haggerstown, Maryland, tended to become poor because they were sick, not sick because they were poor.[9]

Nevertheless, when lower-class persons are asked whether they *feel* sick, they are much more likely than individuals of other classes to say they are in poor health.[10] And this holds true even when the reported number of symptoms or conditions is taken into account. At each level of reported objective conditions, lower-class persons report poorer health than middle-class persons.[11]

Previous researchers, we believe, have not carefully distinguished between *feeling* sick and actually having a condition or a disease. It is obvious, then, that if we are to understand why applicants for psychotherapy present physical symptoms we must understand the subjective as well as the objective dimension.

There are several reasons why lower-class persons tend to feel sicker even when they have the same conditions as others. Of course, it is possible that their objective condition *may* be worse, but this is difficult to verify. Most studies of the distribution of diseases based on reports by physicians of persons hospitalized or seen in outpatient services show that lower-class *patients* are indeed "sicker," thus accounting for the belief that lower-class persons *in the population at large* are also suffering from poorer health. But studies also show that lower-class persons are more reluctant to seek medical care, and hence, when they do come for treatment, they are likely to be sicker than others. Lower-class persons, because they do not understand organized medicine, do not know how to make full use of it, and have less confidence in their own ability to cope with illness, and tend to be more fearful of disease. All studies show more lower-class absenteeism as a result of physical disabilities because many physical ailments which prevent lower-class persons from doing their job would probably not interfere with a white-collar person's work. Loss of work is certainly something for lower-class persons to fear, yet, since they are less involved in their work, they may be less willing to perform when suffering pain or disability. Finally, there is some theory but less evidence to prove that lower-class persons tend to somaticize their emotional problems. That is, their general fears and problems are transformed into physical problems because these are more comprehensible to them and therefore seem more legitimate to complain about.[12] Lower-class persons in the population at large are thus more sensitive to and more concerned about physical illness.

What effects do these facts have on the likelihood that lower-class persons will offer physical symptoms as a reason for seeking psychotherapy? Somatic symptoms have a dual relation to psychiatric sophistication, as the cases we examined in the first chapter suggested. If one is very sophisticated then one recognizes that physical symptoms may indicate the presence of an emotional problem and the need for professional psychiatric help. On the other hand, less sophisticated persons may feel that physical symptoms are legitimate signs of illness and hence are the only excuse for seeing a physician of any sort—including a psychiatrist. In fact, there is no consistent relationship between the number of previous sessions of psychiatry and the likelihood of presenting physical symptoms to the present clinic. Such symptoms apparently neither discourage nor encourage people to continue in psychiatry, nor are they "learned" in the course of treatment. The contradictory relation between psychiatry and physical symptoms is best shown by examining changes between the way applicants for therapy first noticed their problems and the way they now present themselves. Those who read mental health materials are 10 per cent *less* likely than others to present physical symptoms to an analytic clinic if they had originally noticed their problems because of such symptoms. That is, reading seems to result in dropping physical symptoms from the list of complaints. On the other hand, if an applicant did not first notice his problems because of physical symptoms, then reading is associated with a slightly increased chance that these problems will be added to the list of complaints. Further analysis suggests that the effect of psychiatric sophistication depends on one's original level of general sophistication. If an applicant to an analytic clinic is college educated, then membership in the Friends makes him more likely to *retain* physical symptoms as presenting problems; if he is only high-school educated or even less, then he is likely to *drop* these symptoms by the time he applies to a clinic.[13]

Given these opposing trends, and what we know about working-class sensitivity to illness, we would expect that unsophisticated working-class persons would be especially likely to go to psychiatrists because of their physical symptoms, but that otherwise social class would be unrelated to bringing physical symptoms to psychiatrists. Chart VII shows that, indeed, workers applying to analytic clinics who are not members of the Friends are twice as likely to present physical complaints as any other class of applicants.

The chart also shows that expectations of what is considered respectable to present to different types of clinics almost overrides class and sophistication in the presentation of somatic symptoms. Class hardly makes a difference at the Religion and Psychiatry Institute. Because of its nonmedical name unsophisticated applicants do not associate somatic symptoms with this clinic. Unsophisticated applicants to hospital clinics, on the other hand, abound in physical symptoms. Even here, working-class applicants are even more likely than others to present physical symptoms. There are not enough members of the Friends among these applicants for us to be quite certain of the effects of membership, but in any case, when a working-class person *is* a member of the Friends he tends not to apply to a hospital clinic in the first place and not to bring physical symptoms to a psychiatrist.

The sensitivity of lower-class applicants to physical symptoms is shown even more clearly by a special measure of sensitivity which we incorporated into the design of our study. Every applicant for psychotherapy has many emotional and personal problems and many of these have been with him all his life. Yet only some of them are seen as so painful that psychotherapy is required to mitigate them. Given the same experience of a problem such as somatic symptoms, there are sharp differences between social classes in the extent to which these symptoms "hurt," that is, lead a person to seek psychiatric treatment.

After we had asked an applicant to state or write his problems in his own words, we presented him with a standard checklist of problems introduced in the questionnaire as follows: "Here is a list of things that bother some people. Check those that are disturbing to you." Under the heading, "Physical Well-Being," the following psychosomatic types of symptoms and addictions were listed: "Headaches, Fatigue, Ulcers, Heart Palpitations, Drug Addiction, Alcoholism, and Other (Please Specify)."

When confronted with this checklist or with additional oral probes in interviews, applicants admitted to many more problems than they had spontaneously offered. The checklist, presented by a presumed authority, reminds respondents of problems less salient to them; it also makes some shameful problems more acceptable as reasons for seeking treatment. Problems not spontaneously mentioned but later revealed through the checklists must be felt as less acceptable or less self-evident reasons for undertaking psychotherapy. They may be indeed "deeper,"

CHART VII *Proportion of Applicants Presenting Somatic Symptoms, According to Membership in the Friends, Breadwinner, and Type of Clinic*

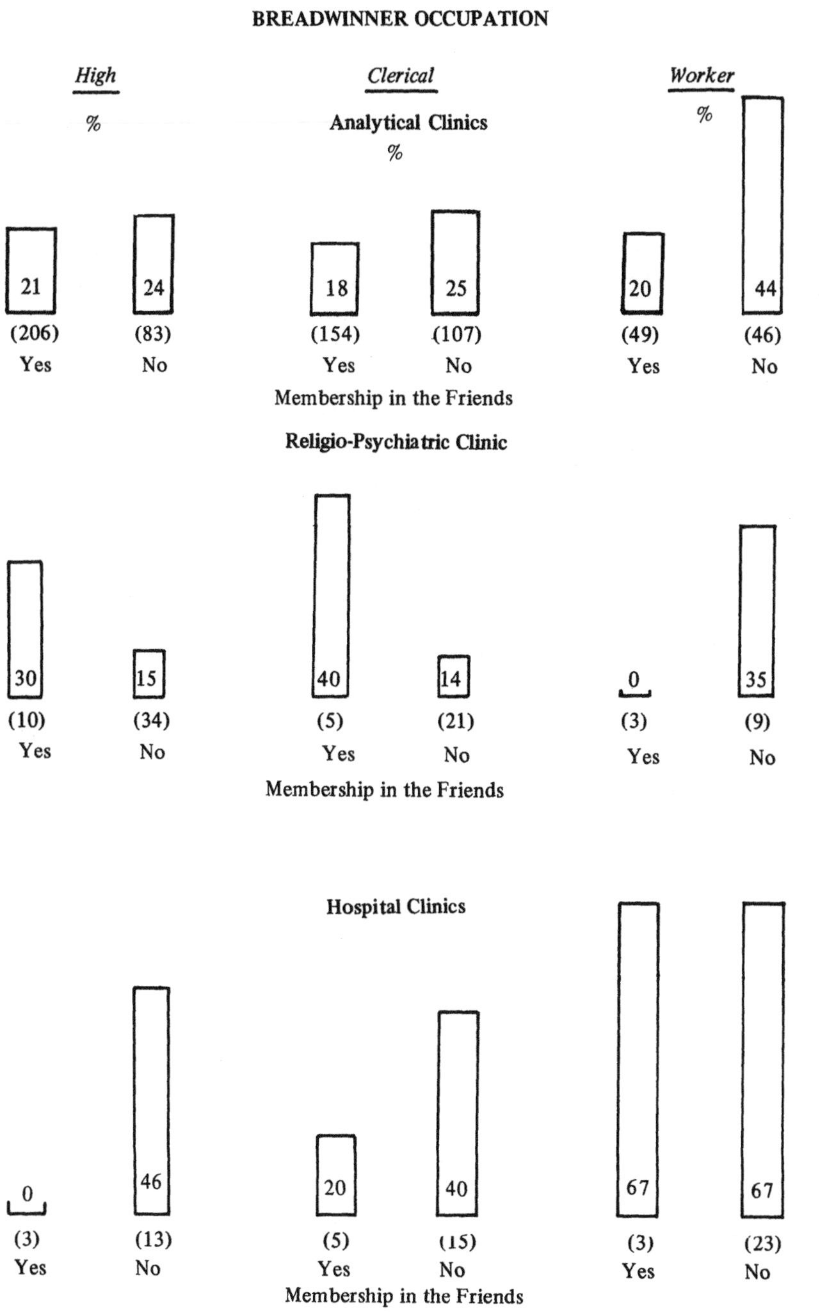

BREADWINNER OCCUPATION

High		*Clerical*		*Worker*	
%				%	

Analytical Clinics
%

21	24	18	25	20	44
(206)	(83)	(154)	(107)	(49)	(46)
Yes	No	Yes	No	Yes	No

Membership in the Friends

Religio-Psychiatric Clinic

30	15	40	14	0	35
(10)	(34)	(5)	(21)	(3)	(9)
Yes	No	Yes	No	Yes	No

Membership in the Friends

Hospital Clinics

0	46	20	40	67	67
(3)	(13)	(5)	(15)	(3)	(23)
Yes	No	Yes	No	Yes	No

Membership in the Friends

Note: Students excluded.

more "profound," or even more private reasons—but they are not as socially legitimate.

For example, a teacher who is a member of the Friends has headaches and fatigue. But she doesn't think these problems appropriate for psychotherapy to handle until we suggest them on our checklist. She is therefore exposed to somatic symptoms, but they are not salient to her. Her main problem, as she sees it, consists in her general inability to get along with people. A working-class man, on the other hand, was referred to the psychiatric clinic because he had "heart trouble." This is his problem. He might also check "Afraid to meet and talk with people" when presented with the checklist, but he would not have thought that problem worth taking to a psychiatrist.

Chart VIII aggregates these examples. The proportion "exposed" represents those applicants of various occupations who checked some of the physical symptoms in the checklist or who spontaneously mentioned them as problems. Among analytic clinic applicants there is obviously very little difference in the exposure to physical symptoms between persons of different occupations. About 80 per cent of each check some physical symptom. "Saliency" indicates the proportion of those who checked some physical symptom who also thought that a physical symptom was their most important presenting problem.[14] It is evident in all cases that working-class applicants are much more likely than others exposed to physical symptoms to feel that these symptoms were the main problem which brought them to therapy.

The evidence is clear. Working-class persons applying to clinics do not *have* more physical symptoms, but they certainly *feel* that these symptoms are more valid reasons for going to see a psychiatrist than do higher-class persons. There may be objective reasons for the greater importance of physical symptoms to the lower class. But the fact that membership in the Friends eliminates the differences between the various classes argues that knowledge and understanding of the role of physical illness in mental health is a major cause of the varying rates of physical symptoms offered as presenting problems.

✿ Marital and Other Primary-Group Problems: A Little Knowledge Is a Dangerous Thing

Marital problems and difficulties with one's family, children, or friends are sources of personal discomfort but they can also be signals of underlying emotional maladjustment. Even more so than physical symptoms, primary-group problems can be interpreted in several ways by persons contemplating therapy. Among supersophisticates, primary-group problems may be regarded as merely symptomatic of other diffi-

CHART VIII *Saliency of Somatic Problems to Analytic-Clinic Applicants of Different Occupations*

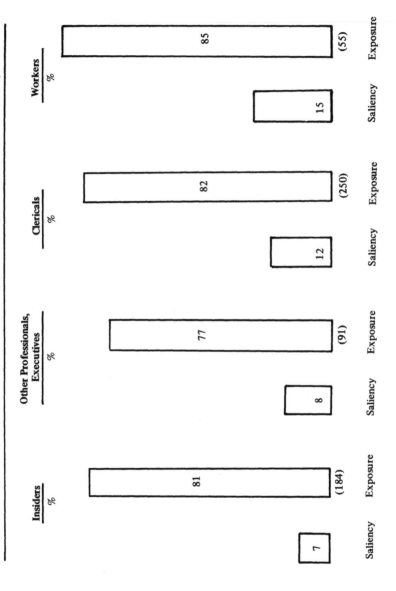

culties; too extensive a focus on the overt problems may to them suggest a lack of "insight." Among those who are newly acquainted with psychoanalysis, however, it may come as a great new truth that family squabbles are the natural lot of mankind and certainly do not indicate a need to consult a psychiatrist.

Unlike physical symptoms, primary-group problems engender a moral judgment, and this may contribute to the ambivalent feeling that prospective patients have about presenting such problems to psychiatrists. Fights with friends, relatives, and one's spouse often fall into the "traffic accident" category of moral evaluation, for it is usually the "other fellow" who is blamed for the catastrophe. At every level of education and among applicants to all types of clinics, persons with primary-group problems are between two and three times as likely as those with other kinds of problems to say that someone else is the cause of their problems. Such an attitude is hardly "insightful" in terms of psychoanalytic ideology.

Besides sophistication, there may be reality factors which make it likely that certain types of persons will experience problems with their spouses, families, or friends. A traditional view of the difference between the sexes implies that women have a greater investment in marriage than do men; if things go wrong, women are more likely to be seriously affected. But this is not now true of a national sample of the population in the United States. Women are not now more involved in their marriages than are men, and there is on the whole only a slight preponderance of feminine marital discontent,[15] though as we shall see, other factors may mask male-female differences. This general similarity of men and women is also true of applicants to psychiatric clinics, with the one exception of young married women under twenty-five who apply to analytic clinics. They seem to have more problems in general than any other group in our study! Early marriage must impose quite a strain on young sophisticated women.

Though economic circumstances are by definition less satisfactory for lower-class than for higher-class families, poverty alone does not seem to produce marital discontent. Nationwide, there is no consistent difference between married persons of different occupational rank[16] or income levels[17] in their experience of family problems. But level of education is another matter. The authors of a national study of the emotional problems of nonpatients summarize their findings:

> The more highly educated people seem to show a greater investment and involvement in their marriages that bring with them a greater sensitivity to both the positive and negative aspects. The greater involvement of the more highly educated people is evidenced in their greater focusing on the relationship aspects of the marriage when they talk of their sources

of gratification, dissatisfaction, problems, or inadequacy. Their greater sensitivity to the positive aspects of marriage is reflected in their much greater expression of marital happiness than that of people with less education. But with this greater happiness there is also an increase in certain stressful aspects of the marriage: the more highly educated people are more self-questioning, they express more feelings of inadequacy.[18]

Among applicants for therapy how much, then, of these effects attributed to education are caused by the style of life characteristic of the better educated and how much difference is directly attributable to greater emotional sophistication?

When both life style (as measured by education) and psychiatric sophistication (as measured by membership in the Friends and Supporters of Psychotherapy) are analyzed simultaneously, the ambivalent attitude toward going to a psychiatrist because of primary-group problems is revealed. For those who are less educated, whose natural life style does not lead to a great investment in marriage, membership in the Friends and Supporters of Psychotherapy vastly boosts the proportion who come to psychiatrists because of primary-group problems. These sophisticated but less-educated applicants are even *more* likely than the better educated to come to a psychiatrist for help with family problems. In fact, it is one of their leading presenting complaints.* Among the better educated, life style—the entire tone of the marital relationship and the degree of investment in it—is responsible for the proportion who come because of primary-group problems. Membership in the Friends does not, in their case, *increase* the proportion of such complaints, though in their natural state, college-educated applicants are somewhat more likely than those with only a high-school education to present primary-group problems. With education and sophistication controlled, women are indeed slightly more likely than men to come because of family problems. The findings are similar when actual contact with psychotherapy or reading about mental health matters replace membership in the Friends as indicators or creators of sophistication.

As with physical symptoms, what one knows about emotional problems determines whether or not a particular symptom will be seen as suitable for a psychiatrist. To the less educated, and hence to the less generally sophisticated, the fact that marital problems are symptomatic of emotional difficulty is a great revelation. But the entire culture of the better educated is already permeated with sensitivity to the emotional nuances of family life. Psychiatric sophistication may add to this sensitivity, but it also creates awareness that family problems should

---

* The generally better educated but psychologically naive applicants to the Religion and Psychiatry Institute also manifest this concern with primary-group problems, for these are the main problems presented to that clinic.

CHART IX *Per Cent of Primary-Group Problems Presented by Married Members and Nonmembers of the Friends Who Applied to Analytic Clinics*

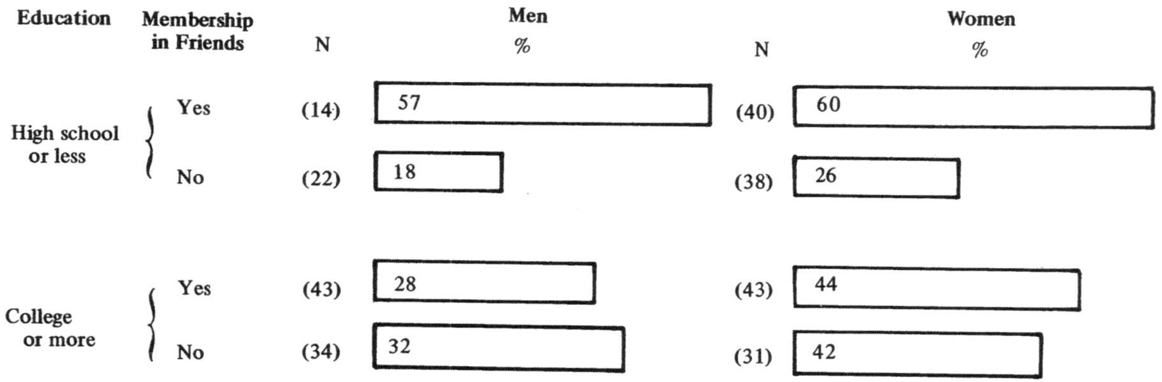

Education	Membership in Friends	Men N	Men %	Women N	Women %
High school or less	Yes	(14)	57	(40)	60
	No	(22)	18	(38)	26
College or more	Yes	(43)	28	(43)	44
	No	(34)	32	(31)	42

Note: Students excluded.

not be taken as legitimate emotional problems in themselves but that they are merely indicators of deeper, underlying difficulties. The "reality" which leads to a greater probability of family problems is mainly a cultural rather than a social structural reality and influences the reaction to the problems rather than directly creating it.

⚙ Sexual Problems and the Avant-Garde

The first two problems we discussed—physical and primary-group problems—were regarded by sophisticated applicants for psychotherapy in an ambivalent way. They saw both problems as symptomatic of underlying disorder, yet felt that neither was altogether the "right" sort of thing to tell a psychiatrist. Because of their ambivalence, membership in the Friends and Supporters of Psychotherapy and other sources of psychiatric sophistication had the greatest effect on those who, without such influences, were *least* likely to be knowledgeable about psychotherapy. But there was certainly no evidence that membership in the Friends directly contributed to the pressures which produced the problems. Newly acquired sophistication had merely made these latter applicants more or less aware of their problems and more or less willing to take them to a psychiatrist.

This is not true of sexual problems. There is no ambivalence about them. Heterosexual (but not homosexual) problems are unequivocally the "right" presenting complaints. All four sources of sophistication (going to a psychiatrist, reading books, membership in the Friends, and high level of education)* produce about 10 percentage points more frequent reports of sexual problems. But the matter does not rest simply with *verbal* accounts of such problems, for membership in the Friends also produces added pressure which leads to a greater frequency of sexual problems for some applicants. Let us see how this works out in detail.

The objective social settings which are related to the largest differences in the number that bring sexual problems to a psychiatrist are not social class alone, but the sex of an applicant, and his or her age

---

* There is some degree of interaction between these variables. By and large, controlling one or several of them reduces the over-all effect of each by about five percentage points. The effects of each are greatest when the others are not present. For example, reading serious books on mental health increases the proportion of *less-educated* applicants who present heterosexual problems from 14 per cent to 32 per cent, but for the better educated there is an increase of only about five percentage points. So they are all, by and large, functional alternatives to sophistication about sexual problems. We shall use membership in the Friends as an indicator of sophistication in the following analysis because it is so clearly related to some social concomitants of pressure which *produce* sexual problems; and it is also closely related to mere increase in *knowledgeability* about sex and emotional problems.

and marital status. For the prevalence of certain sexual practices is jointly affected by being a man or a woman and by social class. Kinsey and his associates find that level of education is related to sexual practices among men but not among women.[19] And despite the fact that we are concerned with sexual *problems* whereas the Kinsey group was interested in sexual *practices*, we too find that level of education does not affect the number of women who present sexual problems but that less-educated men are indeed *less* likely to bring sexual problems to a psychiatrist.[20] But the major difference in rates of sexual problems presented are between men and women, between the single and the married, and between the young and the old.

Since these social positions, and membership in the Friends as well, affect the probability that a person will present sexual problems to a psychiatrist, Chart X takes all of these factors into account. In addition, we have had to indicate where respondents live, for this too affects the nature of their sexual problems. At the top of each section of Chart X are the labels "Live with Parents," "Live with Spouse," and "Live Alone, with Roommates." These are the three major modes of residence and life pattern for applicants to analytic clinics. For the single, sexual problems are a more important reason for entering therapy than for married persons. The one exception is that single as well as married young sophisticated men tend to offer an equal proportion of sexual problems. Single persons living at home show certain unique characteristics. Single women who are sophisticated but live with their parents are not as likely to report sexual problems as their counterparts who live alone or with roommates. The difference between those living with their parents and those living apart is especially pronounced for single women twenty-five or older. Among the latter, sophistication may lead not only to verbal expression of sexual problems but also to a willingness to engage in practices that may result in guilt feelings. These practices cannot be entered into as conveniently by women who live with their parents. Sophisticated single women who do not live with their parents present sexual problems as frequently as men. The following conflict-ridden women are typical.

> A single woman, thirty-four years old, has had two and one-half years of college and comes from a working-class New York City background. She is a Catholic. At present she is secretary to an executive in the entertainment industry, but says she would like to be a housewife. She is both culturally and psychiatrically sophisticated. Her complaint is "Feelings of rejection causing anxiety neurosis. I feel I have not attained any of my goals. Frustration because I'm not yet married after a series of broken romances." She is currently "involved with a man . . . and no chance of marriage is in the offing."

A girl from a small town in the Mid-West, a religious Protestant, is psychiatrically and culturally sophisticated. "I have been getting involved in sex. I have been drinking too much. It is difficult for me to stop drinking after I have taken the first drink . . . as soon as someone reminds me of home I start drinking and usually end up sleeping with someone. While sober I can't stand being touched by a man." In the checklist of problems opposite "Sex life, Other," she wrote, "Immoral."

Advancing age decreases the report of sexual problems among all but men who live with their parents and sophisticated men and women who live alone or with roommates. The decrease is especially noteworthy among the married. Complaints about homosexuality, which form a significant proportion of the difficulties of younger men applying for therapy,* generally decline sharply with age.

Finally, unsophisticated women report sexual problems far less frequently than sophisticated men, though much of the difference is caused by the larger proportion of homosexual complaints among the men. (Kinsey data do show less homosexual *practice* among women, but this in itself need not prove that men have more serious *problems* in their relationships with others of the same sex.) Membership in the Friends almost always has a homogenizing effect: persons of different social position who are members of the Friends come to share similar characteristics. So we note that sophisticated women present about the same proportion of sexual problems as men, despite the fact that they present fewer homosexual problems. Another homogenizing effect is not shown in the chart. Less-educated applicants who are members of the Friends tend to present as many sexual problems as the better educated.

Two factors seem to produce the relationships we have observed: the ability to *talk* about sexual problems and the pressure which *produces* them. Unlike other problems, some social positions are also associated with the cultural fact of freedom to talk about sex, and some sources of sophistication about sex also lead to actual pressures and tensions about sex. Youth, malehood, being a bachelor, having a high level of education, and being a member of the Friends all facilitate greater ease in talking about sexual problems. In addition, youth and being single probably lead to pressures that create sexual difficulties (though sexual

* In 1958-59 the University Psychoanalytic Center ran a special research project with homosexuals. True to our sociological theory of the application process, the "word got around." As a result, 40 per cent (N = 38) of the men under thirty-five who lived alone or with roommates applying to University in that year presented homosexual problems. Data gathered in that year are not presented in the chart, however, since the index of Friends and Supporters was not defined in the questionnaires used in 1958-59.

CHART X *Sexual Problems of Men and Women Applicants to Analytic Clinics, According to Mode of Residence, Membership in the Friends, and Age*

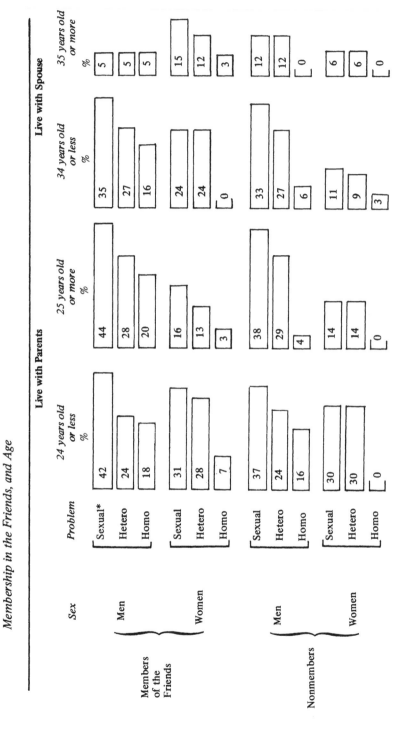

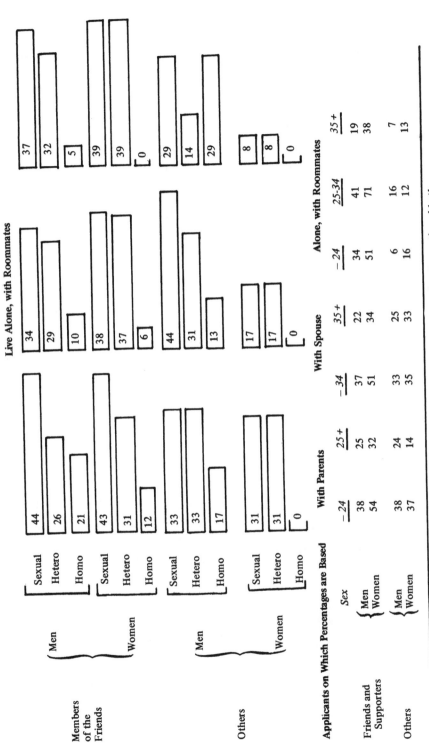

Live Alone, with Roommates

Applicants on Which Percentages are Based	With Parents		With Spouse		Alone, with Roommates		
Sex	*-24*	*25+*	*-34*	*35+*	*-24*	*25-34*	*35+*
Friends and Supporters							
Men	38	25	37	22	34	41	19
Women	54	32	51	34	51	71	38
Others							
Men	38	24	33	25	6	16	7
Women	37	14	35	33	16	12	13

*Sexual problems are less than the sum of Heterosexual and Homosexual problems since some applicants mentioned both.

problems may in turn lead to bachelorhood), for regardless of membership in the Friends the young and the single are more likely to present sexual problems.* Membership in the Friends, aside from making talk about sex easier, also leads to pressures which produce sexual problems, for membership leads to a greater participation in the "sexual revolution." Even if *none* of the practices of the "hip" crowd are *in themselves* emotionally injurious, they may conflict with the sexual mores persons learned as children. These conflicts alone may lead to the sophisticated person's feeling that he or she has sexual problems that ought to be taken to a psychiatrist.

Nevertheless, the essential role of sophistication in the presentation of sexual problems is *not* to produce them, but to make existing problems more salient. It will be recalled that our method for ascertaining the saliency or "painfulness" of problems is to present applicants with a checklist measuring their exposure to these problems after they have indicated in their own words what the problems were that brought them to therapy. Included under a heading "Sex Life" the following problems were listed: "Frigidity, impotence, homosexuality, masturbation, can't get along with opposite sex, Other—What?" The accuracy and utility of this method are shown by comparing it to the results of a psychoanalytic study of homosexuals.

In that study 51 per cent of persons later discovered to be homosexual stated that a sexual problem was their reason for entering therapy.[21] In our sample, 56 per cent of the 85 males applying for analytic treatment who checked homosexuality on the checklist mentioned it as a presenting problem.†

* The relationship between marital status and the presentation of sexual problems holds for all but young married men who are members of the Friends. Here, youth, malehood, and membership in the Friends override the fact of marriage and make such men as likely as the single to present sexual problems.

† Bieber and his colleagues do not indicate in their study whether the "reason for seeking treatment" is the main problem or one of many presenting problems. We suspect the former. His sample of nonhomosexuals indicates about 10 per cent sexual presenting problems, which, taking into account the somewhat older age group in his sample, about matches the 13 per cent of men who did not check homosexuality on the checklist but who did indicate that a sexual problem was their main presenting problem. If only the one main problem is counted, then our rate of initial disclosure of homosexuality drops to only 25 per cent. Assuming that some persons who checked "homosexual" were only fearful of being "latent homosexuals" then our data are still roughly comparable to the Bieber study, and the sensitivity of our method is vindicated.

Fifty-six per cent is a rather high figure, by the way, indicating that homosexuality is much more "painful" to these applicants than are other types of problems. The least salient sexual problem, although checked by more men and more single women than any other problem, was masturbation. Although 46 per cent of the single men checked this problem as bothersome, only 2 per cent of these found the practice a sufficient reason to enter therapy.

TABLE 14 *Saliency of Sexual Problems to Men and Women Applicants to Analytic Clinics*

Membership in the Friends		Now Single		Now Married	
		Men %	Women %	Men %	Women %
Yes	Saliency	20	17	18	9
	Exposure	89	79	75	67
	(N)	(138)	(245)	(60)	(87)
No	Saliency	31	9	24	3
	Exposure	83	67	66	44
	(N)	(77)	(79)	(58)	(71)

Table 14 shows the proportion of main problem to checklist problems or "exposure" for any sexual problem. Marital status and sex of respondent are the social positions taken into account, while sophistication is measured by membership in the Friends and Supporters of Psychotherapy. Men who are not members of the Friends are both much more exposed and much more sensitive to sexual problems than are women nonmembers. Membership in the Friends dramatically reduces the differences between men and women in sensitivity as well as in exposure to sexual problems. It is important to observe that sophistication *increases* women's *exposure* to sexual problems, especially that of married women. Sophistication does not so radically eliminate differences between the married and single. Regardless of sophistication, marriage leads to a reduction in sensitivity to sexual problems for women. Among men, the loss in sensitivity with marriage is negligible.

In summary, sexual problems are presented to analytic clinics more often by the young and single because they are exposed to societal or biological pressures which may generate sexual difficulties. On the other hand, men and the sophisticates present sexual problems only partly because of societal circumstances and pressures. Though their ability to talk more easily about sex and their sensitivity to it may be the most important factors, it must not be forgotten that sophistication also leads many into a style of life and into a social circle that itself creates problems. This sophisticated circle especially affects the women in our sample who may verbally agree with the new sexual mores yet on a deep emotional level may experience a conflict between the values in which they were brought up and the situations in which they now find themselves. These conflicts become important reasons for their entry into psychotherapy.

⚙ The Psychoanalytic Syndrome

In some ways it is comforting to have a problem that one can feel, touch, or point to. Abstract discomfort is more disquieting, for it reduces the opportunity to blame events, one's physical condition, or other people for the pain one is feeling. Evaluative problems—feelings of lack of self-worth and dissatisfaction with one's social or cultural values—are such problems. Applicants who presented them were much more likely than others to mention themselves as the "cause" of their problems. Feelings of being generally unable to relate to other people (as opposed to specific interpersonal fights or difficulties) also fall into this category of abstract malaise. Such evaluative and interpersonal problems are presented by a majority of applicants to analytic clinics. Together with the sexual problems just discussed, these problems comprise the "psychoanalytic syndrome." Not some particular social structure but the way people react to pressure and the way difficulties are verbalized determine whether these problems become reasons for going to a psychotherapist. Sophistication is therefore the key factor which brings these problems to analytic clinics.

Studies of those who do not go to psychotherapists indicate that sophistication rather than the pressures of their social situation or even overt economic pressure is responsible for the appearance of evaluative and interpersonal problems. In the United States, better-educated persons are more likely to see themselves as different from others, to be less self-accepting, to find fault with themselves, and to want their children to be different from themselves.[22] This is also true of professional men and their wives but not of businessmen and their wives, who have the same class standing as professionals.[23]

Applicants to clinics exhibit these same patterns. "Insiders" are more likely than others of the same social class to present problems of self-evaluation. Businessmen, less likely to be members of the Friends, are more attuned to a culture which denies evil and which advocates the assertion of happiness—a point of view expressed in books espousing "positive thinking." (The Religion and Psychiatry Institute, two of whose leaders have written inspirational books, attracts more businessmen than any other clinic in our study.) It is not necessarily the different style of life engendered by the workaday experiences of businessmen and insiders that makes them so different, however. High social class, in itself, does not necessarily lead to self-doubt. Rather, it is the entire social milieu which affects one's willingness to admit to self-doubt.

Considerable evidence supports this contention. Businessmen who are members of the Friends and thus share in this broader milieu are as likely as insiders to express self-doubt or feelings of inadequacy in interpersonal relations. And in both the national study and among applicants to clinics in New York City, education but not occupational level is related to feelings of self-dissatisfaction. Indicative of general sophistication, education sensitizes one to the self while at the same time it enlarges the horizon against which the self is measured. More specifically, the Friends and Supporters of Psychotherapy as well as psychotherapy itself make self-doubt and general inability to relate to others not only legitimate problems but the very prerequisite for entry into therapy. All three factors (membership in the Friends, sessions of psychotherapy, and education) are combined in Chart XI, which shows their effects on the proportion of problems of self-worth submitted to analytic clinics.

The three sources of sophistication are not purely additive in their effect. Rather, as we have earlier seen, they tend to be functional alternatives: among the less well educated, either membership in the Friends and Supporters of Psychotherapy or actual psychotherapy makes these problems especially likely to be given as reasons for going to a psychiatrist. Among the better educated, these specific avenues of psychiatric knowledge are less necessary. Similarly, for members of the Friends, education or actual psychotherapy adds relatively little to the probability of presenting evaluative problems. Social circle member-

CHART XI *Per Cent of Problems of Self-Evaluation Presented to Analytic Clinics by Those with Various Levels of Sophistication*

Number of Previous Sessions	Membership in the Friends	Level of Education			
		High School N	%	College N	%
None	No	(38)	24	(30)	60
	Yes	(36)	42	(67)	58
1-20	No	(41)	32	(45)	42
	Yes	(57)	51	(102)	56
21+	No	(29)	48	(51)	43
	Yes	(48)	50	(122)	62

ship, as indicated by membership in the Friends and Supporters of Psychotherapy, does seem to make for some difference even when other factors are present.* But the most important factor which brings those suffering from self-doubt to psychotherapists is reading. This most specific indicator of psychiatric knowledge produces large differences between those who do and those who do not read (on the order of 20 percentage points) even among the better educated, or those with a good deal of therapy, or members of the Friends. Reading serious psychological literature is thus seen to be especially productive of reports of lack of self-worth. And lest it be said that people read because they feel unworthy, the evidence obtained by comparing changes from the way problems were first noticed to how they were finally presented to a clinic shows that reading accounts for this large difference almost entirely by making applicants more aware of their evaluative problems. Learning about psychotherapy makes people more aware of their feelings of lack of self-worth and teaches them to bring these feelings to psychotherapists. Learning is characteristic of the psychoanalytic syndrome.

Though interpersonal problems show the same general pattern as evaluative problems, there is one special social structural and one cultural aspect which affects the likelihood of such problems being brought to psychiatrists. General interpersonal difficulties are the inverse of specific primary-group problems. Those who live with other people, and especially those who are married, may come to realize that they have psychiatric problems through some specific incident or battle with other people. Single persons living alone or with roommates—that New York City phenomenon which supplies so many of the analytic clinics with patients—do not have this opportunity. They are much more likely than the married (by some 10 to 20 percentage points depending on the sex and age of the applicant) to discover they need a psychotherapist because of some general inadequacy in their dealings with people. Men find sexual difficulties easier to discuss than women, especially those living alone. But women find interpersonal difficulties easier to bring to a psychiatrist than do men. In many ways, these two types of problems are merely different ways of saying the same thing. Men living without families who are not members of the Friends are over 30 per-

---

* Some of this effect may be caused by the tendency of the better-educated nonmembers of the Friends *not* to present problems in the psychoanalytic syndrome. These persons, who persist in shopping from one therapist to another, tend to present only the "sicker" problems such as cognitive and cathectic problems. One suspects that their being more seriously disturbed accounts for their presence in the sample despite the fact that, though exposed to the chance of becoming members of the Friends through their higher education, they have not in fact chosen to do so. They are not going to therapists because they believe in psychotherapy but because they must go.

centage points *less* likely than women in the same circumstances to come to an analytic clinic because of general interpersonal problems. But there is no difference between men and women who are members of the Friends. For men, membership in the Friends *increases* the proportion of interpersonal problems they bring just as for women this circle increases the proportion of sexual problems brought to psychiatrists.

In summary, when it comes to those problems most characteristic of psychoanalytic patients, sophistication rather than social reality seems to make the greatest difference among applicants. Since the difference is always in the direction of producing more problems, it is safe to say that psychiatric sophistication serves to make people more aware of things that might not even be verbalized by other people. Knowledge and understanding make people more sensitive to psychoanalytic problems; it also makes such problems seem more fit to take to psychiatrists. Perhaps most important, membership in the Friends "homogenizes" the circle. Men and women and those of higher and lower education or different class background become alike in their readiness to admit to sexual and interpersonal problems as well as shortcomings in themselves.

❂ The Strong Impact of Reality: Role Performance Problems

There is one area in which social reality rather than sophistication rules supreme. Problems with one's major role—not being able to perform adequately, not being able to get along with people on the job, and worrying about one's future job or employment—seem almost wholly affected by a person's objective social situation, even when various measures of sophistication are controlled. Important differences in the effect of work pressures are closely related to the social positions of sex, occupation, and age. Men are probably more involved in their work, and hence may find problems on the job a good reason for going to a psychiatrist. The same sort of work involvement might be expected to characterize persons with middle-class occupations. Older persons should have become adjusted to their level of performance and so less likely to complain in this area. Chart XII takes all these factors into account, as well as the type of clinic applied to.

The expectation with respect to women is only partially true. Except for students, younger employed women are only somewhat *less* likely than men to find role difficulties a reason to seek psychiatric help, but this is not true for women over thirty-five who may consider their careers as important to them as do men. Housewives are another story.

Analytic Clinics

Age	Own Occupation	N	Men %	N	Women %
24 and Under	Insider	(23)	39	(44)	32
	Student	(77)	49	(87)	46
	Other Prof. Mgr.	(9)	44	(9)	22
	White Collar	(24)	46	(24)	56
	Blue Collar	(16)	38	(5)	20
	Housewife			(18)	39
25 to 34	Insider	(71)	39	(70)	29
	Other Prof. Mgr.	(37)	46	(21)	19
	White Collar	(58)	47	(68)	37
	Blue Collar	(15)	20	(6)	50
	Housewife			(51)	18
35 and Over	Insider	(31)	39	(30)	23
	Other Prof. Mgr.	(26)	46	(10)	40
	White Collar	(32)	25	(53)	32
	Blue Collar	(13)	8	(5)	20
	Housewife			(49)	20

Religio-Psychiatric Clinic

Age	Own Occupation	N	%
4 and Under	Professional, Manager, Student	(33)	33
	White Collar	(26)	19
	Blue Collar	(7)	0
	Housewife	(9)	0
5 and Over	Professional, Manager	(47)	34
	White Collar	(28)	14
	Blue Collar	(7)	14
	Housewife	(31)	3

Hospital Clinics

Age	Own Occupation	N	%
34 and Under	Professional, Manager, Student	(15)	60
	White Collar	(18)	28
	Blue Collar	(15)	0
	Housewife	(20)	15
35 and Over	Professional, Manager	(8)	25
	White Collar	(14)	29
	Blue Collar	(19)	37
	Housewife	(14)	14

*The size of the sample in these clinics does not permit presenting the data by sex as well as age.

We coded housewives' complaints about difficulties in caring for children and running a household as major-role problems, so as to allow for some comparability with employed persons. Even so, housewives aged twenty-five and over are generally less likely than employed women, taken as a group, to present major-role problems. This tendency is even more pronounced among women applicants to the Religion and Psychiatry Institute and to hospital clinics, although the data are not shown in the chart. Among these housewives, complaints about primary-group and general interpersonal relationships are a much more frequent reason for going to a psychiatrist. Role performance—that is, in their case, housekeeping—may not be as important to them, and the adequacy of its performance is more difficult to measure.

The eighteen young housewives under twenty-five applying to analytic clinics, however, are quite different. They have more complaints about everything than any other group of applicants we have been able to single out. The following composite of three cases is typical of the young housewives in this category.

. . . Depressed often, bored, no patience with my two-year-old daughter, often scream at her and lose control of myself. Although I love her, I resent her. I hate to stay home so much of the time. I want to return to day college and teach as soon as possible. . . . General dissatisfaction with being a housewife . . . cannot make decisions . . . dislike my role as a woman . . . feel helpless and worthless . . I find any sort of sexual relationship with my husband unpleasant."

These sophisticated, unhappy young women probably do have many objective problems in performing their roles as housewives and mothers.

Our evidence shows that it is not so much that women generally are not exposed to major-role problems, but that they are not as sensitive to them as men.[24] Not getting one's work done is an experience shared equally by single men and women. Yet even women who are married and employed have similar exposure to work problems. The difference lies in the greater sensitivity of men to these problems. Housewives, however, are generally both less sensitive to major-role problems and less likely to be exposed to them.

Higher-class applicants are more likely to present major-role problems than lower-class applicants. Even among those not applying to psychotherapists, men with more education and with professional or managerial jobs are more likely to say that they have had problems at work.[25] Perhaps this is so because they care more about their jobs, for they are also more likely to report that their jobs satisfy them.[26] But the fact that there is less difference between women of higher- and lower-level occupations than there is for men points to the importance of *involvement* with one's work as a reason for its becoming a psychiatric problem. As we have indicated, women are somewhat less likely to be so completely involved in their work and are therefore less likely to bring these problems to a psychotherapist. The one exception to the social class factor's effect is the high rate of role problems reported by older men applying to hospital clinics. Their large number of physical complaints, rather than their degree of involvement in their work, however, seems to be the cause of their occupational worries.

The actual pressures and satisfactions of work are also factors in bringing work problems to psychiatric clinics, however. One must assume that insiders (educators, professionals in health fields, and those working in the arts and communications) are at least as involved in their work as other professionals, executives, and managers. Yet the image of the harassed, tense businessman seems to be correct. Men who are lawyers, businessmen, engineers or who are in other "square" professions tend to present somewhat more role problems than insiders.

Few jobs place as much emphasis on performance as the occupation of student. A good college always assigns more work than can ever be thoroughly covered, as if to emphasize that any one person's knowledge is necessarily incomplete. Examinations and "quizzes" thus lead, in many colleges, to a sense of continuous pressure. This pressure, plus the lingering problems of adolescence, combined with money problems resulting from a reluctance to use parental financial resources, leads to an enormous proportion of student applicants to analytic clinics. Almost half these students present major-role problems. In fact, students are more likely than any other occupational group to present these problems, and the structured pressure of student life probably falls about equally on young men and women.

Exposure to pressure does make a great deal of difference for students in the presentation of major-role problems, as Chart XIII shows. Exposure is measured by the proportion who checked "can't get enough work done"; saliency, by the proportion of those who were thus "exposed" and who said that difficulties in performing their major role comprised either the most important or the second most important problem that brought them to seek treatment. Students are also more sensitive to performance problems. Among those of equally high occupational rank, the differences between insiders and others of high rank are more a matter of saliency than of exposure to performance problems. The pressures experienced by the businessmen, lawyers, executives, and engineers applying to analytic clinics therefore represent their reactions to these pressures more than they do any essential difference in the perceived importance of getting work done. As for workers, they simply care less about "getting work done." This is only one of the three items in our checklist of work problems. The other checklisted items, "not creative enough," and "have trouble with people on the job," were not nearly as salient. For example, only the insiders found creativity at all a *salient* problem (5 per cent), although over one-third checked it as a problem.

Finally, what is the relation between older age and major-role problems? "Old age" in our study really means middle age—applicants over thirty-five. While evidence from national surveys shows older persons to be less concerned about major-role problems, the fact that this same finding occurs in our data must be interpreted in a somewhat different way. If the really old withdraw from social life and hence find less interest in and fewer problems with their major roles, the same lack of interest in major roles should not be found among men and women in their prime working years. Indeed, there is no decline in interest with age for men who have high-level jobs. The decline occurs only among those with clerical or blue-collar jobs (except for the older men applying to hospital clinics mentioned above). The man over thirty-five performing routine tasks may really find his job less challenging, and therefore less likely to induce worry about it as a psychiatric problem. Executives, managers, and professionals, on the other hand, often find that their most demanding work problems come after they have passed the age of thirty-five.

In summary, applicants who are most involved in their work, whose occupations require the most intellectual effort, are those most likely

CHART XIII *Saliency* of Major-Role Performance Problems to Analytic Clinic Applicants of Different Occupations*

Occupation

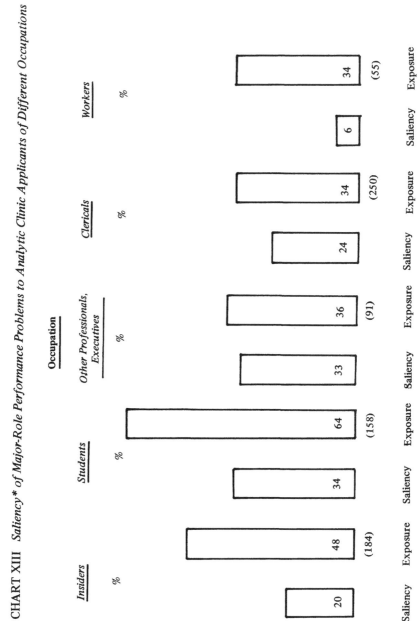

Saliency Exposure Saliency Exposure Saliency Exposure Saliency Exposure Saliency Exposure

Insiders *Students* *Other Professionals, Executives* *Clericals* *Workers*

*First and second most important problems.

to be concerned with psychiatric problems in their major roles. It is therefore probable that men more than women, employed women more than housewives, the young rather than the middle-aged, and persons in higher-class occupations more than in lower-class will present problems with their major roles to psychiatrists.

The same factors that lead to noticing major-role problems also lead to noticing cognitive problems—that is problems in thinking and in general orientation. For it is only when a person is directly confronted with poor performance that he can realize he is not thinking well or is disoriented. So we find college students and young college dropouts exceptionally likely to come to psychiatrists because of cognitive problems. And it is therefore also true that persons of a lower occupational level who nonetheless *aspire* to high-level occupations are more likely than others to present cognitive problems. Finally, cognitive problems are the only ones radically affected by previous experience with psychiatrists, though this is true only of analytic-clinic applicants with less than a college education. In this case, however, it does not appear to be "learning" which is the factor producing more cognitive presenting problems, for psychotherapy contributes mainly to *retention* of cognitive problems from the time they were first noticed to the time of clinic application rather than to *acquisition* of such problems. It may well be that the less educated with a good deal of therapy who otherwise might not wish to continue in therapy are motivated to continue by the severity of these cognitive problems.

✤ Cathectic Problems: Pure Emotion

An entire set of symptoms that loom large in the psychiatric *Diagnostic Manual* have been until now intentionally omitted from our discussion. These are the cathectic problems—those that refer to the level of a person's emotional energy. The level may be too low, in which case a person says he is depressed or immobile. He may have too high or too agitated a level in which case he may suffer from anxieties, fears, tantrums, or other forms of loss of control. Among clinic applicants none of these cathectic problems is uniformly related to any of the measures of psychiatric sophistication, and they are not strongly related to any indicators of social position. There are few special circumstances that serve to trigger the realization that one has such problems, nor do specific events act to throw them into sharp relief. Moreover, there is contradictory evidence about the association of such problems with social position even in nonclinical populations.[27] And unlike problems belonging to the psychoanalytic syndrome these problems are not made comprehensible to those who experience them through membership in the Friends and Supporters of Psychotherapy. Finally, though most applicants experience cathectic problems, they are seen as the most important problem by only 18 per cent of applicants to analytic clinics and 21 per cent of applicants to hospital clinics. Even together with cognitive problems, the traditional symptoms of various mental illness are mentioned as the most important problems by only 23 per cent of analytic and 30 per cent of hospital clinic applicants. Either such problems are hard to notice in oneself because there is no firm foreground or background against which they can stand out, or they tend to be associated with a recognized need for hospitalization rather than for outpatient treatment. And it may be that serious cathectic problems require very strong influence on the part of others in order for them to be taken to a psychiatrist. Very few applicants to outpatient clinics were subjected to such heavy pressure, which may more typically characterize the decision to go to a mental hospital.

❀ Conclusion: Problems That Send People to Psychiatrists

Other things being equal, it is easier to seek professional help for a specific difficulty. Toothaches suggest going to a dentist, lawsuits seem appropriate for lawyers, and broken legs seem to require physicians. But emotional problems by their very nature tend to be diffuse and therefore very difficult for a person to pin down and decide what to do about them. One can recognize emotional difficulties in himself only through some signs or guideposts, and the more vague his sense of unease, the more difficult it is for him to decide that psychiatric help is required. So the role of specific symptoms in the decision to go to a psychiatrist is very important.

We have dealt with four major specific problems: physical symptoms, sexual problems, marital and other primary-group conflicts and difficulties, and job or major role problems. These symptoms are usually clear enough, at least in comparison with other signposts of emotional trouble, and they are often associated with some specific social position or social class. This association means that a person can very likely point to some specific life circumstance or event which caused his problems —another aid in crystallizing the decision to seek help. People with physical symptoms can point to an onset of the symptoms or an exposure to disease or conditions which might have produced ill health. Those with sexual problems usually point to specific events in which their incapacities or difficulties were revealed. And the same holds true for the other specific problems. Nonetheless, with the exception of job or major role problems, we have shown that the major consideration which leads some persons and not others to present specific problems when they apply for treatment is their estimation of the psychiatric relevancy or respectability of these problems. Of the four specific problems with which we have dealt, only sexual problems were unequivocally relevant from the point of view of psychiatry. The more an applicant knew about psychiatry and psychoanalysis, the more likely he was to come to a clinic because of these problems. Physical symptoms were ambivalently regarded, as were marital or primary-group problems. The former, though especially prevalent among working-class applicants, were not induced by poorer working-class health but by their tendency to express emotional discomfort in physical terms, or at least to feel that only physical symptoms were legitimate problems. The presence of primary-group problems among different applicants also appeared to be a function of how blameworthy the other fellow was regarded. Persons of no sophistication tended not to see primary-group problems as at all relevant to psychiatric treatment; the newly sophisticated were usually "converts" to the idea that family strife had psychiatric implications and hence they were especially prone to come with these problems; but those who normally live in a sophisticated milieu, perhaps because they questioned the advisability of presenting such problems to psychotherapists, showed only a moderate tendency in this direction. Finally, some of the specific problems were more narrowly located in a particular group. For a variety of reasons, women without special training were unlikely to present sexual problems. And though unaffected by training or sophistication, job problems seemed to be located mainly among students and men in higher-class occupations. In sum, despite the apparently simple appeal of specific problems, there are definite barriers to their becoming clear and universal signs of mental disorder.

The more universal psychiatric problems are in any case the diffuse ones, for the underlying reason a person needs psychiatric treatment is always that he suffers some inadequacy or breakdown which permeates his every action. A specific problem is therefore a pretext (defense, if you will), rather than a cause. Traditional medical psychiatry, aside from an interest in somatic indications of disorder, has always had a special interest in those diffuse conditions we have called cognitive and cathectic problems. Most of the symptoms described in the *Diagnostic Manual* belong to these categories, and most of the applicants to hospital psychiatric clinics come with these "psychiatric" problems. But neither shows any signs of being the sort of problem which one can learn to identify in himself. Moreover, cathectic problems are relatively unassociated with any major social structure, and hence probably cannot be easily traced to any specific events or occasions in one's life. Although these problems or symptoms are expressed by most applicants to psychiatric clinics (though not as their major problem), their recognition is not aided by training or social circumstance. Thus, despite the fact that cathectic problems are so universal, or perhaps because they are, they do not serve as the best signs of mental disorder, at least to the patient himself. That is why we say people do not go to psychiatrists merely because they are "sick."

This brings us to the diffuse problems commonly associated with an application to an analytic clinic—problems of self-evaluation and general interpersonal inadequacy. Along with the specific problem of inadequate sexual behavior or feeling, these problems were called the "psychoanalytic syndrome." Low self-evaluation and interpersonal inadequacy are problems that have captured the attention of psychoanalysis and psychotherapists, and there is a considerable literature about them. Unlike cathectic and cognitive problems, there is every evidence that people have learned to recognize low self-evaluation and interpersonal inadequacy as signals for the need of psychiatric help. Membership in the Friends and Supporters of Psychotherapy, actual previous therapy, and the reading of books about mental health are all related to an increased tendency to present these "psychoanalytic" problems upon application for psychotherapy. What is more, sophistication tends to make people bring these problems to psychotherapists though they might otherwise not notice or act upon them. Since any form of psychiatric sophistication is associated with higher social class, it is no wonder that higher-class persons are more likely to apply for outpatient psychiatric treatment.[28] They have the "right" problems, in part, because they have been taught to recognize them. In short, "psychoanalytic" problems may not necessarily be the ones which make people feel *worse*, but they are the most effective in recruiting people to psychotherapy simply because people have been taught to conceptualize and recognize these diffuse feelings as indicative of the need for psychotherapy.[29]

The most important thing about psychiatric sophistication is that the several routes to this state are generally interchangeable. For us to point out that previous psychotherapy is related to a greater sensitivity to psychoanalytic problems would be no great discovery. This would be tantamount to proclaiming that the best way to become a psychiatric patient is already to have been one. And while this is in some ways true, the fact casts no light on the entrance of the uninitiated into the system to begin with. Both the reading of certain types of books and membership in the Friends and Supporters of Psychotherapy perform the same task, however, as actual psychotherapy, and for some problems reading is especially effective. Alternative routes to the same state of knowledge about psychiatric problems explain how the uninitiated get into the psychiatric system. Membership in the Friends and Supporters of Psychotherapy is an especially important alternative, because unlike the reading of books, it involves interaction with other people and becomes an important aid in the final decision to go to a psychiatrist. This decision requires social support, and books, of course, cannot give this.

What is especially intriguing about membership in the Friends is that it eliminates differences between otherwise distant groups in the population. One of the major findings about psychiatry in the past 20 years is that both the incidence of mental disorder and treatment are linked to social class. Lower classes are sicker, less sensitive to emotional problems, and less likely to get adequate treatment. Now we can see more clearly why sensitivity and the use of psychiatric facilities are related to social class. Membership in the Friends is highly related to social class and, in any case, many of the sensitivities of the Friends are the natural sensitivities of higher-class persons. Of course, there are some members who are from the lower classes so that the findings about social class and mental illness hold only for nonmembers of the Friends. But membership in the Friends and Supporters of Psychotherapy tends to make lower-class persons as sensitive to psychoanalytic disorders as higher-class persons. This is especially evident when source of *general* sophistication, level of education, is made to stand for social class. Even if one does not have high education, membership in the Friends and Supporters of Psychotherapy is equivalent to a college degree in the understanding of mental disorders! In just as striking a fashion, membership in the Friends eliminates another "natural" cultural difference —that between men and women. In our culture, men are "permitted" to have some problems such as sexual problems, and women are granted the right to other problems such as interpersonal problems. But among members of the Friends women are brought up to the "natural" level of men, and men to the level of women. Membership in the Friends and Supporters of Psychotherapy is therefore a kind of "pre-therapy" which makes people ready for psychoanalytic treatment, for it makes them think about those emotional matters which are central to psychoanalytic treatment.

NOTES

1. See Daniel R. Miller and Guy E. Swanson, *Inner Conflict and Defense* (New York: Holt, 1960), Chapter 8, for a somewhat different definition. See also Otto Fenichel, *The Psychoanalytic Theory of Neurosis* (New York: Norton, 1945), p. 20, and Chapters 8 and 9.
2. See *Webster's New International Dictionary, Second Edition.*
3. The data from our study have been analyzed by Susan E. Flusser, and reported

in her unpublished Columbia University Master's Essay, *The Not So Secret Consultation: The Role of Reading Mental Health Literature in the Decision to Seek Psychotherapy*, 1966.

4. The wording of the questionnaire is given, but the face-to-face interview was substantially the same.

,5. National U.S. samples: "Do you happen to be reading a book at the present time?"—17 per cent (Lester Asheim, "A Survey of Recent Research," in Conference on the Undergraduate and Lifetime Reading Interest, *Reading for Life*, [Ann Arbor: The University of Michigan Press, 1959]). "Have you read a book in the past year?"—60 per cent (NORC Adult Education Study, 1962). New York City, asked the same question, gives a similar percentage, 56 per cent (Elinson, Padilla, and Perkins, *The Public Image of Mental Health Services in New York City*, op. cit., Table 46). When it comes to mental health, 30 per cent of a national sample claimed to have "ever" read in connection with their problems (NORC Survey #272). When asked about *books* read in the last year, 13 per cent of the New York sample said they read books about "psychology, psychiatry, or psychoanalysis" (*ibid.*).

6. For a review, see B. Dohrenwend and D. Crandell, "Some Relations Among Psychiatric Symptoms, Organic Illness and Social Class," *American Journal of Psychiatry*, 123 (1967), 1527-1537.

7. Charles Kadushin, "Social Class and the Experience of Ill Health," *Sociological Inquiry*, 24 (1964), 67-80.

8. E. A. Suchman, *Sociocultural Variation in Illness and Medical Care*, New York City Department of Health, 1963, processed. Thomas S. Langner and Stanley T. Michael, *Life Stress and Mental Health* (New York: The Free Press, 1963), pp. 213, 216, 272.

9. P. S. Lawrence, "Chronic Illness and Socio-Economic Status," in E. G. Jaco (ed.), *Patients, Physicians and Illness* (Glencoe: The Free Press, 1958).

10. Kadushin, *op. cit.*, 76-77. Also, Langner and Michael, *op. cit.* Langner does *not* interpret his data as we do, however. He prefers to believe that lower-class persons really are sicker, but that the data "artifactitiously" make their reports of objective conditions similar to that of middle-class persons. Our reading of the literature on social class biases in reporting of conditions in household surveys leads us to believe that such studies are *not* biased in the direction of underreporting by lower-class persons. See Kadushin, *op. cit.*, pp. 77-78.

11. Ursula Dibble, *Social Factors in Attitudes Towards Health and the Medical Profession*, unpublished Columbia University Master's Essay, 1965.

12. Langner and Michael, *op. cit.*, p. 407, show a higher percentage of lower-class respondents as having psychosomatic symptoms. See also B. Dohrenwend, "Social Status and Psychological Disorder," *American Sociological Review*, 31 (1966), 14-34.

13. Education makes for a 15-percentage-point difference in both retention and generation of physical symptoms.

14. The decision as to which problem was now most bothersome to the applicant was made by simply asking him, "What seem to be the main things about your problem that are bothering you now? Please list them in order of their importance to you." Thus, the *applicant's* point of view is reflected in these tables, not ours.

The ratio used here is similar to the use of effectiveness indexes in communications research. For an explanation of the logic of this procedure, see Paul F. Lazarsfeld, "The Statistical Analysis of Reasons as a Research Operation," *Sociometry*, 5 (1942), 29-47.

15. Gurin, *et al.*, *Americans View Their Mental Health*, Tables 4.12-4.20, pp. 107-111. This is my conclusion, not theirs. They do not accept their clear-cut finding of no difference between men and women in their involvement in marriage, and they tend to emphasize very small and inconsistent differences between men and women in various marital-adjustment indicators. Since our data also show

little difference between men and women in marital-adjustment problems, I am more willing to believe that there really are few or no differences.

16. Gurin, *et al.*, *op. cit.*, *Tabular Supplement*, Table B-34.
17. *Ibid.*, Table B-6.
18. *Ibid.*, p. 116.
19. Kinsey, *et al.*, *Sexual Behavior in the Human Female* (Philadelphia: Saunders, 1953), p. 685.
20. Kinsey and his associates carefully distinguish between sex as an emotional problem and sex as a biological problem. In their *Sexual Behavior in the Human Male* (Philadelphia: Saunders, 1953), they state that only the latter is the "proper" object of scientific work (pp. 57-58). On the other hand, in the second volume on women, some attitudinal data are presented which deal with matters in which widespread anxiety is noted (*Human Female*, p. 65). Only a small proportion of homosexual men or women regret their activities or otherwise find them problematic (*Human Female*, p. 477). More than two-thirds of women over twenty said they were not "worried" about masturbation (*Human Female*, p. 190). Even more said they did not regret premarital coitus (*Human Female*, p. 345). According to these reports, sexual behavior does not necessarily lead to anxiety about sex. Beyond the data just mentioned and a table which shows sources of influence which helped women to "accept" masturbation (*Human Female*, p. 190), Kinsey gives no clue as to which group in the population is more bothered or upset by sexual problems, nor does he indicate whether any of them ever sought help for sexual problems. No studies of mental health in American nonclinical populations have inquired into sexual problems despite their importance to psychoanalytic theory.
21. Bieber, *et al.*, *Homosexuality*, Table II-4, p. 29.
22. Gurin, *et al.*, *op. cit.*, Tabular Supplement, Tables A.1, 2, 3, 4.
23. *Ibid.*, Tables B.22, 23.
24. Data not presented.
25. Gurin, *et al.*, *op. cit.*, Table 6.10, p. 163; Table 6.13, p. 167.
26. Langner and Michael, *op. cit*, Table 12-1, p. 544; Table 12-4, p. 309. The men in the national sample who have better jobs or more education are also more likely to say that they feel adequate to their jobs. The better educated and those with higher prestige jobs who apply for psychotherapy, on the other hand, are more likely than other applicants to feel that they have trouble in performing their jobs adequately. As phrased in the national sample, the question about job adequacy reads, "How good would you say you are at this kind of work—would you say you were very good, a little better than average, just average, or not very good?" (p. 418, question 65b). Answers to this question are not related to the experience of a work problem, whereas feelings of inadequacy in the parental or marriage role were related to the experience of problems. The authors of the national study feel that the job question may not tap a psychological dimension as much as the equivalent question in other areas of social relationship. See pp. 144-148.
27. Some of the most impressive findings in social psychiatry have been the association between degree of mental disorder and social class. The lower classes have been uniformly shown, in all studies, to have a greater likelihood of being mentally disturbed. Many of the symptoms of this disorder are cathectic symptoms. Yet a close examination of these symptoms shows considerable variation in their relationship to class. Many concern physical symptoms (see B. S. Dohrenwend and B. P. Dohrenwend, "The Problem of Validity in Field Studies," *Journal of Abnormal Psychology*, 70 [1965], 52-69, for a critical review of these studies). Of the nonphysical symptoms or syndromes, depression is negatively related to class in Hollingshead and Redlich, *Social Class and Mental Illness* (New York: Wiley, 1958), and in Thomas S. Langner and Stanley T. Michael, *Life Stress and Mental Health*, Table 16-3. On the other hand, earlier studies of the prevalence of manic-depressive psychoses found them more often in higher

classes (C. Tietze, P. Lemkau, and M. Cooper, "Schizophrenic, Manic-Depressive Psychosis, and Social-Economic Status," *American Journal of Sociology*, 47 [1941], 167-175), and "immobilization" symptoms apparently related to depression, are also now found more frequently nationally among higher-class persons (Gurin, *et al.*, *op. cit.*, p. 201). But general unhappiness seems more prevalent in the lower class (*ibid.*, *Tabular Section B*; and Norman M. Bradburn and David Caplovitz, *Reports on Happiness* [Chicago: Aldine, 1965], pp. 20-24). Worries, however, seem not as related to class as happiness (Gurin, *et al.*, *op cit.*); and the general level of emotional feeling in the lower class is low (Bradburn and Caplovitz, *op. cit.*). Nor are self-reports of an "impending nervous breakdown" related to class (Gurin, *et al.*, p. 47). On the other hand, self-reports of "nervousness, feeling fidgety and tense" and "trouble getting to sleep or staying asleep" are strongly associated with lower-class membership (*ibid.*, p. 193). Yet in New York City, evaluations by psychiatrists of survey protocols showed that anxiety, phobias, and compulsions were essentially unrelated to social class (Langner and Michael, *op. cit.*). In short, the evidence in cathectic problems is contradictory, and although psychiatrists may in general find lower-class persons more emotionally disturbed, the subjects themselves do not necessarily concur.

28. Srole, *et al.*, *op. cit.*, pp. 240-246; Gurin, *et al.*, *op. cit.*, chapters 9, 12.
29. For a similar point of view, though conceptualized in quite a different way, see Thomas J. Scheff, *Being Mentally Ill: A Sociological Theory* (Chicago: Aldine, 1966), Parts I and II. Scheff calls the phenomenon we call "training" "labeling" and thinks it is a "bad" thing. But he confines his discussion to "psychiatric" problems, an area where we have found only limited "training."

INTERMEDIATE STEPS
IN THE DECISION
TO SEEK THERAPY
III

Free Advice

8

Personal problems are not the only things that send people to psychiatrists. The influence of other persons is also important, and it can be offered at many stages in the decision to seek therapy. A person with an emotional problem can be told that he has a problem, that he ought to do something about it, to see a professional, or to see a particular professional. The advice may be asked for or it may be unsolicited. This chapter deals with comments, solicited and unsolicited, made by laymen to applicants for psychotherapy. The unsolicited comments of professionals whose advice was sought for other matters are also analyzed. Only comments made in connection with an applicant's *problems* are considered. Chapter 13 deals with advice given in the process of deciding upon a clinic. There, we shall show that the people who give advice about problems are generally *not* the same ones who make referrals to clinics. That comes *later* in the process of seeking help.

❖ *The Data*

Among the data that were gathered in 1959-60, the following questions were asked of all respondents:

> Did anyone ever notice your problem or mention it to you *without* your ever mentioning it to them?
> What did he (she) say?
> Was this helpful?
> Have you ever brought your problem *yourself* to a friend or relative and discussed it with him (her)?
> What did he (she) say?
> Was this helpful?

An additional attempt was made in interviews to ascertain whether or not the applicant would have recognized his problems without intervention. Here are some examples of what applicants said in response:

> A woman born in 1920 in Hungary, married but with no children, has had two years of evening college. She is not a member of the Friends. She works as a legal typist, but wishes to be a free-lance photographer. Her husband is a clerk in the accounting department of an oil company. She is Catholic.
> Her problems: "I have lost all faith in myself and mankind. I feel I am an 'odd-ball' and am completely out of step with the world. I have no goal or purpose in life; I feel lost, unloved and extremely lonely. . . . Uncontrollable sobbing fits that strike without warning when I am alone or with people."
> She noticed her problems "when I found myself crying on my jobs, while I worked. Bursting into tears in the face of a friend, while talking. And finally sobbing so continuously I could not leave the house without sobbing into the face of the first person I'd meet who greeted me with the words, 'Hello, how are you?' After several months of this a neighbor, who was a school teacher, told me to go to a mental hygiene clinic for aid." This advice was judged helpful. Other unsolicited advice came from two physicians, one of whom "told me I had no heart trouble but mental aggravation that caused me pains in (my) chest," and another who "told me I had a deep-rooted problem on my mind that caused vascular spasms." Both of these were judged to be helpful. A close friend "told me to get rid of my husband because he was no good," and this was not helpful.
> She solicited advice from several friends and from her husband. "Friends all advised me to leave my husband. My husband will never listen to me when I talk without ridiculing me."

An applicant to the Religion and Psychiatry Institute, a woman born in 1931, who is a decorator and college educated, as well as a member of the Friends, says she "is shaky and nervous, everyone I work with is a nervous perfectionist." Her boyfriend "isn't the right one."

A close friend mentioned her problem to her about a year ago. "We're very close." He's in Schenectady. "He called attention to the problem especially in a letter he sent me recently. . . . He has the same kind of problem. He feels we shouldn't get too close because we're both shy. He really talked about his own problem."

A lower-class cafeteria worker, whose common-law husband is a janitor, applied to a hospital clinic complaining of "headaches, fullness of the head, back of my neck snapping, boils, lonesome and worrying."

"A couple of months ago" some acquaintances called attention to her problems. "Sometimes if I go out and have a drink they say have a drink and snap out of it; it helps."

She has not herself brought her problem to others, however. "It's a problem that I have and I've kept all for myself." In response to a probe asking whether she talked with her husband about it she said, "No, he knows that I get upset. He's not a citizen and once in a while I get upset I tell him. 'Get back on the boat and go back where you came from.'"

All these applicants had their problems pointed out to them, but they might have recognized them on their own. Some applicants, like the young man in the following case, probably would not have noticed their problems unless others had called attention to them:

A male college student born in 1941 who was applying to Interpersonal Psychiatry, but is not a member of the Friends, comes from a middle-class Jewish family. His presenting problems included: "Have trouble speaking before groups."

"I first noticed the problem while I was in public school. I'm not sure of the exact grade—probably 4th or 5th. One of my teachers kept on harping on the fact that I was nervous when I went up in front of the room to show her my notebook."

Most comments made by influencers were of much more recent origin as in the following case, also of a person who might not otherwise have done much about her problems:

A young woman, born in 1942, applied to Advanced Psychotherapy. A high-school graduate, she would like to become a textile designer. She is a peripheral member of the Friends. Now she lives at home with her parents. Her father is a trucker.

"My problem concerns trying to conform to the usual customs and habits of society. I tried to leave the society and therefore came in contact with the wrong type of people. Generally, some of the individuals were dope addicts."

She first noticed her problem in the following way: "I was somewhat aware of the problem from the start, however, it did not concern me. A while after, my parents became aware of my condition [drug addiction] and immediately confronted me. I started going to a psychiatrist . . ."

A good number of applicants did not report that their problems were noticed by others. Rather, they themselves brought their problems to others for advice.

A Jewish man applying to Interpersonal Psychiatry Institute is a shoe salesman, was born in 1922, and has had three years of high school. He is not a member of the Friends.

His problems include "Intense anxiety—feelings of worthlessness, failure, inadequacy, hopelessness—physically manifested by sleeplessness, indigestion, dizziness, shortness of breath, chest pains, obsessive thoughts."

He spoke to his wife and sister just a month before his application. "Both recommended professional guidance."

❈ Conversations about Problems: Applicants and Nonapplicants

Such examples of conversations are almost universal among applicants. Between 80 and 90 per cent of applicants for psychotherapy reported having previously had conversations about their problems with laymen, initiated either by themselves, by others, or both.[1] Of those who did talk with others, a bit less than 20 per cent received only unsolicited comments, about 40 per cent received only comments they themselves solicited, while a bit over 40 per cent engaged in both kinds of contact. When it comes actually to being given a referral to a clinic (a matter we shall take up in Chapter 13), a considerably smaller proportion of interpersonal contacts was unsolicited. Just talking about problems and actually being told to go to a clinic are quite different sorts of interactions and must be analyzed in different ways.

Giving and asking for advice is universal among other nonapplicants as well. A New York City sample was asked for their experiences: "People sometimes ask others for advice or an opinion about something that matters to them. It may be a serious thing, or just about what to wear."[2] In reply, only 7 per cent said no one had asked them, and only 14 per cent said that they themselves had not asked for advice. About more serious matters, the same sample was asked: "Have you ever been asked by other persons for advice about their own or another's personal problems of mental illness or emotional troubles?" Many fewer, 53 per cent, said they had been consulted on these serious matters. Applicants for psychotherapy, then, are no more likely than other people to discuss general problems, but probably much more likely to talk about serious ones.

Prior consultation with amateurs seems to be almost a prerequisite for entrance into professional therapy. In fact, consultation with laymen goes on even after an applicant enters therapy, for there is no difference between those with no therapy, those with some, and those with twenty-one or more sessions in the proportion who consult with others about their problems. Lay consultation may therefore be an important adjunct to professional psychotherapy.

⚙ *The Functions of Conversation*

Since the conversations are so universal, they must fulfill several different functions for the participants. The examples of conversations given above indicate that they apparently have two basic functions—social support and social control. Each of these in turn has several aspects.

Self-recognition of problems is difficult, and deciding to go to a professional therapist is even more difficult. Social support helps to make these steps easier in two ways. First, some conversations help to confirm the applicant in his assessment of his problem, and to make the problem seem a legitimate one. The young decorator who received a letter from her friend was confirmed in her feeling that she is shy and has trouble getting along with people. Other conversations serve as "warm-ups" for professional psychotherapy. An instance of this is reflected in the report of the shy young mathematician, a member of the Friends, who complains of "fear of girls and fear of social situations." He has brought his difficulties to his friends. "My friends were full of advice. I mostly talked about girls."

Social control of the applicant by others is an extremely important factor in bringing some persons to psychotherapy. After all, the persons in our sample are deviants, and as such are quite likely to provoke the reactions of others. Some social control is merely of the "stop it!" kind, such as that given by the cafeteria worker's drinking friends who said, "Have a drink and snap out of it." Other social controlling conversations provide an applicant with entirely new information about his problems, showing him that they are psychiatric or emotional rather than something else. When physicians told the woman who sobbed "continuously" that she did not have "heart trouble but mental aggravation" they were fulfilling this function. Finally, some social control leads directly to the recommendation to see a psychotherapist or some other professional, as in several of the cases we quoted, although this is by no means the chief consequence of these conversations.

Conversations have functions which help to determine whether they will take place at all and with whom. This reasoning does seem backward, for a conversation obviously can have consequences only after it has taken place. Nevertheless, it is clear from the examples we have given that applicants manage to place themselves in a position to receive certain forms of advice. For example, it is possible that the girl who rebelled against her parents and associated with drug addicts was really hoping that her parents would "become aware of my condition." Of course, only persons who have applied for psychotherapy are present in this sample. Hence our observation point is biased and is affected by the consequences of the various acts that lead up to an application for psychotherapy. For example, without the proddings of neighbors and physicians, the woman suffering from sobbing might not have applied to a psychoanalytic clinic.

Although it is generally possible to ascertain the functions of each conversation from the reports of our respondent, this is difficult to do. We shall, at present, assume that the one who initiates the conversation determines its functions. Later we shall be in a position to support this assumption with data. Completely unsolicited advice is obviously less confirming and also tends to be less supportive than solicited advice. Of course, some unsolicited advice is in effect asked for. Let us, for the moment, assume that persons who asked others for advice and who also received unsolicited advice were in both cases really asking for whatever advice they received, whether they nominally initiated the conversation or not.

☼ Propositions about Conversation

Given these functions of conversations with laymen, we can now try to account for why most persons talked with laymen, whom they talked with, and also why a small minority did not report these conversations. Discussions with others seem to stem from a series of contradictory forces, for the very things that are likely to produce interaction with others are also likely to lead to considerable reluctance to interact, as reflection upon the examples given above should indicate.

A potential applicant for psychotherapy has a certain predisposition to recognize that he has problems. Never mind, for the moment, what produces this predisposition. Now the greater the predisposition to recognize problems, the more likely a person is to recognize them by himself without the interference of others. This, of course, is what is meant by predisposition. But *all* the persons in our sample have applied for psychotherapy, and it follows, then, that almost all of them *have* recognized that they have problems. Therefore, the *smaller* the predisposition to recognize problems, the more likely it is that others have had to intervene to induce potential applicants to realize that they do have problems. Without this intervention they might not have been applicants at all.

At the same time, *whatever* makes one predisposed to recognize a problem also makes a person predisposed to talk about his problems with others. Let us see why this is so.

We have said (Chapter 7) that the more specific and the more socially anchored a problem is, the more *visible* it is to the person suffering from it. Also, the more well defined a problem in psychoanalytic theory is, the easier it is for members of the Friends and Supporters of Psychotherapy to recognize it. For psychoanalytic theory organizes diffuse feelings into a set of "symptoms" and thence to a definable "problem"; it also serves to remove the social stigma from some specific problems which if visible are likely to be swept under the rug. Stigma, visibility, and the degree to which diffuse feelings are organized also affect the likelihood of talking with other people about one's own problems. The less stigma one feels, the more likely one is to talk about problems with others. Similarly, the greater the visibility of a problem, the more likely one is to talk with others about it since they may be already aware of it. And the better organized the feelings, the easier they are to express. Hence, in general, the greater the predisposition to recognize problems on one's own, the greater the predisposition to talk with others about them.

These predispositions are situational, that is, they are related to the occurrence and development of personal problems. What of general psychological predispositions such as those pertaining to trust in other persons? Presumably, those who are more likely to trust others are more likely to have conversed with them. Careful analysis of our data shows, however, that situational factors override any underlying psychological orientations. Applicants were asked to complete sentences beginning with "Most friends," "Most people I know," and "Keeping trouble to yourself." Answers were coded in terms of positiveness or negativeness. We find that there is no difference between the positives and negatives on any of these items, or any combination of these items, in their likelihood of having engaged in conversation with others about their problems. Similarly, reports of conversations considered from only one point of view, that of the applicant, might show a considerable defensiveness. Presumably, no one really likes to be told he has emotional problems. Yet careful analysis shows that reluctance to report conversations with others is almost totally lacking, or at least not systematically present in our data.

At this point we must conclude that theory directs us to two opposing hypotheses: either a high or a low predisposition to recognize problems leads to conversations with laymen about one's problems. The solution, for the moment, seems indeterminate, though we have implicitly accounted for the very high rates of conversations with others, since opposite factors both lead to conversation.

What of the actions of others, the social controllers? Since it takes at least two persons to hold a conversation, we must ask what prompts others to talk with our applicants. Once more, the very things that lead others to intervene and point out an applicant's problems to him are also likely to inhibit such interaction.

Four factors are involved: social distance, interest, nuisance making, and visibility. The first, social distance of others from the applicant, provides the link between the applicant and other persons. The greater the distance, the easier it is for one to tell another that the latter has problems, for the adviser is not intimately involved and has greater objectivity. At the same time, intimacy also produces interaction, if only for the reason that another person is available.[3] The degree of interest another has in either the applicant or in emotional problems in general is the second factor prompting him to initiate conversation. Third, the degree to which the applicant makes a nuisance of himself or otherwise interferes with the activities of other persons is important. Finally, the sheer visibility of an applicant's problems to others is a major factor.

All these related factors produce ambivalence. Others are hesitant to tell a person with emotional problems about them for fear of a negative response from the applicant. The more nuisance a person is, the more obvious his problems; and the more sensitive the observer, the more hesitancy in "telling off" the applicant. Yet for one to wish to interfere in other people's affairs, one has to be sensitive and interested, the problems must be visible and must be a nuisance. Again, the forces at work seem contradictory and the solution indeterminate.

By now it is obvious that the functions of conversations determine which of the several possible outcomes we can expect. In general, a low predisposition to conversation probably reduces the proportion who have talked with others; but a major proportion of those who *have* talked with others, and who nevertheless have a low predisposition to do so, are those for whom conversation resulted in social control rather than social support. Without the controlling actions of others, these less disposed persons might never have become applicants.

These assumptions can be tested, although not directly. Three sets of variables have been introduced: an applicant's predispositions to recognize his problem and to engage in conversation with others about it; the likelihood that others will speak to him; and the functions or consequences which the conversations have. Four sets of other variables which we can measure more directly control the first three and serve as indicators for them. The first indicator is the familiar one of social circles; the second is whom an applicant lives with; the third is the visibility or stigma of problems; and last is who initiated the interactions.

Membership in a circle such as the Friends and Supporters of Psychotherapy is associated with an individual's predisposition to recognize his problems, for a person's norms and general knowledge about psychotherapy are affected, and these in turn affect his sense of stigma and the visibility of his problems to himself. Membership in the Friends also creates a social environment in which sensitivity to emotional problems as well as an interest in them is more prevalent. It thus affects the likelihood that others will speak to the applicant. The person or persons with whom one lives obviously affects the social distance of an applicant from others, as does membership in the Friends. We have already shown that particular presenting problems have various attributes that make for greater visibility to the self and visibility to others.

✿ Social Circles, Predispositions, and Conversation

We may now introduce some propositions about the conditions under which conversations with others take place. Members of the Friends have a greater predisposition to engage in conversations about their own problems; so do the other members in their environment. Members are more likely to engage in conversations which have the consequence of both support and confirmation. That is, as Chart XIV shows, the combination of having received both solicited *and* unsolicited advice is most frequent in all but the Religion and Psychiatry Institute where, as we have previously pointed out, membership in the Friends has a different meaning from what it has in the other clinics. Nonmembers of the Friends are less likely to engage in conversation about problems. If they do talk with others, they are more likely to have received purely unsolicited advice—which serves a more controlling function. Thus, conversation serves different functions for those disposed to psychotherapy than it does for those not so disposed.

When ethnic groups are ranked in terms of favorability to psychotherapy, the same results ensue (Chart XV). Catholics, Puerto Ricans, and nonwhites who apply to analytic clinics ordinarily live in a social milieu in which conversations with others about personal problems are not as free as among Jews and Protestants. Thus, membership in the Friends makes a greater difference for the former than for Jews and Protestants. There is evidence from our data that being tight-mouthed about one's problems is characteristic only of upwardly mobile Catholics, Puerto Ricans and Negroes, for members of these ethnic groups who apply to hospital clinics do not show the same reluctance to converse with laymen about their problems.

CHART XIV *Contacts with Laymen about Problems*

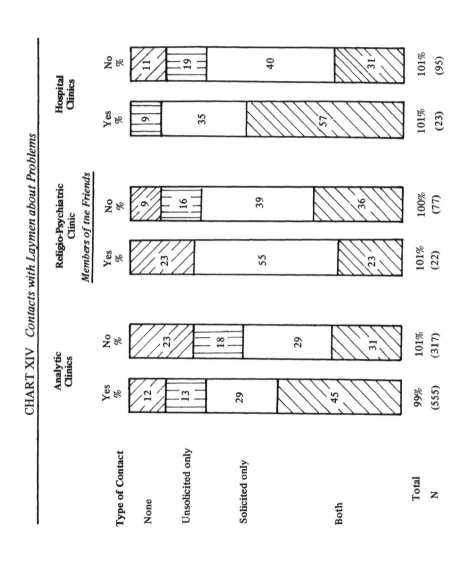

Type of Contact	Analytic Clinics		Religio-Psychiatric Clinic		Hospital Clinics	
			Members of the Friends			
	Yes %	No %	Yes %	No %	Yes %	No %
None	12	23	23	9	9	11
Unsolicited only	13	18		16		19
Solicited only	29	29	55	39	35	40
Both	45	31	23	36	57	31
Total	99%	101%	101%	100%	101%	101%
N	(555)	(317)	(22)	(77)	(23)	(95)

CHART XV *Contacts by Members of Different Ethnic Groups with Laymen about Problems (Analytic-Clinic Applicants Only)*

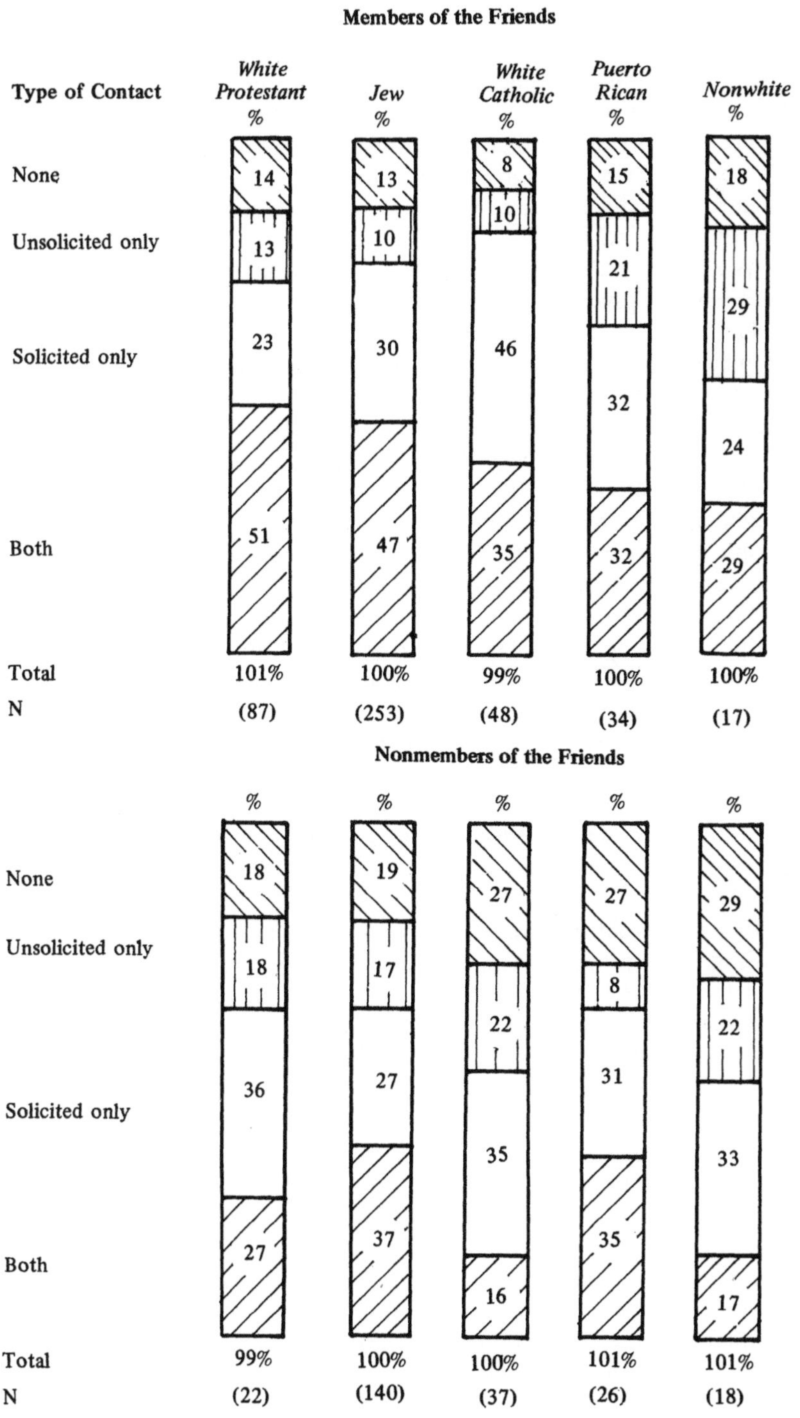

Members of the Friends

Type of Contact	White Protestant %	Jew %	White Catholic %	Puerto Rican %	Nonwhite %
None	14	13	8	15	18
Unsolicited only	13	10	10	21	29
Solicited only	23	30	46	32	24
Both	51	47	35	32	29
Total	101%	100%	99%	100%	100%
N	(87)	(253)	(48)	(34)	(17)

Nonmembers of the Friends

Type of Contact	%	%	%	%	%
None	18	19	27	27	29
Unsolicited only	18	17	22	8	22
Solicited only	36	27	35	31	33
Both	27	37	16	35	17
Total	99%	100%	100%	101%	101%
N	(22)	(140)	(37)	(26)	(18)

Social class is not systematically related to conversation about problems, since among applicants for psychotherapy social class is not as related to the social environment's favorability to emotional problems as are ethnicity or membership in the Friends. In fact, some lower-class groups love to talk about personal problems, as the "True Confession" literature might indicate, whereas some upper-class groups tend to tightly buttoned lips.

We have seen that women in the United States are generally more interested in psychological issues and are the more "sensitive" sex. The data support this appraisal, for the group with a greater predisposition to matters psychological is shown to be the one which talks more about personal problems, as anyone who has spent time with "the girls" knows. Data not shown here also indicate that women are more frequent advice *givers*, as well. Both men and women consult their mothers far more often than their fathers. Moreover, as psychoanalytic theory might indicate, men are more likely than women to consult both their spouse and their mother. Therefore, in addition to membership in the Friends, residence pattern must be considered.

The data generally bear out our hypotheses. Indeed, except among hospital-clinic applicants, unmarried women nonmembers of the Friends are more likely (by 15 percentage points) than their male counterparts to converse with others about their problems. Marriage, on the other hand, is a "feminizing" experience at least in making men sensitive to and interested in discussing personal problems, for there are no real differences between married men and women in these respects. Among the unmarried, membership in the Friends serves to make men and women more nearly alike in their likelihood of talking about personal problems.

In analytic clinics where there are enough cases to demonstrate the finding, it is again apparent that having received both solicited and unsolicited advice is associated with the group which is more predisposed —women; purely unsolicited advice is associated with men—the ones less disposed to discuss problems on their own.

Residence—that is, whom one lives with—determines not only the sex of the person one talks with but also how much control one has over the social circle membership of those in the immediate environment. Obviously, children have little control over the sort of social circle to which their parents belong. Spouses have more control over the affiliations of their partners. Roommates or friends are also likely to have common group affiliations. Thus the immediate social environment of married persons or others not living with their parents more nearly resembles their own social milieu than does that of persons living at home with parents. An environment which concurs with the prejudices of an applicant in respect to conversation about emotional problems merely intensifies his initial proclivities. Thus, members of the Friends living in an environment consisting almost totally of members of the Friends are more likely by an average of 17 percentage points to converse about problems than are nonmembers. But members of the Friends who live at home with their parents are only 4 percentage points more likely than nonmembers to have talked with laymen about their problems. Hence social circle affiliation is more significant for those who live with a spouse or away from their parents than for those who live at home with their parents.

In sum, predisposition leads to conversation about problems, but lack of a predisposition, while generally reducing the frequency of such conversations, also leads to an increase in purely *unsolicited* conversation. Yet an applicant who did not encourage conversation about his problems is like one who was not approached at all. The actions of others, then, serve to explain how many otherwise unpredisposed persons come to be candidates for psychotherapy.

These findings are generally the opposite of those we will report about the decision to go to a clinic (in Chapter 13). Those who are *less* predisposed to psychiatry and psychology tend to go to clinics *only* because of personal influence. Here we have found that conversation (of all sorts) tends to take place with those *more* favorable to psychiatry. But those who, at this stage, are given either no advice or only unsolicited advice about their problems are the ones who eventually are likely to go to a clinic only because someone told them to go. So confirmatory discussion about problems early in the decision to seek help means that the eventual act will appear to be more autonomous.

Whom one talks with is also indicative of the nature of one's circle and is related to the dual functions of control and support. In general, applicants converse with those who are available: with parents if they live at home, with their spouse if they are married, or with friends if they live alone or with roommates. These persons not only are available, but they are the ones most affected by the peculiarities of potential applicants for psychotherapy. Those who live in an environment favorable to psychotherapy do not rely on these "natural" influences. Members of the Friends and Supporters of Psychotherapy, as shown in Table 15 are—not surprisingly—more likely to consult with their friends than with their available relatives. Again, following the principle that free choice accentuates the effect of social circles, the more voluntary the contact, as indicated by solicited as compared to unsolicited advice, the wider the circle of influencers sought out by members of the Friends. Averaging all the differences in Table 15 between members of the Friends and nonmembers, for each of three modes of residence and for each of the key lay contacts, we find that membership in the Friends makes for an average difference of 9 percentage

TABLE 15 *Relationship of Key Contacts to Analytic-Clinic Applicants by Mode of Residence and Membership in the Friends*

	Unsolicited Contact		Solicited Contact	
Relationship	Member of Friends %	Nonmember Friends %	Member of Friends %	Nonmember Friends %
	Living with Parents			
Spouse	—	—	—	—
Parent	27	30	28	60
Close Friend	56	31	82	40
N*	(99)	(74)	(112)	(74)
	Living with Spouse			
Spouse	50	56	55	71
Parent	10	14	16	29
Close Friends	39	15	64	27
N*	(92)	(71)	(113)	(74)
	Living Alone, with Friends			
Spouse	—	—	—	—
Parent	17	9	21	29
Close Friend	57	33	83	42
N*	(170)	(43)	(189)	(38)

*More than one type of contact possible.

points for unsolicited comments but 25 percentage points for solicited comments.

The different functions of solicited and unsolicited advice are apparent. Solicited comments come from persons likely to be congenial to the person asking for advice. Unsolicited comments are made when the respondent has annoyed or otherwise interfered with others. Their reaction is not under his control, and if he is behaving in certain socially disapproved ways, he is likely to hear unsolicited comment from the rather wide variety of persons with whom the average metropolitan dweller comes in contact.

Differences between solicited and unsolicited advice, as shown in our data, suggest that although the data come from the biased source of those who have been influenced (i.e., applicants for psychotherapy), social reality is nonetheless reflected. If our data were merely the projections of our respondents, then the observed differences between solicited and unsolicited advice would not be found.

The scope of one's contacts, that is, the willingness to confer outside the family circle, was shown to be related both to the nature of one's social circle and to the degree to which the advice was solicited. But that general scope referred to all contacts. Whom one chooses as *sole* contact, one's confidant, is equally revealing. Again, if they spoke to only one type of influencer, members of the Friends were much more likely to speak with a person *outside* of their immediate family. The greater scope of even the confidants of members of the Friends does not apply to consultation with a professional. Members of the Friends are only half as likely as nonmembers to have had their problems noticed only by a professional. Their lay social circles are so much more alert to these problems that professionals are less needed.* The confidant relationship is of course one in which the applicant has opened himself to receiving advice. As a more or less voluntary contact it is especially sensitive to structured social circumstances rather than to accidental contacts. It matters little, therefore, who actually initiated the conversation.

❖ *Social Circles and High Pressure*

We have seen how unsolicited advice usually comes from those whom an applicant has annoyed. Such contacts are likely to be controlling rather than supportive. Those who give unsolicited advice are more likely to be responding to their own needs than to those of the applicant. This is especially obvious in the case of unsolicited advice offered by spouses of applicants. One-third of all the unsolicited comments received by married nonmembers of the Friends was given to those whose main presenting problem was a primary-group one—marital problems for the most part. The aggrieved spouse responded by giving free and unwanted advice!

The pressure which unsolicited advice brings to bear on a person will clearly vary in degree or amount. Here we focus on the circumstances that caused an applicant to feel that he had been subjected to high pressures. High pressure is defined as unsolicited comments received under two of the following three conditions: the problem was noticed by others either before or simultaneous with the applicant's realization that he had that problem; another person further specified the nature of the problem; or, in our judgment, the applicant might not otherwise have recognized a problem's existence (see Chart XVI). Pressure to recognize a problem is of course different from pressure to go to a therapist, an influence that generally comes much later in the decision process. By the time a person is told to go to a clinic, he is much more in tune with the idea that he has problems and needs help.

---

* They are also less likely to rely on professionals to give them information about clinics (see Table 29).

CHART XVI *Lay Influence on Problems*

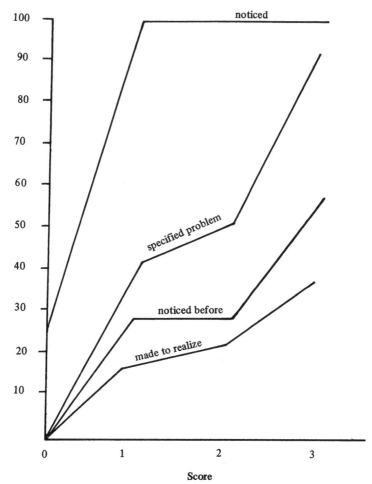

	Problem Noticed by Others	Noticed Before or Simultaneously to Self	Made Respondent Realize Problem	Specified Problem
Score 0	25	0	0	0
1	100	27	15	42
2	100	27	19	50
3	100	54	32	88

Many fewer were subjected to heavy pressure to go to a clinic than were subjected to heavy pressure about their problems.

First, let us see who among the recipients of unsolicited advice is subjected to high pressure of any sort, then we shall examine who is the source of this high pressure. Following the principle that pressure has different functions depending upon whether it is being really called for or not, Chart XVII is separated into purely unsolicited high pressure, and high pressure given to those who also asked for it. Again, unless they really asked for it, members of the Friends, even if given purely unsolicited advice should be less likely to feel that they are being subjected to heavy pressure. In the first place, the kinds of people they know are less likely to be annoyed by their deviant behavior, and second, members of the Friends are less likely to need to have their problems forcefully pointed out to them in order to decide to go to a psychotherapist.

The data confirm our expectations. Nonmembers of the Friends who really did not ask to be pressured were in fact subjected to the most pressure; members of the Friends in similar circumstances were 13 percentage points less likely to be pressured. On the other hand, when

CHART XVII *Per Cent of Analytic-Clinic Applicants Receiving Unsolicited Advice Who Were Subjected to a High Degree of Lay Pressure* to Recognize Their Problems*

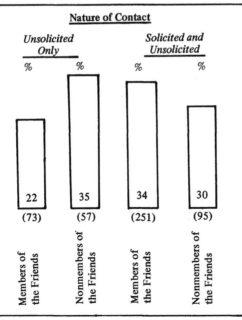

Nature of Contact

Unsolicited Only		*Solicited and Unsolicited*	
%	%	%	%
22	35	34	30
(73)	(57)	(251)	(95)
Members of the Friends	Nonmembers of the Friends	Members of the Friends	Nonmembers of the Friends

*Scores of 3 and 4.

they apparently asked for it, members of the Friends received slightly higher pressure than nonmembers.

In general, persons least disposed to recognize their own problems are more likely to be subjected to heavy pressure from those whom they are annoying or bothering. But *whom* they annoy depends on the sort of social circle with which they are affiliated, as Table 16 shows.

Among members of the Friends who live with their parents or with a spouse, relatively little pressure is exerted by their friends, but parents or spouse and professionals exert high pressure. The reverse is true of nonmembers of the Friends. On the other hand, among those who live alone or with roommates, there is little difference between members of the Friends and others, except for the influence of professionals, who again are likely to have applied heavy pressure to members of the Friends. Yet parents are much more likely than friends to have applied heavy pressure, and this is true of both sophisticates and nonsophisticates.

Those from whom the applicant does not expect to get advice, or those whom the applicant has especially annoyed are those who exert high pressure. Among members of the Friends, relatives are unlikely sources of criticism, and if they do comment, it is probably because they were thoroughly disturbed by the applicant. The reverse is true of nonmembers who live with their "square" relatives. These relatives are

TABLE 16 *Per Cent of Unsolicited Confidantes of Analytic-Clinic Applicants Who Exerted High Pressure (by Mode of Residence and Membership in Friends)*

Influencer	Living with Parents		Living with Spouse		Living Alone, with Friends	
	Member %	Nonmember %	Member %	Nonmember %	Member %	Nonmember %
Spouse	–	–	39	20	–	–
Parent	57	17	100	50	71	67
Friend	19	31	19	50	30	29
Professional	33	17	55	39	39	9
			Number of Cases*			
	–	–	18	25	–	–
	7	12	3	2	7	3
	26	16	16	2	53	7
	12	17	11	13	18	11

*These numbers refer to the base of the percentages in the table. Thus 39% of 18 persons who lived with their spouse, who are members of the Friends and were influenced by their spouse were subjected to high pressure.

expected sources of social control. Personal friends, on the other hand, in nonsophisticated surroundings, would hardly be likely to apply heavy pressure unless they were quite disturbed by the applicant. For those who do not live with relatives, however, friends and roommates are a legitimate source of control, even among nonsophisticates. And parents are equally illegitimate controllers, hence intervene only under special circumstances, and when they do, are perceived as exerting heavy pressure. Professionals are regular intimates neither of sophisticates nor of others, but members of the Friends are expected by professionals to "know better," and they in turn are unlikely to have required unsolicited comment by professionals. Hence, when professionals do apply pressure, it is felt as heavy pressure.

Analysis of who gives advice as well as how much pressure is applied thus confirms our theories advanced on the basis of the mere occurrence of conversation. The "accidents" induced by social structure are an extremely important influence in getting persons to realize their problems. Some pressures are, of course, present in the normal course of events and depend on what sorts of lives people lead. Members of the Friends lead different lives and get different pressures from nonmembers of the Friends. But what really brings matters home are the comments of those who "have no business" giving advice. These "unnatural" sources derive no reward from the conversation except that of curbing the deviance of the applicant. In this view of the process whereby others come to help applicants realize that they have problems, the applicant is seen as moving in a straight line until some unexpected force moves him out of his path and induces him to reconsider his life.

❂ Presenting Problems and Personal Influence

If others influence the applicant, they do so because the applicant himself presents a stimulus to them which induces them to bring the applicant into line. The nature of this stimulus is obviously related to the applicant's problems. Some problems create more disturbances in the environment and therefore are more visible to others. On the other hand, some problems are likely to be so invisible to the self, that only the intervention of others may force the applicant himself to take notice. And some problems, visible to others or not, seem especially shameful to both applicant and his social surroundings, while other problems, not especially shameful, are still best discussed with intimates. In short, the nature of an applicant's problems affects the likelihood that he will have discussed them with other persons.

The social circle to which an applicant belongs affects the response to the applicant's problems in two ways: what they manage to notice, and how they react to what they notice.

Table 17, showing the per cent who talked with laymen about their problem, is divided into the major types of presenting problems, as well as place of residence and membership in the Friends. The numbers upon which the percentages are based are small, but some trends may be seen.

When there is a very low likelihood of a problem being self-recognized, there is a very high probability that applicants had talked with others about the problem. For otherwise, these persons would not be applicants for psychotherapy. Cognitive problems thus override sophis-

TABLE 17 *Per Cent of Analytic-Clinic Applicants Who Talked with Laymen about Their Problems (by Mode of Residence and Membership in the Friends)*

Most Important Problem	Living with Parents		Living with Spouse		Living Alone, with Friends	
	Member %	Non-member %	Member %	Non-member %	Member %	Non-member %
Psychiatric						
Physical	94	58	82	71	67	71
Cognitive	100	100	100	75	85	86
Cathectic	67	93	97	83	87	64
Psychoanalytic						
Sexual	89	7i	92	40	79	50
Evaluative	92	77	77	82	95	71
Interpersonal	94	90	100	85	91	80
Performance	87	86	92	83	87	75
Projected						
Primary group	90	92	87	88	68	83
Situation, no problem	67	70	88	75	87	100
Number of Cases						
	16	12	11	14	12	7
	10	5	4	4	22	7
	15	15	30	29	46	11
	18	17	13	10	38	10
	38	13	13	11	40	14
	18	10	11	13	35	10
	23	22	13	12	31	4
	10	12	32	18	19	6
	3	10	17	16	15	3

tication and place of residence. Those who feel that their main problem is cognitive are extremely likely to have talked with others.

On the other hand, a milieu predisposed to recognize problems pays attention to certain characteristic ones, such as sexual and other psychoanalytic problems. Membership in the Friends both reduces the stigma of these problems and makes them more noticeable to oneself and to others. For example, unsophisticated husbands and wives are especially *un*likely to discuss sexual problems; only 40 per cent of such persons with sexual problems spoke to laymen. In contrast, 92 per cent of married members of the Friends who had sexual problems spoke with laymen.

Psychoanalytic acceptability of problems is not the only determinant of whether applicants have conversed with others, however. The extent to which the problems involve others is also of great importance. First, close social relationships together with a modicum of understanding allow problems loaded with feelings to be discussed with others. Talking about cathectic problems—those concerned with feelings—requires a considerable degree of intimacy. By and large, members of the Friends do feel comfortable in discussing these problems with laymen, provided these available laymen are either their spouse or their friend. For those with cathectic problems need emotional support from others. They get this support if their social circle is a sympathetic one. But our data show that members of the Friends who live with their parents feel alienated from them, while nonmembers do not. Hence members of the Friends who live at home cannot discuss their deep emotional problems with their parents and yet since they live at home they have not developed intimate ties with friends with whom they might be more comfortable. Only 67 per cent discussed problems with others. Nonmembers of the Friends who live at home are probably exceptionally attached to their parents and hence are exceptionally likely (93 per cent) to talk with their parents about cathectic problems.

Second, overidentification by others with the applicant can impede discussion, for the other becomes so involved with the problem that it reflects not only upon the applicant but upon himself as well. Thus, although evaluative problems are of the "psychoanalytic" variety, and more commonly lead to discussions with laymen among members of the Friends, this relationship does not hold true for married applicants. Feelings of lack of self-worth, the typical problem classed under the category of evaluative problems, does reflect on the capabilities of the marriage partner, and this is especially true among members of the Friends because of their greater investment in the marital relationship.

Third, the involvement of others with an applicant's problem affects his likelihood of talking with others when these others have something to gain from discussing the problem with him. Some problems such as interpersonal and marital problems so annoy others that they *must* stop the errant behavior of the applicant in order to maintain their peace of mind. Such problems are especially likely to lead to purely unsolicited comment, that is, the kind of comment usually reserved for those who would not otherwise realize that they had a psychiatric problem. Interpersonal problems generate a good deal of unsolicited advice despite the fact that they belong to the psychoanalytic syndrome, and hence are more prevalent among members of the Friends. Members are usually more likely than nonmembers to have themselves solicited contacts with others. Nevertheless, interpersonal difficulties force others to make controlling comments, of the unsolicited and unwelcome kind. Hence, although members of the Friends are more likely to discuss their interpersonal problems with others, nonmembers are also very likely under these circumstances to talk with others. That is why primary-group problems, not especially indicative of sophistication, show relatively high rates of discussion with others, but are not unusually popular among members of the Friends.

In sum, the attributes of problems affect the probability of conversation in the now familiar two-pronged fashion. Problems which are extremely obvious lead to comment, often unsolicited, which is not supportive or confirming but rather controlling. Problems invisible to the applicant also lead to comment by others. Problems which are in between in their degree of visibility lead to conversation if they interest the social environment yet at the same time are not overly involving or demanding of the would-be helper. The fact that two polar extremes in type of problem do lead to conversation once more demonstrates why so many of those now applying for therapy have talked over their problems with others.

❀ The Nature of Advice

When applicants talk with others about their problems there are consequences beyond mere recognition of problems. Many advisers also suggested things an applicant could do about his problems. These conversations throw further light on the functions of conversations about problems. But it must always be remembered that the advice was given *in the context of discussing a person's problems, not in the context of a person's actively seeking help for his problem.* Advisers tend themselves to be much more diffuse when a person is only beginning to ventilate his problems and more direct when he is looking for a professional source of help. The present analysis concerns this first ventilation. In Chapter 13, we will analyze the impact of other persons at the stage of decision-making when specific overt action—going to a clinic—

is under consideration rather than a general exploration of an emotional problem.

We have said that persons with a low predisposition to recognize their problems generally receive influence which points out new problems or legitimizes the problems an applicant may already have been aware of. Persons with a high predisposition to recognize problems received supporting or confirming comments. The data concerning suggestions on what to do about problems reinforces this interpretation.

Several sorts of things were told to potential applicants. Only 10 per cent were offered the advice to "do something about himself"—change his nature or self. Somewhat less than 10 per cent were advised to "get away from it all," or to take a vacation, or the like. The *least* frequent advice was to talk problems over with other laymen: apparently the lay consultants thought that if they could not help, neither could any other layman! Relatively infrequent among analytic-clinic applicants but given to between 20 and 30 per cent of applicants to other clinics was the advice to take some specific action—such as getting away from one's wife, changing one's job, or the like. But the most popular advice of all, and not surprising since we are dealing with applicants for psychotherapy, was the advice to consult some sort of professional.

Advice to seek professional aid moves the applicant from the stage of merely considering that he has a problem to the stage of considering whether to go to a professional. It is thus from our point of view the logical outcome of conversations about problems and the place where the functions of conversations are most revealed. Two sorts of advice to seek professionals were given. In one type of advice the applicant reported that he was told to see "a professional" of some sort—either unnamed or not a psychiatrist. Other applicants reported that they were told to see a psychiatrist or some other mental-health professional such as a psychologist or social worker. Which advice an applicant was given depended on his needs, as Chart XVIII shows.

Applicants not especially disposed to go to a psychiatrist were more often told to do so. This included both applicants to the Religion and Psychiatry Institute and hospital clinics, and their counterparts among analytic-clinic applicants—nonmembers of the Friends receiving only unsolicited advice. These persons thus received advice that was either new to them or which legitimated action they might otherwise have been afraid to take. Otherwise, solicited advice given to analytic-clinic applicants followed the line of least resistance, for, after all, telling another person what to do is not such an easy thing. Members of the Friends who received purely unsolicited advice really did not need to be told to see a psychiatrist. Hence they were told to seek other professional help. Solicited advice, of course, more exactly fitted what applicants would have liked to hear: if not a member of the Friends, it was

CHART XVIII *Per Cent of Applicants Who Talked with Others about Their Problems Who Were Told to Seek Professional Help, According to Type of Contact and Membership in the Friends*

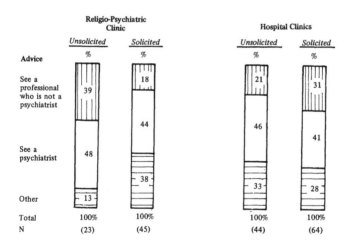

Analytic Clinics

	Unsolicited		Solicited		Both Unsolicited		Solicited	
	Friends	Not Friends	Friends	Not Friends	Friends	Not Friends	Friends	Not Friends
Advice	%	%	%	%	%	%	%	%
See a professional who is not a psychiatrist	42	29	32	42	46	45	31	37
See a psychiatrist	35	39	37	19	20	19	46	19
Other	23	32	31	39	34	36	23	44
Total	100%	100%	100%	100%	100%	100%	100%	100%
N	(76)	(28)	(54)	(26)	(110)	(42)	(95)	(27)

	Religio-Psychiatric Clinic		**Hospital Clinics**	
	Unsolicited	Solicited	Unsolicited	Solicited
Advice	%	%	%	%
See a professional who is not a psychiatrist	39	18	21	31
See a psychiatrist	48	44	46	41
Other	13	38	33	28
Total	100%	100%	100%	100%
N	(23)	(45)	(44)	(64)

to see a nonpsychiatrist professional; if a member, to see a psychiatrist. Thus applicants already disposed to seek psychiatric aid received supportive or confirming advice.

It is important to recognize that at this early stage of the decision to seek professional help, the decision has not yet crystallized. Support or confirmation is of a general nature. So only 20 per cent of analytic-clinic applicants who solicited advice and were then told to see a psychiatrist were told about the clinic to which they presently applied. Only three persons who solicited advice were given the name of a psychiatrist. And less than 10 per cent of analytic-clinic applicants who received unsolicited advice to go to a psychiatrist were given any specific names. A somewhat larger proportion of religio-psychiatric and hospital-clinic applicants were told of specific psychiatrists (generally the clinic to which they are now applying). Again, those less disposed to seek help had to be given much more specific information if they were ever to get to a professional psychotherapist. Finally, lest the reader think laymen are unusually diffuse in the advice they give, it should be noted that physicians do little better. As we shall point out in the next chapter, only one-third of religio- and analytic-psychiatric clinic applicants were told by doctors whom they had visited to see a psychiatrist, and of these only half were given a specific name. Only for those most distant from the psychotherapy system—hospital-clinic applicants—did physicians regularly supply the name of a psychiatrist or a clinic.

❀ *Helpfulness*

The last fact about a conversation is its residue or "aftertaste." Each person who received advice or reported conversations with others about his problems was asked to respond to a checklist question: "Was this (the contact) helpful? Yes; So-So; No." The applicant's own judgment as to which contacts he thought helpful (those who answered with a "yes") confirms our opinion as to the consequences of different types of contacts. Without going into the details of the data, we may report that pressure which we identified as confirmatory and supportive is more likely to be perceived by applicants themselves as helpful, unless it turns out from the later perspective of applying to a psychiatric clinic that the advice was foolish. For example, even high pressure placed upon members of the Friends who asked for the pressure was well received, but high pressure when not asked for was less likely to be thought helpful. In terms of advice as to what to do about problems, the retrospective judgment of applicants proved directly related to our own opinion as to the functions of advice. Those who might not otherwise have come to psychotherapy found advice to seek psychotherapy especially helpful, whereas those who would probably have gone anyway found other advice more helpful, although confirming advice was also highly rated.

❁ Conclusion

Between 80 and 90 per cent of those going to psychiatric clinics have talked with others about their problems, and this amount of conversation about personal problems is considerably greater than that indulged in by the average New Yorker. But there are just as good reasons for not talking as there are for opening oneself up!

Although it does seem reasonable that a predisposition to recognize problems by oneself, an interest in emotional matters, a sense that they carry no special stigma, and the possession of highly visible problems should all lead to conversation with others, these very factors may reduce such voluntary exposure. For after all, a person who knows so much about himself surely does not need the help of others to enable him to recognize his problems. The same type of reasoning holds for the possible intervention of others in the affairs of a potential applicant. Closeness to another person and the degree to which a problem is visible to others and annoys them make it likely that another might intervene—but also make it likely that he would hesitate to intrude.

The solution to these contradictory common-sense notions is found in the fact that there are two types of conversations about problems, each with different consequences or functions. About half the conversations were initiated by others without the applicant's having asked for advice. Somewhat more were initiated at the applicant's own behest. These two types of conversation are empirically unrelated. The majority engaged in both solicited and unsolicited conversation, some engaged in either solicited or unsolicited talk, and a few did not talk with anyone. Purely unsolicited conversation was said to have a socially controlling function aimed at reducing the applicant's deviance, whereas solicited contacts or those unsolicited remarks accompanied by solicited conversation were said to be more supportive or confirming of ideas the applicant already had.

A number of facts revealed later in the chapter supported these imputed functions of conversations. First, solicited advice came more often from persons likely to be congenial to the applicant; unsolicited comment, something the applicant can little control, came from persons that the applicant obviously must have annoyed or otherwise interfered with. For example, members of the Friends and Supporters of Psychotherapy voluntarily consulted their friends more often than their relatives; on the other hand, they were almost as likely to get unsolicited comments from relatives as from friends. And when they did get these unwanted comments, they were perceived as exerting more pressure. Second, those types of problems most likely to disturb others—interpersonal and marital problems—were more likely to lead to unsolicited advice, especially among the less sophisticated applicants. Third, solicited advice, more often than not, turned out to be advice which told the applicant what he wanted to hear; while purely unsolicited advice was less likely to spare the applicant but would urge him to do what appeared to be good for him, at least from the present perspective of going to a psychiatric clinic. For example, applicants to analytic clinics who were of the type one does not expect to find applying to such clinics were more frequently given unsolicited advice to go to a psychiatrist. Finally, the applicant's own evaluation of the advice given to him as helpful or not helpful confirmed our own evaluation of the functions of advice. Solicited comment was generally viewed as more "helpful" than unsolicited comment unless, of course, the advice in retrospect seemed just plain wrong.

Why so many engaged in conversation about problems now becomes obvious. Some persons talked about these matters simply because they and their immediate social circle found them interesting. Perhaps they also needed some support and confirmation in making a difficult decision. Some persons, on the other hand, if they were at all to go to a psychiatrist needed to have others point out their problems to them. They were deviants who had to be socially controlled.

Those who belonged to circles interested in and supportive of emotional problems were more likely to solicit conversation, thus proving the hypothesis. They also engaged in more conversation in general, since their open attitude to emotional matters allowed them to receive unsolicited advice—which they had indirectly asked for in the first place. Such persons were members of the Friends and Supporters of Psychotherapy, as well as Jews, Protestants, and women. Their conversation served as "warm-up" for psychotherapy.

Further proving our point is the fact that those less predisposed to recognize their own problems—the unsophisticated, upwardly mobile Catholics, Negroes, and Puerto Ricans, and men—were more likely to receive purely unsolicited conversation. Those less interested and less knowledgeable about emotional problems "accidentally" ran into someone whom they annoyed. These others responded with socially controlling comment. Without the interference of others, these persons might not have recognized that they had serious emotional problems and might not subsequently have applied for psychotherapy.

Of course, the type of problems an applicant has, or thinks he has, affects the likelihood of others talking with him about them, and also, in part, determines what they say to him. Generally, either highly visible problems, or those such as cognitive problems which the applicant probably would not have recognized by himself, lead to comment. As for other types of problems, it depends on whether they affect others —in which case others are motivated to interfere—or whether they are a matter of interest to others, such as sexual problems which are of interest to the Friends and Supporters of Therapy. Again, just as interest in emotional problems and lack of an interest both lead to conversation with others among applicants for psychotherapy, so polar opposites in type of problem both lead to conversation.

A large proportion of applicants had previously discussed their problems with others because some wanted to and others needed to. In fact, without the interference of others, about 15 per cent of analytic-clinic applicants would not have recognized that they had problems. Conversation about problems early in the decision affects later interactions. Those who got no advice at this stage or only unsolicited advice were more prone to rely on others, to push them into treatment, whereas those whose discussions were more supportive eventually acted on their own.

The importance of casual conversation and its channelling through social groups can better be appreciated if we compare these findings with those of other sociological studies. A number of studies show that persons tend to adopt the political point of view of those they are more likely to come in contact with.[4] These contacts do not occur at random. Rather, they tend to reflect the social groups to which individuals belong. Union members, for example, are more likely to vote Democrat; the more involved a person is with the union, the more likely he is to run into union members and hence the more likely he is to vote Democrat. Discussions about politics thus tend to be confirming, rather than controlling, in the sense in which we have used these words.

Of course, no one completely controls his contacts and associates. Accidents of social interaction do occur, and it is always possible to run into someone of a different social persuasion. As a matter of fact, in a pluralistic democratic society, this likelihood is built into the social structure. When it happens, conversation is likely to be initiated by the other fellow, or so it seems to respondents.[5] Such social control of individuals has an interesting consequence for the society at large. Since by definition one is more likely to run into others who share the majority's point of view, the majority opinion in a pluralistic society is always more stable than the minority point of view.

The data on voting deal only indirectly with social circles. A study showing why the International Typographical Union is democratic, that is, has a two-party system with regularly contested elections for union office, emphasizes the importance of the "occupational community," a unit which well fits our definition of a social circle. Members of the union have common interests fostered by various independent clubs, such as bowling and chess groups, and tend to know a number of other union members whom they see off the job, although they naturally cannot directly know all the union members. The union occupational community serves to bridge the gap between union political activity and the average union member in a fashion analogous to the way membership in the Friends and Supporters of Psychotherapy bridges the distance between therapist and patient. Especially important is the effect on union members who might otherwise be uninterested in union affairs. Because of their membership in social circles, union members come to interact with persons active and interested in the union, thus kindling their own interest as well as providing them with knowledge about union issues.

Our study brings to the fore the different functions of conversation sometimes only implicit in these other studies. When measurements over at least two time periods are available, studies of the effect of mass media and other forms of persuasion show two consequences of influence: "preserving" effects and "generating" effects. The preserving effect is the proportion of persons exposed to the influence who retain the desired characteristic as opposed to those not exposed. The generating effect is the proportion exposed who gain the desired characteristic, who did not previously have it, as compared with the proportion gaining it who were not exposed to the influence. Whenever an attitude or behavior is well entrenched, as is the case with most political attitudes and behavior, the preserving effects are much larger than the generating effects. Political campaigns convert very few; rather, they tend to reinforce latent associations and opinions.

In our study of problems, much more ego involving and much more entrenched than political attitudes, we have seen analogous functions which we called confirmation and control. Again, confirmation is much more frequent than control.[6] There is an important difference over and above the subject matter of the feelings and attitudes. There are socially accepted groups which favor Democrats or Republicans. In the ITU there is an historical tradition of democratic politics. Realizing that one has an emotional problem is inherently unpleasant. Hence the forces operating on potential applicants for psychotherapy must be stronger than those which produce elections. Both confirmation and control must be more powerful than those demonstrated in political studies. But where do they draw their strength?

Confirmation is possible only through the instituting of psychotherapy and analytic psychology. The circle of Friends is thus the sociological equivalent of unions and ethnic groups of traditional importance to American politics. Both confirmation and control—especially control—

draw their strength from an additional aspect of emotional problems: the fact that a person's emotional problems directly impinge upon and annoy others. The motivation to tell someone how to vote is surely weaker than the motivation required to tell someone to "stop annoying me." At key points in the individual's path to psychotherapy, especially among those who are not disposed to this treatment, others' motivations are mobilized to control the reluctant applicant.

Finally, just as chance meetings preserve the stable character of democratic politics—both in the ITU and nationally in the United States—so the accidents of social encounter are especially important in getting those persons to interpret their difficulties in life as "psychological" or "psychiatric" problems. To be sure, these encounters are accidents only when looked at individually. En masse, they form a predictable pattern.

NOTES

1. Sixteen per cent of analytic-clinic applicants, 12 per cent of religio-psychiatric clinic applicants, and 9 per cent of hospital-clinic applicants have had no such contacts. The differences between the latter two types of clinics are insignificant. The higher rate of analytic-clinic applicants is mainly an artifact of laziness in answering questionnaires and probing of all "no" answers in the interviews. About the same proportion as the other clinic applicants checked that they had consulted with laymen, but some of these failed to indicate with whom they had talked. Some were confused by our instructions and thought that we meant professional consultation. Neither those who answered in terms of professional consultation exclusively nor those who failed to report with whom they conversed are included in our figures. Including these persons, however, does not change our results.
2. Jack Elinson, Elena Padilla, and Marvin E. Perkins, *Public Images of Mental Health Services* (New York: New York City Community Mental Health Board, 1967).
3. See Kadushin, "Social Distance Between Client and Professional," *American Journal of Sociology*, 67 (1962), 517-531, for an analysis of the ambiguous role of distance in professional-client relations as well.
4. B. Berelson, P. Lazarsfeld, and W. McPhee, *Voting* (Chicago: University of Chicago Press, 1954), Chapter 6.
5. *Ibid.*, p. 107.
6. Note that our method is different. We used reason analysis; these other studies used panel analysis. We have but one side of the story. It is equivalent to a voting study only of those who voted Democrat. Nevertheless, our results are about the same.

False Starts: Previous Sources of Treatment

9

Long before their present application to a psychiatric clinic, almost all patients had decided to seek professional aid for their problems. In fact, "beginners" who had not previously seen a professional are practically unheard of in most psychiatric clinics. Only 12 per cent of analytic- and 5 per cent of hospital-clinic applicants are beginners. The rest have previously been to at least one professional for consultation about problems related to the very ones now brought to a psychiatric clinic. In only the Religion and Psychiatry Institute are as many as one-fourth of the applicants novices, and this is due to the clinic's anomalous position in the professional referral system. For the fact is that the major role of psychiatric clinics is to take in other professionals' wash.

We are especially interested in the professionals previously seen, not for purely historical reasons, but because one of the major determinants of a person's present choice of clinic is his previous set of choices. Most applicants to analytic clinics had previously been to psychiatrists, psychologists, or social workers; a strong minority had been to physicians.* In contrast, applicants to the Religion and Psychiatry Institute had been either to ministers, to psychiatrists, or to no professional person at all, but had instead read books written by two of the Institute's founders. Most hospital-clinic applicants had been to physicians or psychiatrists. In many ways, then, the current choice of clinic by applicants is simply a repetition of their previous choices.

A significant number of professionals is involved in the process of funneling applicants to psychiatric clinics. About one-third of analytic and religio-psychiatric applicants who had previously seen a professional had consulted with three or more. Hospital-clinic applicants were especially likely to shuttle from one professional to another. Seventy per cent had been to three or more different professionals before applying to a hospital psychiatric clinic.

At each turn, in the progression from one professional to another, psychiatry became, if any changes were made at all, a more likely choice. As a result a very large proportion of applicants had already been to a

TABLE 18 *Per Cent of Clinic Applicants Who Had Been to Various Types of Professionals Before Applying to the Present Clinics*

Former Source of Treatment	Analytic Clinics	Religio-Psychiatric Clinic	Hospital Clinics
	%	%	%
None	12	24	5
Psychiatrists and psychologists	65	35	59
Counseling and welfare services	25	11	25
Nonpsychiatrist physicians	42	44	70
Clergymen	8	35	23
Cultists and healers	1	5	5
Legal services and police	1	6	4
Social improvement	1	4	1
Other, unspecified mixture	1	5	10
N	(1118)	(199)	(135)
Average number of types	1.6	1.7	2.0

* Instead of repeating this qualification throughout the chapter, let it be stated here once and for all: "physician" or "doctor" means nonpsychiatrist M.D. "Psychiatrist" or "psychiatric service" may also mean psychologist. Family and casework agencies, however, are separately referred to as "counseling." Most professionals in such agencies are social workers, although others may also be involved.

psychiatrist before going to the present psychiatric clinic. These previous attempts at therapy were not altogether superficial. Almost 40 per cent of analytic-clinic applicants had had more than 21 sessions; about 25 per cent of hospital-clinic applicants fell into this category; only among Religion and Psychiatry Institute applicants do we find very little previous therapy.

Since we claim that the choice of the present clinic is determined by past patterns of choice, we have indeed a complicated task ahead of us, for tracing multiple patterns of choice can be quite arduous. Fortunately, the very first professional chosen fairly well sets the pattern of subsequent choices. In fact, these subsequent patterns are more likely to be determined by the characteristics of the professions than by the characteristics of the clients themselves. The individual characteristics of clients do, however, determine their very first choice. We need only understand why certain types of persons make the initial choice of professional in order to unravel the essential threads of the entire skein. We shall then analyze typical pathways to each type of clinic from each major starting point. Why applicants left former therapists only to apply to still another will also be investigated. This process of making the rounds from one professional to another, though characteristic, is emotionally wearing, expensive and inefficient. We shall show that one way of estimating the social costs of this procedure is to observe whether lower- or higher-class applicants have had a great deal of psychotherapy in the past. Why this indicates the social costs of shopping and how this class bias varies according to the links between previous therapists and psychiatric clinics will be explained in the last part of this chapter.

❀ *The First Professional*

The first choices of future applicants to the three types of clinics are radically different. These differences are reflected in the different clinics to which applications were later made.

Seventy-five per cent of analytic-clinic applicants chose their first therapist from the medical world. These choices were two to one in favor of psychiatry rather than nonpsychiatric medicine. The situation is reversed among hospital-clinic applicants, who most often chose nonpsychiatric medical professionals. Religion and Psychiatry Institute applicants were about equal in their choice of psychiatrists and other physicians. In addition, they were much more likely than either analytic- or hospital-clinic applicants to choose clergymen first.

These first choices depend upon the social situation and circle of applicants. This is true despite the fact that we are dealing with persons

TABLE 19 *First Professional Sources Chosen by Those Who Had Been to Other Professionals before Applying to a Clinic*

Professional Source	Analytic Clinics	Religio-Psychiatric Clinic	Hospital Clinics
	%	%	%
Outpatient psychiatry and psychology	44	24	16
Inpatient psychiatry	1	0	6
Counseling and welfare services	19	6	11
Nonpsychiatrist physicians	29	32	45
Paramedical	1	5	5
Clergymen	4	20	9
Cultists and healers	1	34	2
Legal services and police	0	1	1
Social improvement	1	4	1
Other, unspecified mixture	0	4	4
Total	100	100	100
	(968)	(147)	(165)

who are all now applying to psychiatric clinics. Higher social class, membership in the Friends, motivation to pay for psychotherapy, and especially living in a milieu in which others go to psychotherapists and in which one can ask for possible sources of treatment are all related to going to psychiatrists first.*

Except for the most "crazy" symptoms—complaints about inability to think clearly, or at the extreme, inability to know where one is, drug addiction or alcoholism—the kind of symptoms applicants have are *not* related to having been to a psychiatrist first. Such a wide range of symptoms and problems are dealt with by psychiatry that few specific maladies can be singled out as naturally leading to its being chosen first. Accordingly, except among Religion and Psychiatry Institute applicants, psychiatric diagnosis is *not* related to having gone to a psychiatrist first.

Counseling as first choice follows the same rules as psychiatry—except that because it is cheaper, social class factors are not as important. Students and housewives are more likely than others (10 to 15 percentage points more) to pick counseling first. Students do so probably because counseling is readily available on campuses; housewives may be more interested in family matters congenial to social work counseling and may also prefer it because they can go on their own and not ask their husbands for money.

* All the differences reported here range from 10 to 15 percentage points, although some differences, especially those relating to going to physicians, are around 20 percentage points.

Low class and low sophistication produce physical symptoms which lead to the physician as first choice.

Belonging to a religion which is interested in the religion and psychiatry movement or which has special and strong attitudes toward matters that are a problem to many applicants, such as homosexuality, seems to make clergymen a more likely first choice. Thus Catholics and Protestants consult clergymen much more frequently than do Jews, who do not view rabbis as experts in psychotherapy. This accounts for the low frequency with which analytic-clinic applicants had consulted clergymen first, since most of these applicants are Jews.

These findings are certainly congruent with our view that therapy-seeking depends upon the nature of one's social circle. Since the first professional chosen has so much to do with the ultimate choice of clinic applicants, it is easy to understand why the different clinics draw upon applicants with such different social backgrounds.

There are a couple of puzzles here, though. Let us try the easier one first. Lower-class persons tend to choose medicine first. But they also are more likely, as we know, to have physical presenting problems. What causes what? Does choice of physician merely reflect the fact that lower-class persons think they have physical symptoms (which later turn out not to have an evident physical basis), or do they simply trust physicians more? The data show that if a lower-class applicant does *not* complain of a physical symptom, then his pattern of first choices is just like everyone else's. On the other hand, among people who *do* have physical presenting problems, lower-class persons are much more likely to try a nonpsychiatrist physician first. Even though they may experience physical symptoms, more sophisticated applicants more often attribute these symptoms to emotional problems. Since they made their own diagnosis that their physical pains were "only apparent" these sophisticates by-passed the internist or the physician and went directly to a psychiatrist.

The second puzzle concerns money, social class, and sophistication. All are related to seeing a psychiatrist first. But do higher-class people try psychiatry first because they have more money and feel they can pay for psychiatry, or is it because higher-class persons also tend to be more sophisticated and are more often members of the Friends?

The findings which relate going to psychiatrists first to higher social class *still* hold when nonprivate psychiatry is considered, thus tending to eliminate mere money as a causal factor (although private care makes up more than three-quarters of all care previously given to clinic applicants). Second, if class factors such as occupation and education are controlled for by membership in the Friends, then among members of the Friends there is no relationship between class and having had previous therapy. Class differences are accentuated among nonmembers of the Friends where solid support for psychiatry is less evident. Ability to pay seems a factor only when one is less than enthusiastic about psychiatry.

We have perhaps oversimplified matters. To psychoanalysts, money is an extremely important part of therapy. It is a question of attitude as well as of cash.

> A very important problem in the setting up of the original contract [between patient and psychiatrist] is the question of money. Freud reminded us of how hypocritical and evasive we all are about payment for getting and giving help. . . . The analysis will not go well if the patient is paying less than he can reasonably afford to pay. It should be a definite sacrifice for *him* and not for someone else.[1]

Being able to afford therapy is not only a matter of how much money one has, but how much one is willing to sacrifice in order to pay for therapy. To a clinic applicant, money is one of the most sensitive aspects of life. The issue is so delicate that we have had to discard responses to our question on income as being either evasive or untruthful. This is the only part of the questionnaire or interview we feel has been willfully distorted by respondents. For example, we frequently had cases of professionals in well-paying industries reporting very little income, or of students refusing to estimate the income of their parents, giving us instead, a ridiculously low figure. Consequently, we have had to rely on education and occupation as measures of social-class standing rather than income. Since money is so obviously related to going to a psychotherapist, we had best have a closer look at money, class, and attitude as they interact in determining whether one goes first to a psychotherapist or only later as a last resort.

We asked all applicants (in the 1960 version of the questionnaire and interview) the following series of questions about therapy and money.

What is the maximum fee you could possibly afford per week for treatment? (Remember these answers *will not* affect your fee at this clinic.)

$ 0– .99	$10.00–14.99
1.00–1.99	15.00–19.99
2.00–3.99	20.00–24.99
4.00–5.99	25.00–29.99
6.00–6.99	30.00
7.00–9.99	

Which of the following would you consider doing to help pay for treatment? (Check all that apply.)
—use your savings or loans.
—forego family expenditures such as for clothing and vacations.
—make major changes in your life such as changing jobs, or moving your place of residence.

—ask for financial help from others (friend or relative).
—would you expect the clinic to alter its policy of fees to take you.

In view of the ambiguous responses applicants gave when asked about their incomes, these questions about money probably reveal the intensity with which an applicant approaches psychotherapy rather than measure the extent of his personal financial resources. There are, however, important differences between the responses to the questions about size of fees and the extent to which one might make sacrifices. When both are treated as ranked measures (the fee question is already in that form and the sacrifice question merely requires, in order to arrive at a score, that we add up the total number of sacrifices a person is willing to make, excluding, of course, his expectation that the *clinic* change its fees), there is some correlation (Tau $\beta = .110$) between the amount of fee one could pay and the number of sacrifices one might make. Though statistically significant (past the .001 level using Kendall's S) the association leaves considerable room for unexplained variance. It is therefore quite possible that a willingness to pay higher fees may be more related to social class, whereas a willingness to make sacrifices may be more related to social circle membership and sophistication about psychotherapy. The chart below tests this hypothesis, using occupation of breadwinner (student excluded) to stand for social class, and membership in the Friends to stand for circle affiliation and sophistication about psychotherapy. Also included is level of education (students excluded) though it is a somewhat ambiguous variable, since it is indicative of both social class and sophistication.

The three independent variables—occupation, education, and membership in the Friends—are of course all intercorrelated,[2] though education and breadwinner occupation are the most highly related. What is most important to observe is that occupation is not truly correlated with a willingness to make sacrifices, since the observed correlation of .109 is reduced to .06 (not significant) when education is controlled. Hence occupation of breadwinner is linked to a willingness to make sacrifices only through its link with education. Similarly, membership in the Friends and Supporters of Psychotherapy is barely related to a willingness to pay higher fees to begin with (d = .082, significant at the .05 level) and the association is reduced to practically nothing (d = .025, not significant) with occupation controlled. Education demonstrates its ambiguous nature by maintaining a relation with willingness to make sacrifices which is quite independent of its link with the Friends and Supporters. The latter, indicating circle membership is, of course, related to willingness to make sacrifices quite independently of level of education. Education and circle membership are thus independently related to a willingness to make sacrifices. On the

CHART XIX *Model of the Relationship (Sommers D) for Analytic-Clinic Applicants between Social Class Variables, Social Circle, and the Motivation to go to a Psychiatrist*

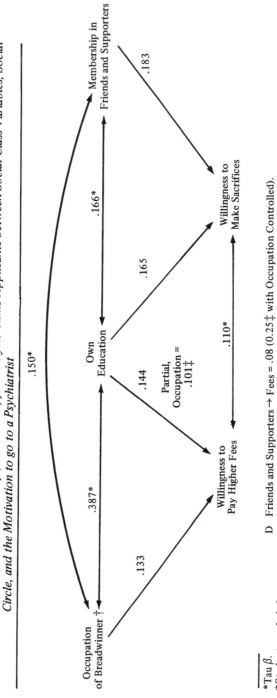

*Tau β.
†Students excluded.
‡Average D over all classes of third variable.

D Friends and Supporters → Fees = .08 (0.25‡ with Occupation Controlled).
D Occupation → Sacrifices = .109 (.06‡ with Education Controlled).

other hand, although education is also related to a willingness to pay higher fees, this relationship is less strong than its relationship to a willingness to make sacrifices. Moreover, the relation between education and higher fees drops when occupation is controlled. In sum, though it is relevant to both social class and circle membership, education is more closely allied to sophistication than it is to sheer personal income.

The hypothesis is confirmed; we conclude that the size of a fee a client is willing to pay for therapy is more related to his actual money resources, whereas his willingness to make sacrifices to pay for therapy is more related to his attitudes about psychotherapy.

Given these facts we might expect that willingness to make sacrifices should be related to trying psychiatry first, but that willingness to pay a higher fee should not predict going to a psychiatrist first. Indeed, money does not lead to try psychiatry first, but our direct measure of attitude makes a difference of almost 20 percentage points. Only 30 per cent of those who did previously try some kind of professional before going to analytic clinics and who are unwilling to make sacrifices chose psychiatry first. However, fully 48 per cent of nonbeginners willing to make three or more sacrifices went first to a psychiatrist. (We deal with nonbeginners only because the more sacrifices a person is willing to make, the more likely it is that he has previously been to *any* professional.) Among the nonmembers of the Friends there is an even greater relationship between making sacrifices and trying psychiatry first.

In sum, although we are dealing with a clinic population, and thus by implication with persons who are either impoverished, "cheapskates," or merely prudently looking for a good buy, their *actual cash* solvency and ability to pay for therapy were *less* important in their going first to a psychotherapist than their *attitude* about money and their membership in the social circle of Friends and Supporters of Psychotherapy.

❄ *Pathways through the Helping Professions*

Now that we know some of the determinants of first choice of a professional, what happens next? In most cases, a person goes to still another professional before applying to a clinic and becoming a member of our sample. Various complex paths were possible to him. To simplify matters, we shall focus our analysis on the relationship between the first and last place a person went to, as well as other intermediate ones without distinguishing the order of these intermediate places. Table 20 indicates these paths. We shall look at the paths from a teleological point of view: how many steps does it take for a person to be placed in his present position—an applicant to a psychiatric clinic.

All roads do lead toward our "Rome"—psychiatry—with fairly little

TABLE 20 *Patterns of Previous Treatment*

				ANALYTIC-CLINIC APPLICANTS	
Began with	Also Tried*	N	Last Visited	Per Cent With This Pattern	N
Psychiatry 44%	No one else		Psychiatry	46	174
	Other psychiatrists		Psychiatry	22	84
	Counseling / Medicine / Clergy / Other	21 / 40 / 8 / 2	Psychiatry	19	71
	Medicine / Clergy / Other	3 / 1 / 1	Counseling	4	15
	Counseling / Clergy / Other	4 / 1 / 1	Medicine	7	26
	Medicine	1	Clergy	1	4
	Medicine / Clergy	3 / 3	Other	2	8
			Total	101	(382)
Counseling 19%	No one else		Counseling	42	71
	Other counselors		Counseling	12	20
	Psychiatry / Medicine / Clergy / Other	14 / 5 / 1 / 2	Counseling	10	16
	Medicine / Clergy / Other	6 / 3 / 2	Psychiatry	29	48
	Psychiatry / Clergy	5 / 1	Medicine	6	10
	None		Clergy	2	3
	None		Other	0	0
			Total	101	(168)

TABLE 20 (continued) *Patterns of Previous Treatment*

	ANALYTIC-CLINIC APPLICANTS				
Began with	**Also Tried***	**N**	**Last Visited**	**Per Cent With This Pattern**	**N**
Medicine 33%	No one else		→ Medicine	30	84
	Other medicine		→ Medicine	2	7
	Psychiatry / Counseling / Clergy	11 / 3 / 1	→ Medicine	5	13
	Counseling / Clergy	6 / 3	→ Psychiatry	52	146
	Psychiatry	6	→ Counseling	8	24
	Psychiatry	2	→ Clergy	1	3
	Psychiatry	3	→ Other	2	5
			Total	100	(282)
Clergy 4%	No one else		→ Clergy	6	2
	Medicine	1	→ Clergy	3	1
	Medicine	2	→ Psychiatry	61	20
	Psychiatry / Medical	1 / 3	→ Counseling	15	5
	Psychiatry	2	→ Medicine	12	4
	None		→ Other	3	1
			Total	100	(33)
			Grand Total		(865)

*The actual number of persons consulting the intermediate sources other than the first and last ones is indicated. The data do not show the number of intermediate sources of the same type. Thus if a person went to a psychiatrist, and then to a physician who was not a psychiatrist, then to a psychiatrist and then to another psychiatrist, his starting point is shown as psychiatrist, the intermediate source as physician, and the last source as psychiatry. The intermediate source of psychiatry is not listed separately. Only persons for whom the entire sequence could be properly unravelled are shown. Because of the small number of cases in the other clinics, intermediate sources are shown only for analytic clinics.

TABLE 20 (continued) *Patterns of Previous Treatment*

HOSPITAL-CLINIC APPLICANTS

Began with	Last Visited	Per Cent With This Pattern	N
Psychiatry 23%	One psychiatry source only	37	9
	More than one psychiatry source	21	5
	Counseling	8	2.
	Medicine	21	5
	Clergy	8	2
	Other	4	1
	Total	99	(24)
Counseling 12%	One counseling source only	8	1
	More than one counseling source	16	2
	Psychiatry	23	3
	Medicine	38	5
	Clergy	0	0
	Other	16	2
	Total	101	(13)
Medicine 56%	One medicine source only	36	21
	More than one medicine source	10	6
	Psychiatry	41	24
	Counseling	3	2
	Clergy	3	2
	Other	7	4
	Total	100	(59)
Clergy 9%	One clergy source only	*	3
	More than one clergy source		0
	Psychiatry		6
	Counseling		1
	Medicine		0
	Other		0
	Total		(10)
	Grand Total		(106)

TABLE 20 (continued) *Patterns of Previous Treatment*

RELIGION AND PSYCHIATRY INSTITUTE APPLICANTS

Began with	Last Visited	Per Cent With This Pattern	N
Psychiatry 24%	One psychiatry source only	41	12
	More than one psychiatry source	21	6
	Counseling	7	2
	Medicine	17	5
	Clergy	14	4
	Other	0	0
	Total	100	(29)
Counseling 8%	One counseling source only	*	5
	More than one counseling source		2
	Psychiatry		1
	Medicine		0
	Clergy		1
	Other		0
	Total		(9)
Medicine 43%	One medicine source only	37	19
	More than one medicine source	8	4
	Psychiatry	21	11
	Counseling	6	3
	Clergy	17	9
	Other	12	6
	Total	101	(52)
Clergy 25%	One clergy source only	53	16
	More than one clergy source	7	2
	Psychiatry	20	6
	Counseling	0	0
	Medicine	13	4
	Other	7	2
	Total	100	(30)
	Grand Total		(120)

*Base figure too small for per cent.

digression. Those who first went to a psychiatrist were most likely to stay with it. Those beginning with other professions were more likely to abandon them even before they applied to a clinic. The number of steps taken and the number of false moves made do vary with the type of clinic to which persons are now applying, for, as analysis throughout this chapter indicates, analytic clinics are most closely linked to previous sources of help, but hospital clinics and the Religion and Psychiatry Institute are further removed. As will be recalled, in terms of the sheer *number* of professionals previously seen, hospital clinics are indeed the furthest removed from the starting point, since over 70 per cent of their applicants had previously been to three or more professionals.

Applicants to analytic clinics most consistently chose psychiatry. Sixty-six per cent who first chose psychiatry stayed with it all the way, compared to only about 40 per cent for the religio-psychiatric and hospital clinics. In terms of number of professionals subsequently seen, a first visit to a psychiatrist is the shortest route to an analytic clinic, and even to a hospital clinic, but a much longer road to the Religion and Psychiatry Institute. In fact, among analytic-clinic applicants sticking to psychiatry, two-thirds had previously been to only one psychiatrist. Some applicants began with psychiatry, flirted with other professions, and then returned to psychiatry before their present application. About 20 per cent of those beginning with psychiatry followed this path. The proportion does not vary from one type of clinic to another. But even these flirtations were mostly with professions allied to psychotherapy—medicine and counseling. Among starters in psychiatry, medicine was the only other major profession which immediately preceded the present application. About 20 per cent in nonanalytic clinics traveled this reverse route—specialist first and general medicine later. Only 7 per cent of analytic-clinic applicants who started with psychiatry ended with medicine, however. In short, relatively few applicants to analytic clinics regretted their first choice of psychiatry. More bouncing around was evident among applicants to other clinics, but by and large, the patterns of those who first chose psychiatry are quite similar in all types of clinics.

Counseling and welfare agencies form an interesting contrast to psychiatry, for they are feeder routes to psychiatry. Few who chose psychiatry first went to a counseling or social agency later. But counseling led to psychiatry in 20 to 30 per cent of the cases in each type of clinic. Among analytic and religio-psychiatric applicants it seemed to be a question of timing—when one made the switch to psychiatry. Most who began with counseling made the switch to psychiatry with their present application (60 per cent of analytic and religio-psychiatric applicants who began with counseling stayed with it until their present application). In fact, among analytic-clinic applicants, counseling is as direct a route to the present clinic as psychiatry. Those who wandered back and forth from counseling went no further afield than psychiatry. Counseling is the least direct route among hospital-clinic applicants, most of whom went to a large number of professionals—generally doctors or psychotherapists—before applying to the present clinic.

Medicine as first choice had similar consequences in all three types of clinics. The relationship of medicine to psychiatry is perhaps the most stable. About 40 per cent began and ended with medicine before their present application. Of these, three-fourths tried no other profession. Nonetheless, there was considerable switching from one doctor to another before applicants eventually settled upon psychiatry. Those who began with medicine were very likely to have tried a great number of professionals of all sorts. On the other hand, if persons who began with medicine did not end with medicine before applying to a psychiatric clinic, it is simply that they made the switch to psychiatry much earlier: 40 to 50 per cent of those beginning with medicine switched to psychiatry even before coming to the present clinic, with the exception of religio-psychiatric applicants who on their exit from medicine, turned either to psychiatrists or to clergymen. With this one exception, other professions were simply not likely to follow upon a first choice of medicine.

The link between the present clinic and clergymen determines whether applicants abandoned clergymen long before their present application or stayed with this profession until now. Few stayed with clergymen among analytic-clinic applicants, more among hospital-clinic applicants, and over half among Religion and Psychiatry Institute applicants. Amongst the last, the clergy represent the most direct route to the clinic. But among analytic-clinic applicants, clergy produce the most indirect path to the clinic. Over 60 per cent of those who began with clergymen, among analytic- and hospital-clinic applicants, then went to a psychiatrist. Only one-fifth of Religion and Psychiatry Institute applicants who began with clergymen saw a psychiatrist before coming to the religio-psychiatric clinic.

As we said, the paths between the various professions appear to be set by the structure of the professional world of healing and represent the influence of professionals upon clients rather than the individual characteristics of the clients themselves. What pattern appears is determined in part by our vantage point. If we are observing from the point of view of the Religion and Psychiatry Institute, which is linked to the healing professions largely through clergy and only indirectly through medicine, counseling, and psychiatry, then a person who began with ministers took the most direct path to the clinic. In view of his current position, his first choice of minister was the "right" one. This choice was largely conditioned, it may be recalled, by his religious background. If one observes choices from the point of view of the analytic clinics, then going to a minister first was a "bad" choice for a future analytic-clinic applicant. Only by passing from one professional to another would he eventually be likely to go to an analytic clinic. That is, he needed considerable socialization to the role of analytic-clinic applicant if he began with a clergyman.

The role of medicine in the healing professions seems the most constant, since the channels into which it led patients appear the same from the point of view of all three types of clinics. If one starts with medicine, then one is unlikely to go to any profession other than psychiatry. It is true that a fair proportion of Religion and Psychiatry Institute applicants gave up on the medicine-psychiatry axis altogether and went then to clergymen—which explains how they got from medicine to the relatively distant religio-psychiatric clinic. The real question with medicine, though, is not where potential psychiatric patients go from there, but how long it takes them to get into the psychiatry system. When we first gathered data in 1957-1958, tranquilizers were relatively new to most persons. Even then, most physicians gave them to those of their patients who eventually came to the Religion and Psychiatry Institute. The same is true today of applicants to all clinics. But there seems to be a difference in reaction. In the earlier period giving tranquilizers was associated with going to still more physicians. Apparently, patients interpreted the pill as meaning they were physically ill. In our 1960 sample no such association between pills and continuing with nonpsychiatrist physicians is evident. Tranquilizers have perhaps become instituted as "mental" pills! It remains true that despite medicine's good connections with psychiatry, it takes quite a long time for a person to transfer from medicine to psychiatry. One factor is the apparent unwillingness of physicians to make referrals to psychiatrists. Only one-third of those analytic-clinic and religio-psychiatric applicants who had been to physicians reported that they were told to see a psychiatrist, and of these only half were actually given the *name* of a psychiatrist or psychiatric clinic. Two-thirds of hospital-clinic applicants were told to see a psychiatrist, generally by the medical clinic of the same hospital in which the psychiatric clinic is located. Without this direct push they probably would never have entered the psychiatric system. In many ways, then, it is up to the nonpsychiatrist physicians to send patients to psychiatrists, and if we are to take applicants' present actions as indicating need of psychiatric treatment, the majority of physicians are not doing this job. A study of HIP patients and physicians, relying on records and interviews with patients and physicians, confirms this finding. Yet the medical orientation of the patients who first chose a physician means that even if not referred, after having been to a doctor they do tend to choose the psychotherapy system rather than the clergy or other healers. In conclusion, we may state that while going to a non-psychiatrist physician proved to be a direct route to psychiatry, it nevertheless took considerable travel from one physician to another until the move to psychiatry was taken.

As we pointed out, beginning with psychiatry is, aside from actually starting at a clinic, the shortest route to all psychiatric clinics except to the Religion and Psychiatry Institute. It is something of a false start for applicants to that clinic because the Institute is not well linked to psychiatry. Which brings us to the question, if psychiatry was the "right" choice for most applicants to begin with, why did they leave their former therapists and come to a clinic? This topic deserves special investigation.

❖ Why Applicants Left Their Last Psychotherapist

There are many reasons for leaving a therapist, not all of which are clear to the applicant even in retrospect. To surmount this difficulty, we gave all our respondents who had been to psychiatrists or psychologists a checklist of possible reasons for leaving, which included both voluntary and involuntary reasons. Among the involuntary ones was referral, although of course one may have asked to be referred. Voluntary reasons allowed for respondents to indicate a change in their self-evaluation, complaints about money, and complaints about the therapist himself. By giving a checklist and allowing for answers in a number of dimensions, we feel we obtained more truthful and meaningful answers. Table 21 shows how applicants to the three types of clinics compared in their answers.

Although, as we have seen, analytic-clinic applicants are more closely linked to the clinic via psychiatric sources, still only 30 per cent said they had left their previous therapist because they were referred elsewhere. It is interesting to note that the other reason involving action by the therapist rather than the patient ("He said I no longer needed treatment") is offered twice as frequently by hospital-clinic applicants. Therapists may have tended to dismiss these lower-class persons without a referral. The third involuntary category may reflect a rationalization, but it is true that higher-class persons, especially young professionals such as compose the analytic-clinic sample, are more likely to move about. Hence "he moved or I moved" is found more frequently among the clinics with wealthier clientele. Cross-tabulation of the reasons by social class confirms that moving is a more common reason among higher-class applicants.

Dissatisfaction with the therapist—indicated either covertly by saying that one's problem had changed and was no longer suitable for a particular therapist, or overtly by assenting to one of the two specific

TABLE 21   *Reasons for Leaving the Last Therapist: "Why Did You Leave (or Why Do You Want to Leave) the (Last) Psychiatrist or Psychologist? (Check All That Apply.)"*

Reason Checked or Offered	Analytic Clinics %	Religio-Psychiatric Clinic %	Hospital Clinic %
Involuntary reasons			
"He referred me elsewhere"	30	7	21
"He said I no longer needed treatment"	7	7	15
"He moved or I moved"	18	21	6
Other	1	0	2
Voluntary reasons			
"My problem was no longer suitable for a psychiatrist or psychologist"	15	32	21
"It was too expensive"	41	21	27
"He didn't help the problem" and/or "He didn't answer my questions"	26	32	21
Other	5	4	4
Total	(505)	(28)	(52)

complaints against therapists we allowed for—was less frequently a reason for leaving among analytic-clinic applicants, but was found among almost one-third of Religion and Psychiatry clinic applicants. The analytic applicants are again "closer" to psychiatry even before their application, while one reason for the religio-psychiatric clinic applicant's choice may be his dissatisfaction with orthodox psychiatry.

Money, of course, is the chief problem of analytic-clinic applicants. Either they cannot or will not pay the fees of private psychiatrists to whom they might otherwise go. Hence they are the chief complainers in this area. Money is less of a factor to religio-psychiatric applicants, because it is not the money involved which bothered them about therapy, and hospital-clinic applicants do not conceive of themselves as being able to pay for any medical treatment of long duration.

Aside from moving, reasons are *not* systematically related to applicants' background characteristics. Their class standing, for example, as measured by education and occupation does not relate to their complaints about money as a reason for leaving therapy, which again suggests that therapists are correct in saying that money does represent lots of things besides money. Of course, we do not have anyone really wealthy in our sample, and that might make a difference.

The most important determinant of reasons for having left a previous therapist is the nexus between applicant and therapy, that is, social position not in the world at large but in the therapy system. For example, we can make analytic-clinic applicants "look like" applicants to other clinics simply by sorting them according to the way they heard of the analytic clinic to which they are now applying. Those who heard of a clinic through psychiatric sources were more likely to say either that they had left the previous therapy because they had been referred elsewhere or because it was too expensive. In fact, they were probably referred because they felt they could not pay for private care. Those who heard of a clinic through friends were more likely to say that they had been dissatisfied with their previous therapist. One supposes that they had to rely upon their friends for a referral to a clinic for this very reason. Finally, those who heard about a clinic from other than these two sources were those most likely to say that they or the therapist had moved, that he was no good, or other voluntary reasons besides expense.

Persons closely linked to a clinic via psychiatry give reasons which do not reflect negatively on their previous relationship with psychiatry. Overt dissatisfaction is more apparent from those who came to a clinic via their friends. Covert as well as overt dissatisfaction are both more evident among those who come to a clinic less directly—neither from psychiatry nor from friends knowledgeable about psychiatry.

The determinants of reasons for leaving therapy appear to be like the general determinants of the entire pattern of previous care. The social institution of psychotherapy itself and the way one stands in relation to it are the major factors.

✵ Social Class, Social Distance, and Previous Therapy

The relationship between a clinic and other sources of treatment determines the type of applicants it receives. Generally, the reason analytic clinics receive better-educated applicants who are more likely to be members of the Friends is partly that these clinics receive more referrals from private psychiatrists. The social-class composition of clinics tells a good deal about their function. Clinics can become repositories for middle-class patients who do not want to pay the fees of private therapists, as the reasons for leaving prior therapists among analytic-clinic applicants suggest, or they may be places which receive discontented patients, which the data for the religio-psychiatric and hospital clinics seem to suggest. Clinics can also represent a *continuation* of therapy for those who, for various other reasons, were referred by their former therapists. One imagines that clinics, as well as the tax-paying public which supports many of them, would prefer this last function.

The number of previous sessions received by clinic applicants of different social-class standing is a good indicator of whether a clinic is receiving the failures of other therapists or acting as a natural continuation of therapy. Here we are talking not of the first therapist chosen, as we did before, but of the total amount of therapy received. As a cohort of persons moves from one therapist to another through some of the complex paths we described, the original predominance of higher-class persons decreases. The better-educated and wealthier more quickly find what they want and can afford to pay for it; the less advantaged are forced to move on. In fact, we know that lower-class persons are much more prone to drop out of therapy, even when cost is not a factor, as in clinics. It stands to reason then, that the weaker the link between a clinic and other sources of psychotherapy, the more likely that its lower-class applicants have had appreciable amounts of previous therapy. Because of their social distance from other sources of therapy, some clinics may draw applicants who are themselves socially distant from therapy.

Analysis of applicants to the Religion and Psychiatry Institute in 1958 showed that the clinic indeed received lower-class applicants who had failed in previous therapy.[3] The clinic had at that time even less connection with psychiatric sources than it had in 1959 and 1960 when further data were collected. Hence all who had been to therapists previously came to the clinic strictly on their own without a referral. This lack of continuity with previous therapy insured a higher proportion of those who had not gotten along in therapy or had not found what they wanted as opposed to those who simply ran out of money. By the way, money seems more of a factor to higher-class persons who first think in terms of private therapy than it does to lower-class persons who did not consider private therapy and have gone mainly to clinics.

In the clinics in our 1959 and 1960 sample there is only a small association between social class and having been to a psychiatrist, psychologist, or social welfare or counseling agency, a fact congruent with the hypothesis that the number of higher-class persons who go to psychiatrists decreases as patients travel from one therapist to another. In the analysis that follows, education will be used as an indicator of social class. Education is the most sensitive of the class indicators for our present purposes since it measures patient interest, acceptability of a patient to a therapist, and the amount of money a patient has. Most important, it is a good measure of the amount of social distance between therapist and patient. The total number of sessions of therapy attended, whether given by psychiatrists (the large majority), psychologists, or counselors will be used to measure the amount of previous therapy a person has had—grouped as none, one to twenty sessions, and over twenty sessions.

There is indeed a small positive relationship (Tau $\beta = .10$) between high education and more previous sessions of therapy for applicants to both analytic and hospital clinics, as we might have predicted from the clinics' links to psychiatry. The religio-psychiatric clinic has improved its position since 1958 (when there were *no* referrals from psychiatrists in our sample of 110). Now there is only a negligible negative association (Tau $\beta = -.02$) between education and the number of previous sessions among its applicants.

More interesting is the fact that the pattern of relationships between education and the number of previous sessions of therapy closely follows our predictions when the link between clinic and prior therapist is taken into account: a good link means that better-educated applicants had more therapy, and a poor link means that *less*-educated applicants had more therapy. The relationships remain small and are generally not statistically significant in each individual case, but their pattern is suggestive and does match our prediction. The last source of information about the clinic is divided into three—psychiatric sources, friends or relatives, and other sources. If a person heard about the clinic from psychiatric sources or from his friends, then among *both* religio-psychiatric and analytic-clinic applicants there is a *positive* relationship between the number of previous sessions and level of edu-

TABLE 22 *Tau Beta between Education (Grammar School, Some High School, Some College, College Graduate, and Postgraduate) and Previous Number of Sessions (None, 1-20, 21 or More)*

| | Source of Information about Clinic | | |
	From Psychiatry	*From Friends*	*Other*
Analytic clinics			
Tau β	.09	.07	.00
S.D.	(2.0)	(1.48)	–
N	(432)	(295)	(132)
Religio-psychiatric			
Tau β	.15	.13	−.10
S.D.	(.58)	(1.16)	(1.14)
N	(13)	(61)	(101)
Hospital clinics			
Tau β	.18	−.04	.05
S.D.	(1.04)	(−.21)	(.55)
N	(26)	(20)	(77)

cation, that is, high education means more previous therapy. Other sources of information about the clinic result in a *negative* relationship for religio-psychiatric applicants between education and prior therapy, and no such relationship among analytic-clinic applicants. That is, when there was a positive link to the clinic—and either psychiatric sources or friends who are "fans" of the clinic count as positive links —then higher-class persons are the ones who appear to have had more therapy. The "other" links are weaker and in fact still predominated in 1960 among religio-psychiatric clinic applicants, thus accounting for the slight over-all relationship in that clinic between *low* class and previous therapy. Psychiatric links to hospital clinics also produce a positive relationship between previous therapy and high education. If friends were the source of referral to hospital clinics then there is only a slight likelihood that poorly educated applicants will have had more therapy. The reverse is true of other ways of hearing about hospital clinics for among them there is a slight likelihood that better-educated applicants will have had more therapy. These other ways include the hospital's own medical clinics which are, of course, a direct link. Friends and relatives can hardly be "fans" of hospital clinics in the same way that they are of the religio-psychiatric and analytic clinics. Thus, even the exceptions among hospital clinic applicants seem to suggest the importance of the quality of the link between past therapy and the present clinic. The poorer the link, the more likely that the original relationship between high class and psychotherapy disappears or is even reversed. Given the present state of psychiatry, any lack of the expected relationship between past therapy and higher class is a sign that a clinic is getting patients who were either disgruntled or who otherwise could not get along in therapy. But this statement needs to be qualified.

One more important factor influences the flow of former psychiatric patients to clinics. To begin therapy again a former patient must be motivated to do so. Willingness to make financial sacrifices is associated with going to still another psychotherapist, as well as with going to one in the first place. Therefore, only among those who are less motivated do we find the "natural" association of high class with previous therapy. As Table 23 shows, the trend is even reversed among those with high motivation. Less educated persons who are highly motivated have indeed not only been to therapists but have the courage to try again. These unusual lower-class persons are of course an exception to the rule that a great deal of previous therapy among lower-class clinic applicants is a sign of failure in therapy. Not surprisingly, these findings about class and motivation apply more to private psychiatrists previously visited than to public or clinic facilities.

When all these factors are put together—education, previous therapy, motivation, and source of information about the clinic, we can

TABLE 23 *Per Cent Who Had Previously Been to a Psychotherapist*

Level of Education	Number of Sacrifices Willing to Make to Pay for Therapy			
	None %	*1* %	*2* %	*3 or More* %
Some high school	35	60	77	87
High-school graduate	39	50	65	77
Some college	40	76	66	79
College graduate	71	61	46	82
Postgraduate	63	70	62	68
	Number of Cases			
	17	62	22	8
	13	91	37	17
	15	98	44	29
	7	62	39	23
	8	50	37	25

clearly specify the conditions under which lower-class patients with a good deal of previous therapy tend to pile up in clinics. Motivation affects our story in the following way. Relatively poor motivation yields two "natural" associations: (1) *high* class is associated with a good deal of therapy among those with *good* links to analytic clinics (psychiatrists and Friends, and (2) *low* class is associated with a good deal of therapy among those with *poor* links to the clinics (other sources).*

Relatively *high* motivation tends to cancel out these "natural" relationships, as Table 24 shows. Therefore, our statement about class, previous therapy, and links to clinics must be modified as follows: Given the present state of psychiatry, a lack of relationship between high education and previous therapy *among applicants who are less than highly motivated* is a sign that a clinic is getting disgruntled or otherwise unsuccessful therapy "retreads."

The unhappy retread business takes up a good deal of clinic time among all clinics in our sample. But one's attitude toward this characteristic of clinic applicants may vary. For example, in the years when most of the field work was done at the religio-psychiatric clinic the chief psychiatrist delighted in picking up lower-class applicants who had not done well elsewhere. He felt that providing help "at the end of the line" was an important function for a religiously oriented clinic. These sorts of patients are very expensive to deal with. Since they are less motivated as well as being poor, they not only pay little

* We have too few cases to test this with other types of clinics.

TABLE 24 *Relationship (Tau β) between Education (HSG vs. College) and Number of Previous Sessions for Applicants to Analytic Clinics*

Number of Sacrifices Willing to Make to Pay for Therapy	Last Source of Information about the Clinic		
	From Psychiatry	From Friends	Other
One or none			
Tau β	.27	.14	.03
S.D.	3.15	1.57	.25
N	(176)	(146)	(68)
Two or more			
Tau β	.00	.06	.01
S.D.	.02	.46	.06
N	(131)	(95)	(44)

but also tend to drop out in any case. In later years, beginning in 1959, the Religion and Psychiatry Institute changed its fee policy because of financial exigencies, and fewer of these types of persons applied. And in general, most training clinics do not accept persons with a good deal of previous therapy, unless they come highly recommended by a psychotherapist associated with the clinic.

✿ Summary and Conclusion

In this chapter we looked at the psychotherapy system and saw that most people have already entered the therapy system by the time of their application. Their present application is not so much a product of their own personal characteristics and actions but of their position in the therapy system of psychiatric clinics. Most of this book shows how the individual characteristics of clinic applicants and the social circles to which they belong influence the way they go about deciding to enter therapy. Here we showed how the institutional structure of medicine, psychiatry, and psychotherapy play a vital role in preserving the original decision and in structuring the paths to psychiatric clinics as well as being a factor in determining the quality of applicants.

Four separate but related studies of past choices of clinic applicants were undertaken. The first one showed how the first choice of professional is indeed related to the social circle of an applicant, to his motivation to pay for psychotherapy, and only to a small extent to the nature of his problems. The second study investigated the paths applicants followed once they had made their initial choice of professional. These paths were not dependent upon the characteristics of the applicant but on the starting point they had chosen and on the clinic to which they eventually applied. Beginning with a clergyman means that unless one goes to a Religion and Psychiatry Institute, many more steps must be taken before an application to a psychiatric clinic is made. Beginning with psychotherapy is of course a direct route to a psychiatric clinic. Psychiatry sends practically no one to see other professionals but the movement from counseling to psychiatry is quite strong, and generally takes place even before a person's present application to a psychiatric clinic. Medicine is closely connected with psychiatry, but does seem to hold on to its patients until they eventually go to psychotherapists. Most of them went *not* because they were sent to psychiatrists by their physicians but because psychiatry seemed the "natural" choice after nonpsychiatric medicine.

The third study concerned the reasons patients gave for leaving their former therapists. Those for whom the clinic represents a continuation of former treatment gave expense and referral by their former therapist as their reasons for leaving. Those who found a clinic through the lay referral system were more often overtly dissatisfied with their previous therapy. Others were not as likely to complain about expense but indicated either covert or overt disapproval of their last experience. Once more, the nature of the therapy system itself, especially the nature of the links between one part and another, determines the reasons given for leaving former therapists. Individual characteristics of respondents are less important.

The last study was an attempt to evaluate the consequences of this rather extensive travel from one professional to another which characterizes clinic applicants. In one sense, all professionals previously seen failed: if their patients had been satisfied they would not have applied for more treatment. Yet experience is a teacher of sorts. Previously we showed that those who had had more therapy before applying to a clinic "learned" what were the "right" problems to have. Unsatisfactory choices in the past might suggest to applicants what they really want. Finally, not all changes are failures. Going from a once-a-week therapist to a daily psychoanalyst might represent a promotion.

Generally, a lack of association between high education and a good deal of previous therapy means that clinics are receiving the failures of other therapists, since the better educated, who are more numerous candidates for therapy to begin with, tend to be better patients and to remain in therapy, rather than going from one therapist to another.

There are other factors, however. First, a direct link between former therapist and present clinic generally represents a continuation of therapy rather than an interruption. Some referrals even represent a "promotion" into analytic treatment, since "pull" by one's former therapist gives applicants to some analytic clinics a distinctly better chance of being accepted. Second, high motivation to continue may mean that more lower-class applicants who might otherwise drop out of treatment and not try to get further help will continue to seek therapy. We found that if the links are poor and the motivation low, then failures in previous therapy tend to come to clinics. This finding matches the conclusions one might draw from the reasons patients themselves gave for leaving former therapists. Failures constitute only the minority of analytic-clinic applicants but the majority of Religion and Psychiatry and hospital-clinic applicants. Again, whether or not the clinic receives "good" or "bad" applicants depends on its position in the therapy system.

Our sample of clinics is skewed in favor of the analytic clinics, since they represent more closely the private practice of psychotherapy. On the basis of our data, however, we might guess that most of the public facilities for outpatient mental care are receiving the failures of other therapists, rather than patients who come for a continuation of former treatment. This may well represent half the load of applicants to public facilities in a big city such as New York. Taking in other people's dirty linen is always a nasty business, and might be a dubious role for public facilities. On the other hand, some place must represent the end of the line. We doubt whether public clinics at present really have the funds, the motivation, or the capacity to serve as that "end of the line," though performing that function may be an important public service.

NOTES

1. Karl Menninger, *Theory of Psychoanalytic Technique* (New York: Basic Books, 1958), p. 32 (author's italics).
2. All reciprocal relations are measured with Tau β. All asymmetrical relations are measured with Sommers' d. Tau β is the geometric mean of the Sommers' d when the d yx and d xy are averaged. Tau β is identical to Phi which is identical with Pearson R for the case of fourfold tables. In Chart XIX, occupation of breadwinner was divided into professional and executive, semi-professional, white collar, and blue collar and service. Education was measured as eighth grade, some high school, high-school graduate, some college, college graduate, and post graduate. Membership in the Friends and Supporters was dichotomized. Since rank correlation measures are used, partial correlations cannot be calculated by the usual means, and tables must be actually partitioned according to the values of the third variable, and the association between the two variables must be actually measured for each table created by partitioning the third variable.
3. Kadushin, "Social Distance Between Client and Professional," *American Journal of Sociology*, LXVII (1962), 517-531. Contrary to expectation, this clinic's lower-class patients were more likely to have had therapy than its higher-class patients. Higher-class patients came for reasons related to the religion and psychiatry movement, but lower-class patients came because they had failed in previous therapy but nonetheless felt they still needed help.

From Bartenders to Psychiatrists: Images of the Professions

✹

10

In the last chapter we analyzed the various paths taken by applicants through the maze of professions on the way to a clinic. In this chapter we look at the residuals of this experience: the images applicants have of the range of alternative sources of help. Though images of the world of professions are shaped by one's experiences with practitioners, actual previous visits to a professional tend to understate the variety of healing agents persons considered as possible sources of help. The fact that a Christian Science practitioner was at least considered by applicants to a psychiatric clinic means that the present choice of a more conventional profession was not automatic. In fact, 5 per cent of analytic-clinic and 18 per cent of Religion and Psychiatry Institute applicants at one time or another considered going to a religious healer. We need therefore to understand the determinants and consequences not only of the actual choice applicants made but also their fantasy choices. These fantasies, some of which are more fantastic than others, will prove the best way of ascertaining the image of the professional world harbored by clinic applicants.

In order to ascertain the fantasy choices of the clinic applicants we tried the usual attitude questions about professionals. Some of these questions were selected because they had been used in other surveys which could then be used as a source of comparative data. We found, however, that our sample was too heterogeneous to make the same questions meaningful to all respondents. Questions which hospital-clinic applicants did not even understand were considered silly by the very sophisticated analytic-clinic applicants. The answers therefore did not scale very well or lend themselves to meaningful analysis. Yet when applicants did respond in terms of actual professions they had considered going to, interesting and meaningful results ensued.

First, we shall check on the size of the vote for these fantasy alternatives. Then, we shall show what types of professionals are more instituted than others—which are more firmly anchored in real choices. We will also want to know which professions applicants thought best as well as the social characteristics of those who made various types of choices. Then, we will chart some which show how professions are related to each other, and we will conclude by showing how these pictures affect the choice of clinic.

❀ The Size of the Vote

Applicants to psychiatric clinics were presented with these instructions for filling out a checklist of professions:

> Here is a list of places people sometimes go to with problems. Check below those places you have ever *considered* going to yourself—whether or not you actually went there.

Some thirty-one items followed, ranging from police to psychiatrist to bartender. The items were grouped in the following way:*

Psychiatry	Cultist
Mental hygiene clinic	Spiritualists
Psychiatric clinic	Hypnotists
Psychiatrist	Yoga
Psychoanalyst	Theosophy
Psychologist	Astrologist
Mental hospital	Fortune Teller

* They were not presented in this fashion in the questionnaire, however. See Appendix for exact order. Items written in by respondents were fitted into the appropriate category.

Medicine
  Doctor
  General hospital

Counseling
  Social service agency
  Welfare department
  Social worker
  Vocational guidance center
  Alcoholics Anonymous

Clergy
  Minister, priest, rabbi

Healing
  Christian Science practitioners
  Other religious practitioners

Law
  Lawyer
  Police

Social Improvement
  Dale Carnegie or other person-
    ality training program
  Dance studio
  Friendship club
  Marriage broker or introduction
    center

Mass Media
  Radio, TV, newspaper advice
    programs or columns

Chiropractic, etc.
  Chiropractors

Bartenders, miscellaneous

Items were administered as "split halves," that is, the list was split in two, turned around and presented to half the respondents in an opposite order so as to minimize the chance that the first items on the long list would be checked more often than items lower on the list. Table 25 shows the per cent who checked one or more items in each category.

Obviously, with the exception of a few "no answers," almost all who

TABLE 25 *The Size of the Vote: Per Cent Who Considered Different Institutions*

Institutions Considered	Analytic Clinics %	Religio- Psychiatric Clinic %	Hospital Clinics %
Psychiatry	95	76	73
Medicine	41	49	64
Counseling	40	30	33
Clergy	22	57	36
Social improvement	17	22	12
Cultist	12	10	13
Mass media	7	10	7
Legal	7	14	14
Healing	5	18	4
Chiropractic, etc.	3	2	6
Bartenders, miscellaneous	2	3	7
Average number	2.5	2.9	2.7
Number	(1118)	(199)	(135)

applied to an analytic clinic said they had considered psychiatry. Not so with the Religion and Psychiatry Institute and hospital clinics, however, where only 75 per cent had considered psychiatry. But how can one apply somewhere without having considered it? One answer to this seeming inconsistency is that not everyone who applies to the Religion and Psychiatry Institute, as we shall later see, views it as a psychiatric organization. Many see it as a religious one; hence, almost 60 per cent of those applying there said they considered clergy as a resource. Almost all those not considering psychiatry had considered clergy. Similarly, many applying to a hospital clinic see it as a medical institution. Over 60 per cent said they had considered medicine. Both these choices are much less frequent in clinics that do not "specialize" in either religion or medicine. Counseling and welfare services are considered by 30 per cent or so—about the same frequency as medicine among analytic-clinic applicants, and less frequent than medicine among applicants to other clinics. Counseling, medicine and the clergy, then, are the main professions which are perceived as direct alternatives to psychiatry—the same four which were actually the chief prior choices of applicants.

Other professions lag behind these big four. Yet surprisingly popular are various social improvement devices such as dance studios, personality improvement courses, and introduction centers; they are considered by about 15 to 20 per cent of clinic applicants. The cultists, mass media advice columns, legal services (conventional choice for persons with marital problems), religious healers, chiropractors and bartenders round out the list with popularities running from about 2 to 10 per cent of clinic applicants. The point is not that so few considered these professions, but that among psychiatric-clinic applicants, *any* of these offbeat channels of help were considered at all.[1]

❂ The Established Professions

Because an applicant had considered a professional does not mean he had actually visited him, although there is a high correlation between considering a professional and going to him. The percentage of persons who actually visited the type of professional they had considered is a measure of the degree to which a particular profession is instituted, that is, socially entrenched as "the thing to do." If persons consider a religious healer but do not actually visit one, then such a professional is not well instituted. Table 26 shows a ranking of professions according to the proportion who visited them among those who had considered that source.

Among analytic-clinic applicants, psychiatry and medicine are equally instituted; over two-thirds of those who had considered these professions

TABLE 26 *Instituted Rank of Sources of Treatment* (Per Cent of Those Considering It Who Had Actually Gone, Beginners Excluded)*

Rank Order	Analytic Clinics	%	Religio-Psychiatric Clinic	%	Hospital Clinics	%
1	Psychiatry	69	Medicine	76	Medicine	83
2	Medicine	66	Clergy	66	Chiropractic	63
3	Counseling	47	Psychiatry	54	Psychiatry	60
4	Clergy	34	Law	42	Clergy	58
5	Chiropractic	14	Counseling	25	Counseling	55
6	Law	13	Chiropractic	25	Bartenders	50
7	Cultist	8	Bartenders	25	Cultist	33
8	Bartenders	6	Healer	25	Healer	17
9	Social improvement	5	Social improvement	20	Law	16
10	Healer	5	Cultist	17	Social improvement	6

*Mass media omitted, since these were not tabulated as a profession which could be visited or consulted.

had actually visited them. (Psychiatry, of course, is really 100 per cent instituted in our sample, since all are now applying to a psychiatric clinic. To minimize this effect, only persons who had actually been elsewhere before are included in the figures.) Counseling and clergy then follow. There is a sharp gap again between these "big four" and the rest of the professions. At best, only about 15 per cent who even considered them went to them; at worst, the figure drops to 5 per cent.

The picture among religio-psychiatric and hospital-clinic applicants is radically different. Medicine is the best instituted profession among applicants to both types of clinics. Psychiatry is third on the list. The aura of medicine carries over to the paramedical professions such as chiropractic among hospital-clinic applicants. Clergymen are given as high a rating among religio-psychiatric applicants as are doctors among analytic-clinic applicants. Their rating is quite high among hospital-clinic applicants as well. In general, the less popular professions are given higher ratings among applicants to nonanalytic clinics. That is, if applicants to nonanalytic clinics had considered these more offbeat professions, then the chances are greater that they had actually visited them. Analytic-clinic applicants are more focused in the range of professions instituted among them. Other applicants are more catholic in their tastes.

Among all these professions medicine is in a somewhat different position. First the popularity of "doctor" as a place considered is highly affected by its position on the list. When "doctor" was placed further down the list on one of the split-half forms, 20 per cent fewer checked it. This is the only profession so affected. Further, when "doctor" was placed further down the list, only half of those who had actually been to see a doctor checked "doctor" as a place they considered. But 90 per cent of those who visited clergymen indeed checked them as a place they had considered, regardless of whether "minister, priest, rabbi" was high or low on the list. "Doctor" and medicine are apparently so well instituted that they elicit an "oh, yes" or "of course" sort of response; yet persons do not spontaneously think of them. They are in the peculiar position of being so well entrenched that they are taken for granted.

❀ Who Is Fairest?

A final measure of the status of a profession among those who are seeking help for emotional problems is the proportion of applicants who think that the profession "can do the most good for people with problems like your own." Applicants were asked to select the three best places from the checklist provided. The opinion they expressed is, of course, a different matter from actual visits to a professional. In fact, simply *because* they have visited a certain type of professional, applicants may now feel him *ill*-equipped to help them.

Psychiatry was thought best by 99 per cent of those applying to analytic clinics—hardly surprising in view of their present choice. But psychiatry was *not* thought best by all who applied to other types of clinics. Thirteen per cent of those applying to the religio-psychiatric and 20 per cent of those applying to hospital clinics did *not* list psychiatry as one of the three best sources of help. Instead, almost half of religio-psychiatric applicants said they thought clergymen were among the three best, and one-third of hospital-clinic applicants said doctors were best. Only 10 per cent of analytic-clinic applicants shared these opinions. The last member of the "big four," counseling and welfare sources, does not do very well in any setting. Between 10 and 20 per cent of clinic applicants list such sources as among the three best ones. In short, analytic-clinic applicants view former choices and other professions considered as a mistake; applicants to other clinics are not so sure that professions other than psychiatry are useless.

This point of view is reflected in the legitimacy accorded to the various professions considered, for one can consider a profession and try it out without thinking it best for solving one's problems. A profession is "legitimate" in solving mental problems if those who considered it thought it actually among the three best. Despite the fact that not everyone had considered psychiatry, and not everyone who had considered it actually had previously been to a psychiatric source, between 95 and 99 per cent of those who considered psychiatry thought it among the three best sources. And this is true of all types of clinics. This means that even among applicants to religio-psychiatric and hospital clinics, if a person viewed the clinic as a psychiatric institution, he then thought psychiatry the best source of help for him.

Second and third places in legitimacy are especially interesting. Among analytic-clinic applicants there is an enormous gap between psychiatry in first place, with 99 per cent of those who considered it thinking it best, and second place, with 30 per cent of those considering clergymen thinking *them* best. Other professions are also in this lower range— from 23 and 22 per cent for counseling and medicine, respectively, to only 4 per cent of those who considered the mass media thinking them best. The situation is quite different for religio-psychiatric and hospital-clinic applicants. True, psychiatry is in first place by a wide margin, but other professions are given considerably more legitimacy than analytic-clinic applicants are prepared to grant. Clergy are in second place among religio-psychiatric applicants (63 per cent of those who considered them thought them best), closely followed by counseling and, surprisingly, by religious healers! Medicine is ninth on the list: only 16 per cent of those who considered it thought it among the three best. Another surprise is that hospital-clinic applicants also place clergy in second place (with 55 per cent) and drop medicine to third place, for only 42 per cent think it best.

In sum, analytic-clinic applicants are consistent: first, they have primarily considered psychiatry, and even though they may have considered or tried other sources they do not think such places can help them. This finding matches their actual behavior in being most likely to begin with psychiatry. Applicants to other types of clinics are generally similar to analytic-clinic applicants in the *range* of possible healing professions considered, except for clergy and medicine. Applicants to the religio-psychiatric and hospital clinics are not as completely sold on psychiatry, however, as their counterparts applying to analytic clinics. If psychiatry fails them, they may well try professions that psychiatry might consider offbeat. Perhaps their grant of legitimacy to other professions explains their choice of a clinic not so intimately linked to psychiatry.

Are the images of the various professions merely afterthoughts and rationalizations made after the choice of a clinic? We think not, for among those who had never been to any professional previously, the same factors which produce the choice of a particular type of clinic are also related to considering different types of institutions in general. Applicants seem to have different "world views" which lead both to considering different types of institutions to solve their problems and to acting in different ways. For example, the social-class–education–membership-in-the-Friends axis of background characteristics correlates, among "beginners," with professions considered. The better educated, higher class and more sophisticated were more likely to have considered psychiatry but the less favored were more likely to have considered medicine, the clergy, and the various offbeat professions. Since members of the Friends and the more educated are more likely to apply to analytic clinics, this does seem to match the general picture of analytic-clinic applicants as compared to those applying to other clinics. And the picture is borne out by the data on the first professional consulted among those who actually had been to other professionals.

The major difference between analytic-clinic applicants and those applying to the Religion and Psychiatry Institute is not social *class*, but social *circle*, especially as linked with non-insider occupations and religious Protestants. It is the religious beginners who considered the clergy, and even with religiousness taken into account, non-Jews in general were more likely to consider the clergy. Differences between clinics thus seem to be caused by the factors which produce choice of clinic rather than by the consequences of having made the choice.

These same findings occur when the degree to which professions are instituted is measured. The less sophisticated in all clinics rank medicine even above psychiatry. Non-Jews and especially religious persons in general grant much higher rank to the clergy. And the same occurs for those professions considered best.

Views of the professions are associated with making decisions in the first place rather than merely being a rationalization of the decision.

❂ Applicants' Map of the Professions

By calling some types of professionals "offbeat," at least from some persons' point of view, we are not only implying a value judgment but are grouping professions into categories. It certainly seems that some professions ought to "go together" in contrast to others which are quite different. Clergymen and psychotherapists both engage in "talk." Medicine and chiropractic have in common a physical view of problems. One can continue to attempt a classification of professions on *a priori* grounds. But it does seem from the data just presented that applicants have their own ideas about what professions belong together in the same category. Since the average applicant considered between two and three professional areas, we can see whether applicants who considered one profession also considered another related one. By grouping together those professions which were likely to be chosen by the same persons we can gain some understanding of applicants' views on which professions go together. Moreover, we would like some measure of how far counseling is from, say, psychiatry. Is it felt to be quite similar to psychiatry or much more like the clergy?

A recent development called "nonmetric multidimensional scaling"[2] makes it possible to give answers to these questions when the data consist of items such as ours. For we do not wish to assume that we can *measure* how similar medicine and psychiatry are as compared to psychiatry and the clergy, but merely that one pair is closer together than the other pair. We do not know exactly *how much* closer. The logic of the procedure is quite simple. We wish to depict our eleven types of professions on a chart in such a way that the distances between them correspond to the rank order of their similarity to one another. That is, if medicine is more highly correlated with the choice of psychiatry than it is with choosing clergymen, then the point which represents psychiatry should be closer to the point which represents medicine than to the one representing the clergy. An analogous problem would be to reconstruct the map of a given area when presented only with a table of the distances of its cities from each other. Maps, of course, are drawn in two dimensions but when we try to group professions we are not limited to two dimensions, for applicants may have had more than two criteria in mind when they considered the professions.*

Let us see how well we can arrange the 55 correlations between the 11 professions with the aid of this technique. Figure 1 shows the result if two dimensions are chosen. The figure at the bottom which indicates "stress = .20" shows us how well we have been able to meet the objective of arranging the points so that the distances between them correspond to the rank order of the 55 correlations. A figure of .20 is said to be poor, .10 is fair, .05 is good and .00 is perfect.[3] But these criteria have been developed with physical properties in mind, not social-science material. Our configuration of points is poor largely because considering a healing profession is indeed more complex than merely the two considerations which a configuration of two dimensions implies. But this is always the case in survey research—our data are always an approximation and we are happy if we can do as well as "poor" and yet, more important, have a configuration whose meaning we can understand. Most social-science applications of this technique have stresses similar to those shown in our data.

This brings us to the question of meaning and interpreting the two dimensions we have chosen to depict the configuration. The important thing about the configuration is *not* the axis or dimensions, for they are quite arbitrary. Given the placement of the points in the plane we

---

* Since the map problem just given seems so easy, the reader who thinks he can easily solve it might try to arrange 11 or so cities in the fashion suggested. He had better save the task for a very long ocean trip, however, for he'll probably be at the task for several years and still be unsuccessful! Fortunately, along with the theory of multidimensional scaling comes a computer program to do the work. (Yes, we have tried the program on the map problem—it works!)

Figure 1   *Total Sample Configuration of Institutions Considered†*

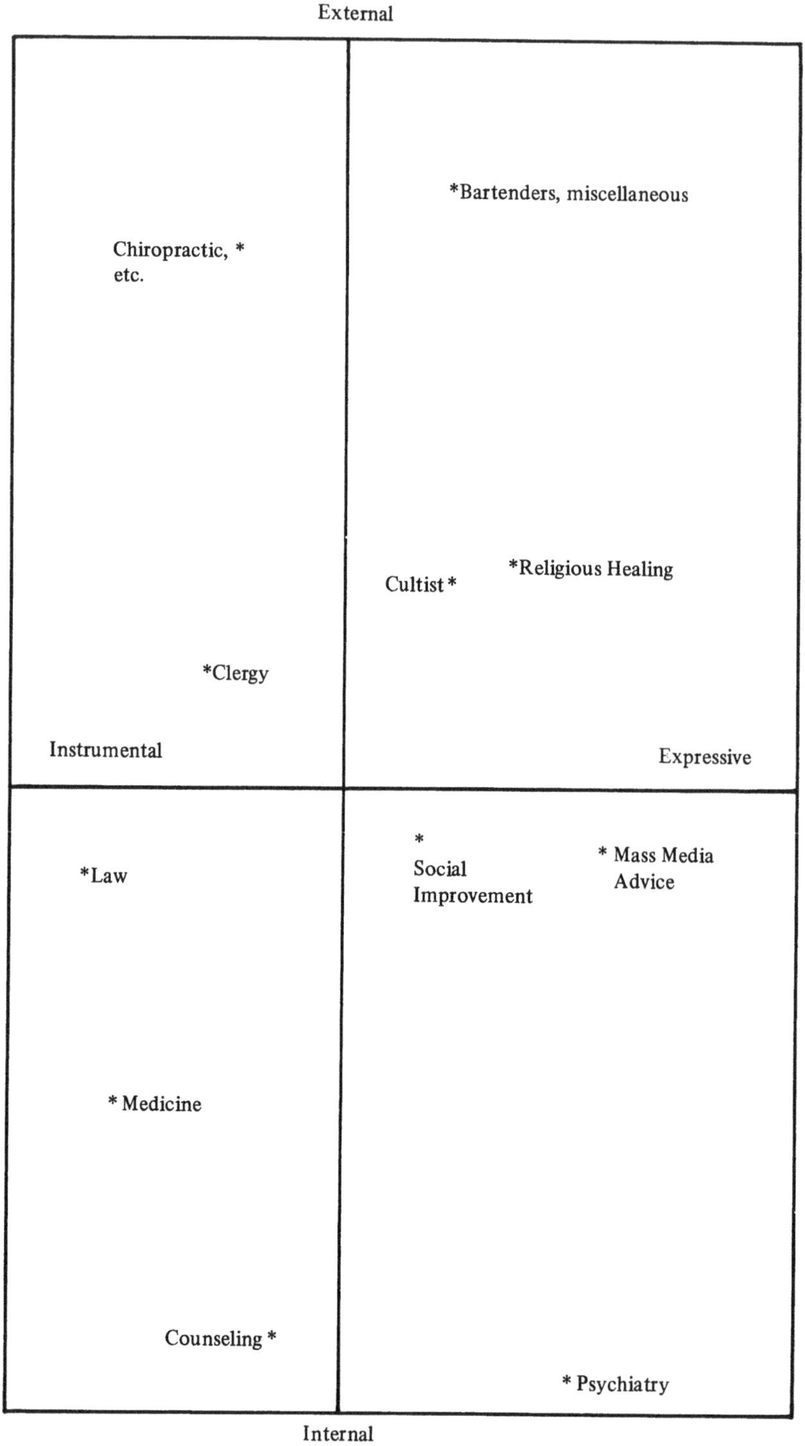

External

Chiropractic, *
etc.

*Bartenders, miscellaneous

Cultist *   *Religious Healing

*Clergy

Instrumental   Expressive

*Law

*
Social   * Mass Media
Improvement   Advice

* Medicine

Counseling *

* Psychiatry

Internal

†stress = .20

could draw the lines anywhere we wanted to. The aim in drawing axes is to display the points in a way which most easily leads to "understanding" of the configuration. To avoid complete subjectivity in performing this transformation, we used what is known as a "normalized Varimax rotation."[4] In this system a computer attempts to place the axes, at right angles to each other, in such a way that they account for as much of the variance of the points from the axis as possible. A varimax rotation tends to place a few points near each axis with the other points quite removed. It thus becomes possible to "understand" the configuration by noting what sorts of points have been placed near one axis but far from another. In our charts we have also "reflected" the axis to make sure that the same orientation in space is preserved for each chart. The important thing to remember is that the axes are *our* "invention" and are not "inherent" in the data. Only the *relationship* of one point to another is determined by the data. And that relationship is further dependent on the number of axes *we choose* to use to depict the relationships.

With this word of caution and explanation, let us see what the configuration in two dimensions for our total sample seems to indicate. The lower righthand corner shows psychiatry in splendid isolation. It is quite distant from other points. It is different. The point nearest to it is counseling, which in turn is not too far from the traditional professions of medicine, law and the clergy. On the other hand, clergy is fairly close to a cluster composed of less traditional healing professions: cultists, religious healers, social improvement agencies such as Dale Carnegie, and mass media advice columns. Chiropractors are "out in left field," and bartenders and the like are in the outer pastures on the right. This picture seems to make intuitive sense.

The placement and interpretation of the axes is an attempt to explain analytically why the picture appears sensible. The location of religious healers and mass media at one end of the horizontal axis and law at the other end suggests that what separates them is an instrumental-expressive continuum. The instrumental professions are those whose emphasis is on objectivity and on "getting things done." The expressive ones are those which emphasize the more emotional and experimental aspects of life.

The other axis can be said to represent an internal-external dimension. Thus, psychiatry is most concerned with the inner man, but chiropractors and bartenders with his external appearance.[5]

Use of these axes helps to explain the way the professions are grouped. From the point of view of a person with problems who seeks solutions for them, psychiatry, mass media, religious healers, and to a lesser degree, cultists, bartenders and social improvement agencies, focus more on emotional expression than on instrumental manipulation. But psychiatry is much more internal and relevant to the "psyche," while social improvement, mass media, advice columns, cultists, religious healers and so on deal more with manipulation of appearance and with action in the environment. Bartenders and the like are most external, and most different from other sources of help. Psychiatry is most concerned with integration of the self. Counseling is almost as internal a concern as psychiatry, but it is more instrumental, although not as much so as law. This is reasonable since counseling is supposed to be more concerned with "reality" problems. Medicine too is clearly instrumental; it deals with cause and effect. Of the professions in the lower lefthand box, counseling is most internal, medicine less so, and law the least. And the same order holds for these three on the expressive and instrumental dimension. Yet all are concerned with maintaining the basic personality patterns of an individual, hence they are grouped together. Clergy, almost as expressive as counseling, is more concerned with the exterior than even law.

All this is presented from the point of view of the sample as a whole. The reader may "disagree" with this clustering which is empirically derived. Let us now look at a group of persons who may be more like the average reader—applicants to analytic clinics. Things look different from their point of view (see Figure 2).

Psychiatry is even more isolated than before. We saw that psychiatry was practically the only profession completely instituted and legitimated among analytic-clinic applicants. It does indeed stand alone. But compared to the view of the sample as a whole, psychiatry is seen as much more instrumental—much further removed from religious healing and the like, and much more akin to the traditional liberal professions which emphasize "scientific" and rational approaches. Counseling is seen as much more expressive and also less internal—perhaps the Freudian's view of "superficial" marriage counseling! And the clergy, as one might expect from the rather low esteem in which they are held by analytic-clinic applicants, have been removed from the proximity of law and medicine and placed closer to mass media advice and religious healing. To these persons, the clergy are more like "quacks" in the field of mental health.

The "quacks" themselves—cultists, mass media advice, and religious healers—are more or less grouped together in the quadrant representing expressiveness and externalism, as indeed they are seen by all types of applicants. As we pointed out, even clergymen and counselors are placed by analytic-clinic applicants in this same general area. Perhaps this lack of differentiation is caused by their not really caring or thinking about anything but psychiatry. Bartenders and chiropractors are again placed in "left field," but this time bartenders are seen as furthest away from the expressive "quacks," whereas chiropractors are more expressive and the most external.

Figure 2 *Analytic Clinics Configuration of Institutions Considered†*

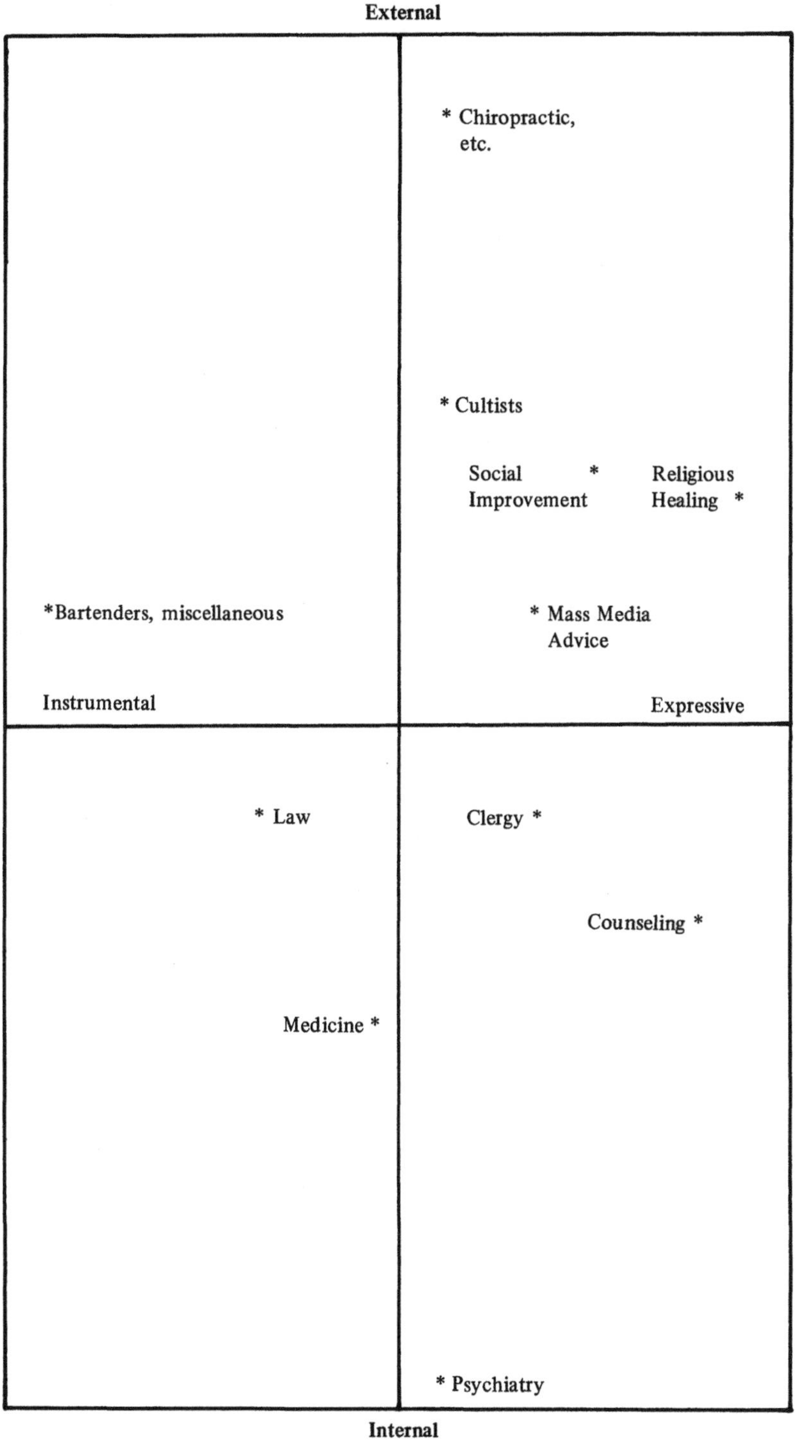

External

* Chiropractic,
  etc.

* Cultists

Social   *   Religious
Improvement   Healing *

*Bartenders, miscellaneous   * Mass Media
                                           Advice

Instrumental   Expressive

* Law   Clergy *

                              Counseling *

Medicine *

* Psychiatry

Internal

† stress = .1 5
  Origin moved to x = −.2

These views are, of course, just what might seem reasonable to expect from "psychocentric" analytic-clinic applicants.

Religio-psychiatric applicants have still another point of view (see Figure 3). They group the clergy tightly together with the liberal professions of law and medicine, and at the other extreme from cultists, healing, mass media, and social improvement. This is somewhat surprising in view of the religion and psychiatry movement. One might have thought these applicants would view the ministry as expressive along with religious healing. But not so. Analysis of data previously collected[6] shows that more religio-psychiatric applicants who had consulted with clergymen before applying to the clinic had initially expected them to be instrumental, and that this expectation was confirmed by the treatment they received. Moreover, these persons grant clergymen high prestige, and this is reflected by grouping them with the traditional liberal professions. Psychiatry is seen as much more expressive—and this too matched previous detailed interviews on expectations concerning psychiatrists by applicants to the Religion and Psychiatry Institute. Psychiatry is also somewhat less differentiated from other healing professions. Counseling is felt to be more "inner" even than psychiatry—perhaps because of the concern of religio-psychiatric clinic applicants with marital problems. Curiously, the small number who considered bartenders and the like view them in the same league as marital counselors! The shift in position may, however, merely represent the instability of the small numbers involved. Both chiropractic and the social-improvement–cultist–religious-healing–mass-media-advice group retain relatively the same position as with analytic-clinic applicants. They are somewhat more highly grouped together.

The chief difference between religio- and analytic-psychiatric clinic applicants, then, concerns the role of counseling, the clergy, and psychiatry.

Finally, we have the radical view of the professions typical of the lower-class applicants to hospital clinics. In common with all other applicants they do see mass media, cultists, and social improvement as being of a piece—somewhat internal and definitely on the expressive side of things. But religious healing, Christian Science, for example, is much nearer to both medicine and psychiatry. The latter, still the most internal, is moved sharply over to the instrumental side. Hospital-clinic applicants expect formula and authority from psychiatry. Both clergy and counseling are placed sharply toward the external end of things. The clergy, to these persons, are rule-setters; so are counselors, most of whom are associated with the welfare department and other controlling agencies (see Figure 4).

Figure 3   *Religio-Psychiatric Clinic Configuration of Institutions Considered†*

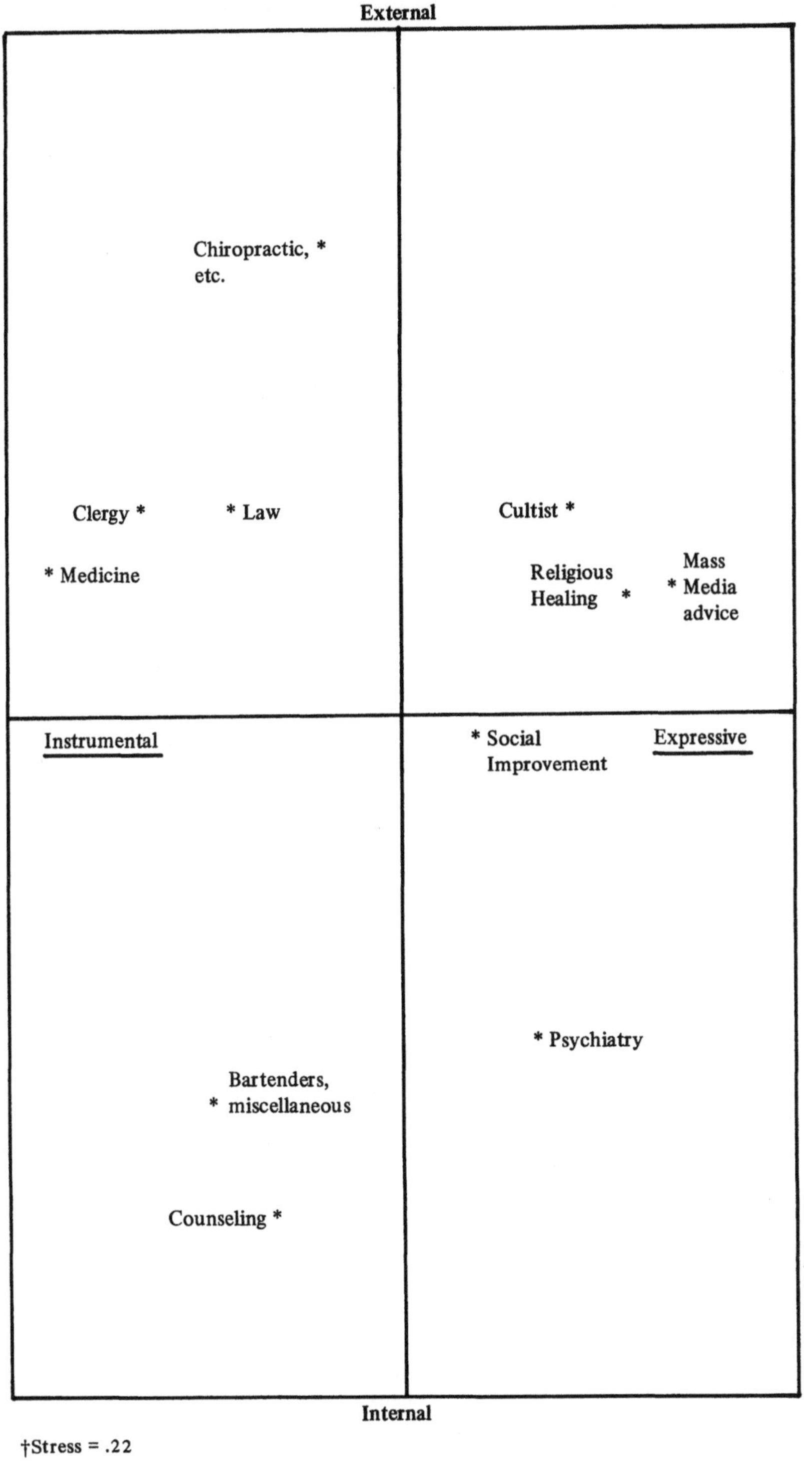

External

Chiropractic, *
etc.

Clergy *   * Law   Cultist *

* Medicine   Religious   Mass
                                           Healing   *   * Media
                                                           advice

Instrumental   * Social   Expressive
                    Improvement

                                           * Psychiatry

            Bartenders,
          * miscellaneous

          Counseling *

Internal

†Stress = .22

Figure 4 *Hospital-Clinics Configuration of Institutions Considered†*

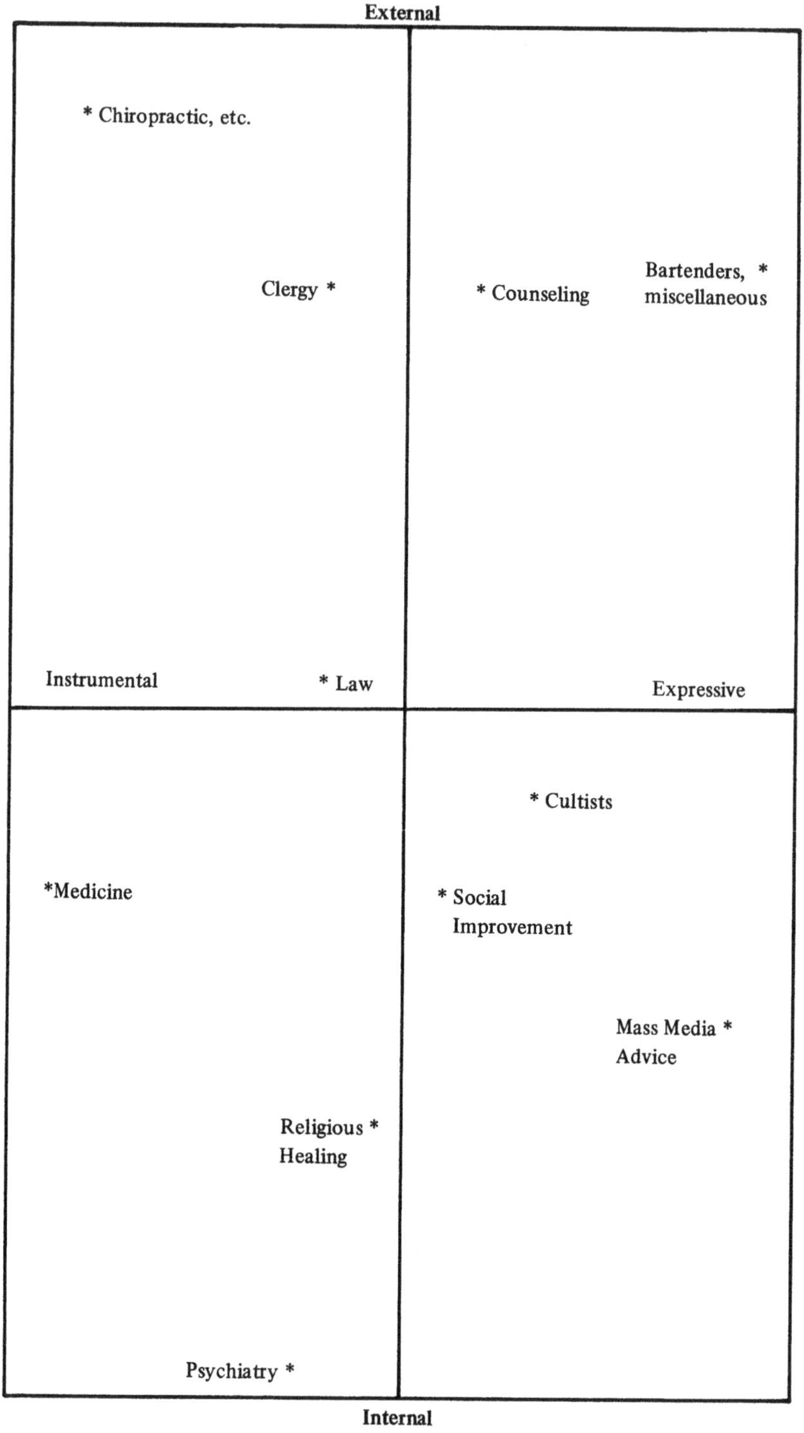

External

* Chiropractic, etc.

Clergy *   * Counseling   Bartenders, *
                                        miscellaneous

Instrumental   * Law   Expressive

                                  * Cultists

*Medicine   * Social
                   Improvement

                                  Mass Media *
                                  Advice

          Religious *
          Healing

          Psychiatry *

Internal

†Stress = .20

⚙ Summary and Conclusion

The figures we recently viewed and the frequency distribution of choices show that the professions have no automatic or guaranteed position. Their position depends on the way their clients view them. How they are perceived depends on the particular subculture of which potential clients are members. Our data indicate that the applicants to the three major types of clinics are indeed members of different subcultures or social circles. The very choice of clinic may have been in part determined by the view applicants have of the professional world.

Applicants came to analytic clinics in part because they viewed professions other than psychiatry as illegitimate and not instituted to deal with their problems. We see from Figure 2 that psychiatry does share, in their view, some things with other professions—notably counseling and clergy. It differs in being radically nondirective. More than anything this trait makes psychiatry unique to these applicants.

Religio-psychiatric clinic applicants are primarily interested in psychiatry yet they also grant clergymen a goodly measure of legitimacy. By going to them, if they considered clergymen, they also indicate that the clergy is instituted among them. Yet because they may associate the clergy with the instrumental ministry of pastors who emphasize "self-help," they tend to see all clergymen as instrumental and dealing with the external. In contrast, psychiatry is internal and expressive. Their choice of clinic, then, may be the result of their ambivalence toward the quite different things they themselves feel religion and psychiatry represent.

Hospital-clinic applicants also grant legitimacy and institutional validity to a profession other than psychiatry. But the main difference between medicine and psychiatry is that the latter, together with religious healing, deals more with the internal. As such, it is different in this one respect from medicine, for in their eyes both medicine and psychiatry are instrumental. Psychiatry, to them, represents a mere shift in emphasis. Hence when the resident in internal medicine at the hospital clinic sends them over to psychiatry, this is seen as a natural continuation of the medical process.

The map that applicants have in mind of the world of the professions, though not a consciously articulated one, is nonetheless apparent from their fantasy choices. There is a reason and coherence to these choices even though most applicants do not usually think in terms of "institutional areas." The choice of most professionals is an "obvious" choice to them. To a given respondent it is "obvious" that for some difficulties one goes to a doctor, for others to a lawyer. Taken collectively, however, the way these choices cluster illumines the meaning of the various healing professions, their relations one to another, and serves to explain why one type of clinic rather than another was chosen.

NOTES

1. See Lee Steiner, *Where Do People Take Their Troubles?* (Boston: Houghton Mifflin, 1945).
2. J. B. Kruskal, "Multidimensional Scaling by Optimizing Goodness of Fit to a Nonmetric Hypothesis," *Psychometrika*, 29 (1964), 1-27; "Nonmetric Multidimensional Scaling: A Numerical Method," *Psychometrika*, 9 (1964), 115-129; "How to Use MDSCAL, a Multidimensional Scaling Program," Bell Telephone Laboratories, Inc., Murray Hill, New Jersey, n.d., multilith.

   Dr. Kruskal graciously supplied the Bureau of Applied Social Research with a copy of his program.
3. Kruskal, "Multidimensional Scaling . . .," *op. cit.*
4. William W. Cooley and Paul R. Lohnes, *Multivariate Procedures for the Behavioral Sciences* (New York: Wiley, 1962), pp. 161-163.
5. These two dimensions are also used by Talcott Parsons to define the two major axes which differentiate social structure (in "General Theory," *Sociology Today*, Merton, Broom, and Cottrell, eds. [New York: Basic Books, 1959], pp. 5-7). In this and all figures that follow, the placement of the four basic functions is the same as depicted by Parsons, beginning with the Latency cell in the lower lefthand corner and proceeding clockwise to Adaptive, Goal Attainment, and Integration cells. Our cluster of professions does not, however, correspond to Parsons' location of them, as implied in his "Definitions of Health and Illness in the Light of American Values and Social Structure" (in his *Social Structure and Personality* [New York: Free Press, 1965], p. 270). For one thing, our system reference is not American value and social structure, but rather an individual with his problems. Second, no one expects the average person applying to a psychiatrist to view the professions in the same way as a sociologist. In fact, that is why an *a priori* "scientific" classification of professions can be quite far from the subjective experience of persons deciding upon them. What therefore is especially surprising is that Parsons' dimensions are nonetheless useful and implied by the grouping of the professions in the figure, despite the fact that in detail their placement does not agree with Parsons' own classification.
6. Kadushin, "Social Distance Between Client and Professional," *American Journal of Sociology*, LXVII (1962), 517-521, 527; and "Steps on the Way to a Psychiatric Clinic," unpublished Ph.D. dissertation.

THE DECISION TO GO TO A CLINIC

IV

Searching for Information
and Acquiring Knowledge

❂

11

With the exception of a few applicants, mainly to the hospital and religio-psychiatric clinics, almost no one accidentally stumbled into applying to a clinic. It was a conscious decision, and although much about the decision remains subterranean, a great deal can be discovered by asking people why they came to a clinic, for the applicant to a psychiatric clinic is a buyer even if he pays no money. At the very least he invests himself—his time and his ego—and that is certainly a great deal. Why should a person go to a psychiatric clinic? Some of the answers have already been given in terms of the previous stages in the decision. An applicant has his ticket of admission, his problems. Moreover, he has probably talked these problems over with laymen in order to gain a better idea about them. And further, half the applicants had read books about psychiatry and psychology. Additional preparation for the role came through visiting various professionals previous to applying to the present clinic. Many had even had some prior "training" in psychotherapy itself. As a result of these experiences, an applicant has, by and large, put psychotherapy in a category separate from the other healing professions and has chosen it in preference to ministers, doctors, and other helping professions. Now he is ready to apply to a clinic. But why now and not some other time? How does he get the names of places to which he can apply? How much pressure is put upon him to go? And what does he really expect of therapy?

These questions are not unlike those that might be asked about any decision—including buying a house, a car or even a TV set. For some elements are common to all decisions and constitute the formal aspects of an "accounting scheme" for studying decisions.[1] First there is the matter of knowledge. What does a person know about the alternatives? Then there is the question of a precipitating incident, the last straw. In the case of all decisions, one can ask whether a person was pushed into his ultimate action or whether he made it on his own. In medical situations this question brings up the matter of "referral," a rather confused idea which we will have to unravel. Further, no one buys even a car without having some idea of what its qualities are and what is expected from it even if he does not know the difference between a sparkplug and a manifold. The qualities of therapy and the clinics must also be cognized and evaluated. Finally, in every decision there are deterrents to action, and these too must be examined.

Despite many similarities, deciding to go to a psychiatrist is obviously different in at least one crucial respect from buying a car: Though it is true that a person's self-concept and his very ego are involved in the sort of car he buys (or so research tells us), car buying can hardly be compared with trying to change one's very life; and that is what our data show most applicants actually expect from therapy. Besides, it is not shameful to buy a car (unless one is Amish), but even among applicants to a sophisticated psychoanalytic clinic like University Psychoanalytic Center, 90 per cent said *yes* to our question, "Do you think that some persons think there is something wrong with a person who goes to a psychiatrist?" Though "something wrong" is ambiguous, popular usage points to a pejorative connotation. These two related factors, self-involvement and shame, plus a few others we shall discuss, tend to make this decision different from others; and we shall have to keep these matters in mind.

Knowledge, a key to all decisions, is seldom purely matter-of-fact and devoid of social or emotional content. In the decision to undertake psychotherapy, knowledge is intimately connected with a host of personal emotional factors, as well as with institutional arrangements. Something as simple as the name of the clinic to which a person is now applying and the names of other clinics or other psychotherapists is so important to professional-client relations that it has been given a special name—"referral." A referral is usually a transaction between two persons in which one of them gives the other the name of one or more professionals he might visit. A great many elements are involved in this transaction, all of which are related but all of which are also capable of separate analysis. In fact, so many factors are involved that in the introduction to this book we suggested that the concept was altogether useless for scientific research in spite of the fact that it has some meaning to practitioners (for they almost invariably ask on a client's very first visit, "Who referred you to me?").

Suppose a client reports to Dr. Baker, "Dr. Able referred me to you." What is involved in this brief exchange? In the first place, Dr. Able told his client that Dr. Baker exists, and perhaps also told him how to get in touch with him. Second, there is an implied imperative on Dr. Able's part—"to see Dr. Baker." Third, there is also an implied evaluation, "Dr. Baker is a good doctor." And fourth, there is an implied connection between Dr. Able and Dr. Baker. Dr. Baker may not have been very happy about a patient referred by Dr. Clark, for Dr. Clark may usually refer only patients who cannot pay their fees. Separate analysis is required for each of these four implications of a referral: sheer information, personal influence, evaluation and weighing of qualities of clinics, and the institutional connection between the person making the referral and the clinic to which the referral was made. Typical statistics of referrals kept by clinics themselves also include the category "self-referral." It is difficult to know just what is meant by this term and we shall not use it. It cannot mean referral by laymen, for the records usually include such categories as "relatives," "former patients," and the like. It has been suggested that it really covers instances where no discernible pressure was brought to bear upon the patient to come to the clinic, in which case the source of information is confused with the *pressure* to go.[2] The person listed as "self-referred" might merely have read about a clinic, but more often he was in fact told about it by someone else, and then made up his own mind to apply there.

The acquisition of knowledge about sources of treatment is emotionally tinged for applicants. Even the most purely cognitive aspect of a referral, learning the names of sources of treatment, is a complex and dynamic process. We shall show that the person who acquires more such information than others is a very different sort of person from one who does not garner much information; in short, knowing many alternative treatment sources has important consequences for the decision process. Although we cannot prove it conclusively with our data, we suspect that the very process of acquiring information changes both the applicant and his self-concept. Asking for the names of psychiatrists or psychiatric clinics is therefore a vastly different thing from asking for the name of a reliable automobile dealer.

Of course, there are more things to be known about psychiatry than mere sources for treatment and these, too, are socially and emotionally tinged. There is the entire process of therapy—what takes place, how does it happen, how long does it take, and what are the goals of psychotherapy. What areas of life can be changed and who is to be changed in this process. We inquired into what applicants expected in these areas, and the relationship between what they expected and what clinics actually offered. Then there is the matter of private psychiatry versus treatment in a clinic—which of course hinges on money but also on other things. Applicants ascribed their delay in applying for therapy to lack of money but gave many other reasons as well. And then there is the question of which clinic is best for a particular person. All of these matters require evaluation by applicants, for some sort of evaluation has to occur in all decisions that are not wholly impulsive. In this decision, perhaps because it is so important, there is a tendency to make evaluations even without very much knowledge of what is being evaluated. Nevertheless the same people who go about acquiring information tend to be the ones who know best what to expect of therapy, are most concerned about quality, yet are also those most worried about costs. Other than direct previous experience in therapy, the best teacher is, of course, membership in the Friends and Supporters of Psychotherapy.

Pressure to go to a clinic is implied in all referrals. We shall find, however, that though the pressure applied to applicants is much less than most people think, still, some personal influence is a crucial last straw for a great many persons. Influence is less important a factor for those who have *previously* discussed their problems with others, or who have asked for information, or who generally know more about therapy—in short, it is less important for the Friends and Supporters of Psychotherapy. This social circle constitutes a latent source of personal influence exerted by a group rather than by individuals.

The most remarkable thing about the referral system is that it works at all and that there is a fairly good match between the expectations of applicants and the expectations of clinics. This must mean that referrals are a complex social process which have as much to do with the structure of psychotherapy as they have with the needs of individuals.

In this chapter we shall take up the problem of knowledge of sources of treatment; in the next chapter the question of cognitions of therapy itself and evaluations of clinics; and Chapter 13 will deal with the issue of pressure and personal influence.

❂ *The Importance of Knowledge*

Ordinarily one would imagine that decisions consist of choosing from among available alternatives. In fact, people make all sorts of decisions without much knowledge of possible alternatives or without expending any effort to acquire that knowledge. For example, one study concluded "that [only] about a fourth of durable-goods buyers [TV sets, refrigerators, etc.] displayed most of the essential features of deliberate decision-making—planning, family discussions, information-seeking, as well as choosing with respect to price, brand, and other specific attributes of the commodity. Another fourth of the purchase decisions shows almost a complete lack of deliberation."[3] Decisions to buy sport shirts were even less deliberate.

Buying psychotherapy is, of course, quite different from buying a TV set or a sport shirt, though perhaps not nearly as different as one might expect. The major differences lie, as we have said, not so much in the greater deliberateness of the decision to "buy" psychotherapy as in the greater consequences of such a decision for the individual ego. Self-involvement and shame are the crucial differences between the decision to undertake psychotherapy and the decision to buy a TV set. Those who *ask* about sources for psychotherapy and those who *know* of alternative sources are therefore altogether different sorts of people from those who do not inquire or know, for they belong to quite different social circles. Even more important, merely *asking* for sources of help at once puts people in touch with an entirely different social system. As a result of these contacts, persons who ask for and know of alternative sources of psychiatric treatment tend to go to different types of clinics. This will explain the "magic" whereby members of Friends and Supporters of Psychotherapy tend to go to analytic clinics whereas other persons go to hospital clinics or the religio-psychiatric clinic.

In the 1960 data collection we asked this question: "Here are ways some persons get information about psychiatrists, psychologists and psychiatric clinics. Have you ever done any of the following?" A checklist of various sources of information then followed. We found that types of clinics differ sharply in the proportion of their applicants who said they had taken steps to gain information. Almost all (91 per cent) of analytic-clinic applicants, but only about half of the others (53 per cent of religio-psychiatric and 44 per cent of hospital-clinic applicants) said they had taken some action to get information. Moreover, the more "analytic" the clinic, the more likely applicants were to have asked others for information. One of the best predictors of who will apply to an analytic clinic, therefore, is whether or not a person has inquired about sources of treatment. These figures become even more meaningful when they are compared with the extent of information-seeking engaged in by durable-goods buyers. Eighty-four per cent of such buyers took some action to gain information (asked friends, visited stores, or read). Thus analytic-clinic applicants rank slightly higher than durable-goods buyers in their rate of information-seeking, but religio-psychiatric and hospital-clinic applicants rank much lower than the durable-goods purchasers.

Asking for information is of crucial import—even if an applicant gains no additional knowledge as a result of his intrepid action. Philosophers, especially those in the American pragmatist tradition, have extolled not only the virtues of knowledge, but also the importance of merely *searching* for knowledge. Dewey pointed out that persons learn best when they themselves are actively engaged in the search for knowledge and are not merely passive in the consumption of information. Here we will show the mechanisms which lend support to Dewey's contention. But the process is a social one, not simply a psychological property of learning. A major thesis of this book is that the very process of deciding to enter psychotherapy is itself part of the psychotherapy. Since fear of exposure of one's illness or condition is no doubt the crucial deterrent to gaining information about psychotherapy, searching for information about therapy itself helps one to overcome the feelings of shame. In addition, the very interactions with others which are part of and the result of this search clarify the nature of one's problems, as we have seen. Further, these interactions begin a chain of interactions which in turn lead an applicant to the psychiatric clinics we are studying. How all this comes about is a paramount concern of this chapter.

By overcoming shame and by putting persons in touch with others who can help them, information-seeking facilitates the decision to undertake psychotherapy. These are aspects of the decision that are tied to individual psychology and action. But there are other reasons for the importance of information-seeking which are intimately related to the structure of the institution of psychotherapy. Psychiatry is a relatively invisible institution. Private psychotherapists are not permitted to advertise, and although public clinics can be mentioned in mental health publicity campaigns, they too are relatively invisible. Private psychiatrists appear in the classified telephone directories merely as M.D.'s and are thus indistinguishable from other types of physicians. Psychologists, who are listed as such, have some advantage in this respect, though most psychologists do not engage in private therapy. Ninety-six per cent of a sample of New Yorkers was not able to name a psychotherapist when asked to do so.[4] The open character of the consumer-goods market is so different from the obscurity in which psychiatry operates that the study of consumer habits quoted above did not even bother to ask whether buyers knew of alternative brands or goods or stores. Moreover, durable goods are present all around us. About 60 per cent of those buying these goods recalled having inspected various models in friends' homes. Only 16 per cent of New York's population knows someone who is now in therapy.[5] Even among those analytic-clinic applicants who made vigorous attempts to gain information, only 60 per cent have friends in therapy (the equivalent of having already seen the "goods"). Only one-third of the applicants to other clinics knew someone who had been in therapy. As a result, it should come as no surprise that even among persons entering therapy, a great many did not know what alternative sources of psychiatric treatment were available. Nearly two-fifths of analytic-clinic, one-half of hospital-clinic and one-third of religio-psychiatric clinic applicants said they did not know of any other clinic besides the one to which they were now applying. This is not much better than the one-fourth of New Yorkers in general who could name a mental health clinic.[6] And despite the fact that so many of these applicants had already been to psychiatrists, there was still a goodly proportion who said they did not know any private psychiatrists, except, presumably, the one whom they had already seen. And of these applicants, many seemed so dissatisfied with their experience of psychotherapy that they did not even list their previous therapist as an alternative.

Asking about sources of treatment is not only a therapeutic activity but becomes almost a necessity when we consider the difficulty of finding therapy sources. Those who asked for sources, in fact, did get answers. For example, of those applying to analytic clinics who had asked their friends for information, over 40 per cent now know the names of at least three private psychiatrists, whereas only 15 per cent of those who did not ask know as many as three psychiatrists. Similarly, almost 70 per cent of those who asked their friends for the name of a psychiatric clinic now know of at least one other clinic besides the one to which they are at present applying, and 25 per cent know of at least three, but only half of those who did not ask know of another clinic, and less than 10 per cent of them know of as many as three other clinics. These facts suggest that most people who did not ask about clinics did not do so because they *already* knew, but because they were *afraid* to ask. Gathering information is the key to acquiring the data necessary for a rational decision to undertake psychotherapy.

General information does not automatically lead to a decision, however. Increased information is associated with getting a referral from a source closely affiliated with a *particular* type of clinic. This means getting a referral from a psychiatrist if one is applying to an analytic clinic, from a minister in the case of religio-psychiatric clinic applicants, or from a physician for those going to hospital clinics. Knowledge thus has a social consequence and meaning. It puts a person in touch with a referral system not otherwise available to him. In particular, this explains why members of the Friends go to analytic clinics. Let us look into this entire process in greater detail.

❖ Who Asks Whom?

First, what types of persons are more likely to search for information about psychiatry? In general, persons of higher social class more often ask for information about anything—whether about consumer goods or for traffic directions—though they are also the ones who need this knowledge least since they presumably know the most.[7] But the type of social circle to which one belongs is even more related to asking and to knowledge than sheer social class, especially in the decision to undertake psychotherapy. It will be recalled that over 70 per cent of those culturally and psychiatrically sophisticated asked their friends for a referral to a clinic or a private psychiatrist, almost 60 per cent of those only psychiatrically sophisticated did so, but only 10 per cent of those who were not psychiatrically sophisticated asked friends for a referral.[8] Membership in the Friends (psychiatric sophistication), however, is not as strongly related to making other inquiries, such as asking doctors, psychiatrists, or other professionals for a referral or looking up the names of doctors or clinics in a directory. Asking friends for a referral is clearly more sensitive a matter since it is more likely to expose a person to shame. To ask them for information about psychiatry one must have understanding friends who know enough to give some useful answers about sources of therapy. These attributes—sympathy and knowledge— are so significant that asking friends for a referral was one of the most important defining characteristics of the Friends and Supporters of Psychotherapy.

Strangely enough, asking friends for a referral is a key indicator not only for the personal, emotional reasons we have just mentioned but also because of the structure of psychiatric referral. As Table 27 shows, friends were the most frequently consulted sources for information, especially among analytic-clinic applicants; professionals, on the other hand, were *less* often consulted: of those who asked for information, about 20 to 30 per cent inquired of doctors, approximately another 20 per cent turned to other professionals; mental-health associations, and various directories accounted for considerably fewer. The hypothetical sources of information volunteered by a general sample of adult New Yorkers who said they would consult some mental-health professional if they had personal or emotional problems are quite similar to those actually used by clinic applicants—with two glaring exceptions. Friends

TABLE 27 *Sources Consulted for Information about Psychiatrists or Psychiatric Clinics*

	Analytic Clinics	Religio-Psychiatric Clinic	Hospital Clinics	New York City nonpatients*
	%	%	%	%
Asked				
Friends for psychiatrist	38	19	37 ⎫	10
Friends for clinic	43	23	23 ⎭	
Doctor for psychiatrist	23	25	33 ⎫	37
Doctor for clinic	18	9	23 ⎭	
Minister, nurse, or other professional	23	23	17	12
Mental-health association	16	4	17	1
Looked up				
Private psychiatrists	14	27	10 ⎫	18
Clinics	4	17	6 ⎭	
Other	4	11	4	
Average number of types of sources	1.8	1.3	1.7	1.3†
Total number who made a search	(709)	(53)	(52)	(324)

*Selected comparable *hypothetical* sources mentioned by those who *would* have consulted a mental-health professional for emotional or personal problems. See Elinson et al., *op. cit.*, Table 71. Figures are approximate because the categories used in the New York City study are not exactly comparable.

†The nonpatient study allowed for many more sources of information than did our study. Hence the *opportunity* for a person to be coded as mentioning many types is *greater* than in our study.

and mental-health associations are more important among those who actually asked for information and went to psychiatrists. Again, this is symptomatic of shame in asking about psychiatrists. Those who actually went to psychiatrists were better able to overcome shame and ask their friends or an impersonal nonprofessional counselor.

Because friends are a key first source of information, membership in the Friends and Supporters of Psychotherapy is the key determinant in asking for information. Once membership is taken into account, social class largely fades out as a factor. (One suspects that if a "Consumer Union" type of social circle were isolated for durable-goods buying, the relationship between class and information-seeking would largely disappear there too.) Even with membership in the Friends (and type of clinic) controlled, however, being a woman or being in the 25- to 34-year-old age group is especially associated with asking for information.

Women in general are more psychologically concerned, and the age group noted is the one which composes the bulk of analytic-clinic patients. In short, it is psychological sophistication or special interest which allows persons to expose themselves to others by asking for the names of psychiatrists or psychiatric clinics.

The ability to see oneself as especially needing help is also a factor in asking for information. Those who feel that their problems are of the "sicker" kind—cognitive problems, loss of control, and depression—more frequently asked for information.* Similarly, those who were especially anxious to gain information from reading (whom we classified as having read only because they needed help with their problems) were also those most likely to have asked others for information. And naturally, those who were especially *unwilling* to see themselves as having problems and had to be told so by others in the form of purely *unsolicited* comments were *less* likely than others to have searched for information.

Both an orientation to matters psychological and a willingness to see oneself as especially needing help are therefore traits related to asking others for information about psychiatrists and psychiatric clinics. Which comes first is really hard to say, on the basis of our data. But no doubt a search for information contributes as much to developing psychological sophistication and seeing oneself as needing help as these feelings contribute to wanting to know more.

❂ How Questions Lead to Answers

We have seen that special kinds of persons are more likely to ask questions and that asking questions may be related to their emotional growth. But why does asking lead to going to an *analytic* clinic?

First, the more sources an applicant has consulted for information, the more likely he was to have previously visited a psychiatrist or a psychiatric clinic. Seventy per cent of analytic-clinic applicants who consulted three or more sources had previously been to psychotherapists, but only 50 per cent of those who did not ask for information had been in therapy. The differences among applicants to other types of clinics are even greater. The reason for this is simple. We asked applicants if they had "ever" searched for information. Over one-third had done so at least six months before filling out our questionnaire. They had considerable opportunity to get some answers and to be referred to a private

---

* Merely asking for information seems less self-revealing than actually consulting one's friends about personal problems. Problems like depression and fear led to consultation with laymen only if friends and relatives were sympathetic, intimate, yet not overly involved.

psychiatrist or another clinic. Merely having been somewhere before also boosts the number of alternative sources of treatment one knows— in part because the very professionals previously seen were sometimes counted by applicants as "other" psychiatrists or clinics, and in part because they learned of other sources through the professional already seen.

Second, the more likely a person was to have been to a psychiatrist previously, the more likely he was to be an applicant later to an analytic clinic. To understand why this is so, we have to know the system of psychiatric referral. The sources through which applicants hear of the clinic to which they are now applying vary according to clinic type, as we have previously suggested (Chapter 3). Analytic clinics are closely linked to the psychiatric profession. The most analytic of these clinics received 60 per cent of its referrals from psychiatrists. Social-service agencies tend to refer to the more "psychotherapeutic clinics" (as distinguished from analytic), and the hospital clinics (other than St. Francis) receive the bulk of their patients through referrals from medical sources, usually within their own hospital. The Religion and Psychiatry Institute, isolated from both medical and psychiatric sources, receives some referrals from ministers, and a large number through the mass media. Though family and friends are important sources of referral for analytic clinics and the Religion and Psychiatry Institute (but less important sources for hospital clinics), professional sources generally overshadow the number who were referred by friends. Thus, applicants to analytic clinics are more likely to hear of the clinic through psychiatric sources, applicants to the Religion and Psychiatry Institute hear through the clergy or books written by people in the religion and psychiatry movement, and applicants to medical clinics are sent by medical sources. The interesting thing about the flow of referrals is that the very last professional seen is unrelated to the source of referral to a clinic. That is, an analytic-clinic applicant who had just previously been to a minister was *not* likely to have been referred by the minister to the clinic. But if a person had applied to a religio-psychiatric clinic and had last seen a minister, he was quite likely to be referred to a religio-psychiatric clinic. This means, as we have already seen, that for those who ultimately go to an analytic clinic, a visit to a doctor or a minister is a disjuncture, for they are ultimately likely to ignore his recommendation and seek a referral or help from another source. It is easier to go to the place recommended by the last professional seen, for if one does not follow his advice or recommendation then it takes a further search and more effort to find an alternative.

For these reasons, anything that disposes a person to go to a psychiatrist puts him in the psychiatric system and makes him more likely to go to an analytic clinic. Anything that makes a person go to a minister places him in the religious orbit and makes him more likely to go to a religio-psychiatric clinic (though it is less popular among ministers than analytic clinics are among psychiatrists). And going to a doctor, especially to a hospital medical clinic, predisposes one to go to a hospital psychiatric clinic. We also should add that anything which predisposes one to contact with the Friends and Supporters of Psychotherapy also makes it more likely that one will be referred by them to an analytic clinic.

Asking for information leads to going to psychiatrists which in turn makes people more likely to be referred to an analytic clinic. But merely knowing more sources of treatment has consequences for the referral process. Among analytic-clinic applicants the more sources of treatment an applicant knew, the more likely he was to have been referred by a psychiatrist. But the results for applicants to other clinics are especially interesting and show the important relationship between knowledge and social environment.

Knowing alternatives means that one is referred by professionals who are closely and systematically linked to the particular type of clinic to which one is applying, as Table 28 shows. Among religio-psychiatric clinic applicants the more alternatives a person knew the more likely he was to have been referred by a minister rather than through contact with the environment or through the mass media. And among hospital-clinic applicants, greater knowledge also decreased reliance on casual sources (the hospital, in their case) and increased reliance on psychiatrists, psychiatric clinics, and friends. By initiating interaction to gain knowledge, applicants enter a social system. Which social system they enter may in part depend on their starting point, though it is usually a psychiatric social system. Knowledge of alternative sources implies a tendency toward a referral from a more responsible professional source no matter what the source. Wider horizons obtained in the first place by engaging in social interaction bring applicants into contact with some social circle. Most often with future psychiatric patients, it is the circle of Friends and Supporters of Psychotherapy. But as Freidson points out, there are other types of referral networks and circles.[9] Knowledge can bring one into the professional religious referral network or into the combined lay and professional network which characterizes general medical referrals.[10]

Knowledge and the search for it represent an entry into a social system which has the possibility of changing the life of an individual. In this respect, asking about sources of referral initiates a chain which is quite different from that initiated by asking about TV sets or washing machines. We now need to know what parts of the chain are causal for other parts, and what parts can be short-circuited. For example, is membership in the Friends and Supporters sufficient guarantee that one will

TABLE 28 *Per Cent Hearing about a Clinic from a Given Source (by Type of Clinic and High or Low Knowledge of Alternatives)*

Source of Information	Analytic Clinics Knowledge of Alternatives		Religio-Psychiatric Clinic Knowledge of Alternatives		Hospital Clinics Knowledge of Alternatives	
	Low %	High* %	Low %	High* %	Low %	High* %
Mass media	2	4	47	38	1	0
Environment, prior contact with institution	1	2	19	8	60	24
Private psychotherapist	18	34	3	4	2	14
Psychiatric clinic	9	10	0	0	6	24
Social agency	16	11	4	8	6	3
Private doctor	6	3	2	4	7	3
Other medical	1	2	0	0	4	3
Other agency	10	12	0	0	1	3
Clergyman	1	1	10	29	2	3
Other professionals	0	1	2	0	0	0
Layman (friends and family)	44	40	38	42	15	35
Average number	1.1	1.2	1.3	1.3	1.00	1.1
N	(372)	(394)	(68)	(24)	(82)	(29)

*Three or more psychiatrists and/or psychiatric clinics.

get a referral from a psychiatrist (or a member of the Friends) to an analytic clinic or does one also have to ask and initiate interaction? Which is more important, the search for knowledge or the knowledge itself? That is, even if one does not get many answers, is there a gain from merely having asked for sources of treatment? And if one already knows a great deal is it still important to ask? To answer these questions we need simultaneously to look at the effect of membership in the Friends, asking for information, and knowledge of alternatives on the sources from which applicants heard about analytic clinics. These sources will be divided into three:* psychiatrists and other psychiatric sources, laymen, and sundry other sources (Table 29). A referral from a therapist indicates that a person came to the clinic through the psychiatric system. So does a referral from a layman, if one is a member of the Friends and Supporters of Psychotherapy. The major question before us is which counts the most in producing a referral from the psychiatric social system —membership in the Friends, asking for information, or knowledge of alternatives.

The results are not quite as simple as the question, for which factor is most important depends upon one's alliance with the Friends and Supporters of Therapy. First, membership in the Friends and Supporters of Psychotherapy is almost like an ascribed status. The proportion of members referred by laymen (presumably other members of the Friends) hardly varies whether a member asked for information or knew of other alternatives. Membership in the Friends makes knowledgeable laymen available whether or not one asks for their help and regardless of the state of one's knowledge of various sources of treatment. But as far as being referred by a therapist is concerned, it is knowledge that counts, especially among members of the Friends. If a member of the Friends knows many alternative sources, then unless he has already relied upon a layman for a referral he is likely to know a therapist who can refer him to an analytic clinic. Among nonmembers of the Friends, however, merely asking does produce more referrals from therapists. The more one asks, the less one relies on casual sources. But knowledgeable laymen are not as available to nonmembers of the Friends. They therefore tend much more than the Friends to utilize professionals as referral sources. (Even when they do ask they generally receive a smaller number of alternatives.) Finally, if an applicant is not a member of the Friends and does not ask and does not know alternatives, in order to go to an analytic clinic he must depend on a variety of incidental and casual sources or those not firmly connected with the analytic movement—all here grouped under the label "other." In this respect he is just like ap-

* There are not enough cases in our sample from other clinics to produce such a four-variable table.

TABLE 29 *Per Cent Hearing about an Analytic Clinic from a Given Source*

Number of Sources Consulted	Heard of Clinic From	Membership of Friends Knowledge of Alternatives		Nonmembers of Friends Knowledge of Alternatives	
		Low %	High %	Low %	High %
None	Therapists*	18	35	23	39
	Laymen	49	50	33	39
	Other	33	15	44	22
	Total	100	100	100	100
	N	(33)	(20)	(57)	(28)
One	Therapists	27	55	31	48
	Laymen	59	35	24	28
	Other	14	10	45	24
	Total	100	100	100	100
	N	(80)	(87)	(62)	(52)
Two or more	Therapists	22	35	56	60
	Laymen	53	48	30	21
	Other	25	17	14	19
	Total	100	100	100	100
	N	(113)	(174)	(27)	(33)

*Private or other clinics.

plicants to nonanalytic clinics, except that sheer chance (i.e., something we have not taken account of) has sent him to an analytic clinic. Needless to say, such persons are in the decided minority of analytic-clinic applicants.

In sum, the answers to our questions about the relative importance of (1) membership in the Friends, (2) searching for knowledge, and (3) actually having knowledge is roughly as follows: the search for knowledge is not especially important to members of the Friends for they are already in touch with the psychiatric social system. Sheer knowledge, however, does lead them to a more professional part of this system. On the other hand, among nonmembers of the Friends, asking is even more important than knowledge, for what they lack is contact with the psychiatric system and mere asking for information is a way of putting them in touch with the system. But they must in any case rely more on the formal and professional parts of the system rather than on the informal channels available to the Friends.

✿ Summary and Conclusion

The chart below summarizes the major factual argument of this chapter. Pressure and need lead to asking for information. So does sophistication, especially as represented by membership in the Friends, for membership also may lead directly to a referral by laymen to an analytic clinic. For nonmembers of the Friends, asking can lead directly to a referral by a professional even if the applicant has made only a nominal visit to him. Generally, however, asking questions leads both to going to psychiatrists and to gaining knowledge of alternative sources of treatment. Both of these—going to psychiatrists and knowing alternatives—tend to lead to a referral to an analytic clinic.

The implications of these facts suggest, we believe, why knowledge and the search for it are so important to depth decisions. Such decisions involve so much of the ego that the decider will in the end be a different person from the one who began the decision process. A person must begin to change himself even before he begins extensive psychotherapy. Searching for knowledge and getting answers bring him in touch with the social system that will eventually change him, and the search is especially important if he is not a member of the Friends and therefore entirely out of touch with this system. A person does not therefore acquire mere facts by asking for sources of help. He also gets partly through the door of a new community. Perhaps these social aspects of searching for knowledge are what Dewey had in mind when he stressed the importance of the search for general education. All of this makes the issue of knowledge and its discovery a different matter in the deci-

CHART XX *How Asking for Information Leads to Going to an Analytic Clinic*

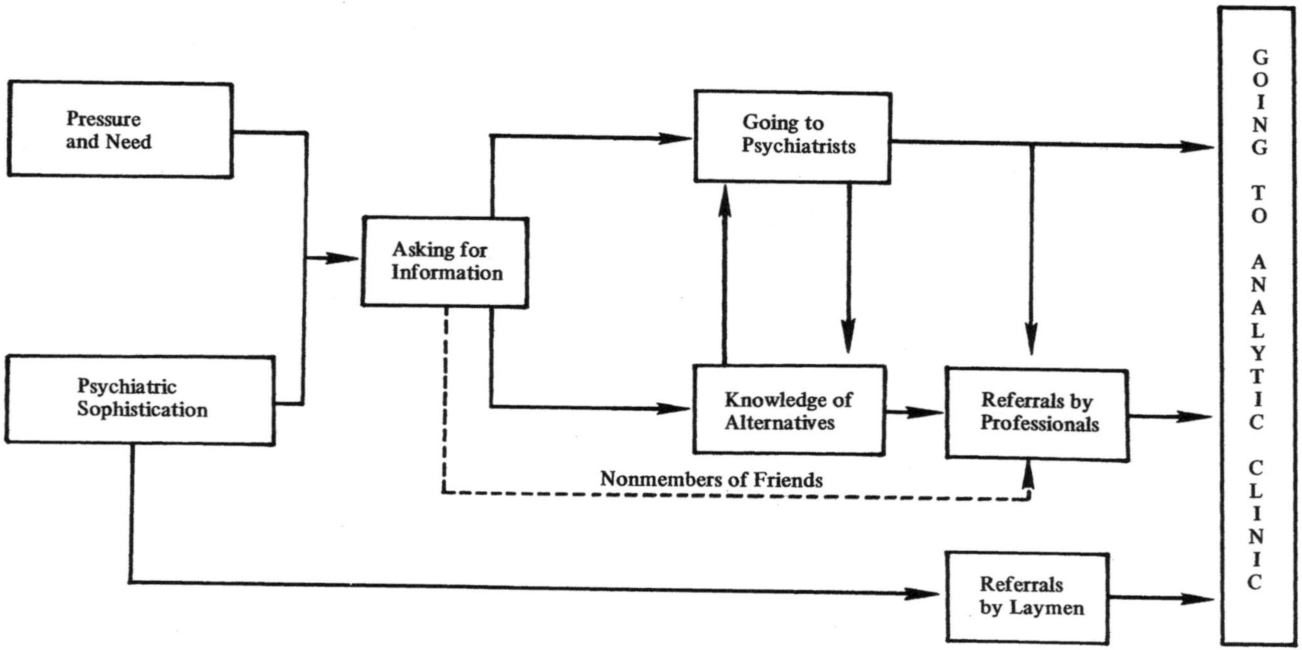

GOING TO ANALYTIC CLINIC

Referrals by Professionals

Referrals by Laymen

Going to Psychiatrists

Knowledge of Alternatives

Nonmembers of Friends

Asking for Information

Pressure and Need

Psychiatric Sophistication

sion to undertake psychotherapy from what it is in the decision to buy a TV set. Yet our argument also indicates that rationality has a social basis, and that implication carries over even to the buying of TV sets. Those who know more alternatives tend to go to analytic clinics. Does .this make these clinics the best ones? Is an application to them the sign of the rationality which must accompany greater knowledge? According to social perspective the answer is yes. For the culture which dominates the mental-health system in New York City is the culture of the Friends and Supporters of Psychotherapy and *they* hold psychoanalysis to be the preferred method of treatment. And the more analytic a clinic is, the "better" it is. But the exceptions to this rule show us the social basis of knowledge. Some persons who know a good many alternatives applied not to analytic clinics but to the religio-psychiatric or hospital clinics. They tended to be referred to these clinics by professionals who believed these sources to be best for their clients, since these professionals were themselves institutionally allied to these clinics. A rational decision, then, is that which is made in full knowledge of the "correct" alternatives provided by one's cultural and social setting.

NOTES

1. See Kadushin, "Reason Analysis," *Encyclopedia of the Social Sciences,* 2nd ed. (New York: Crowell-Collier, 1968), vol. 13.
2. Norma Jacob, "Referral Sources and Methods in Community Psychiatric Clinics in New York State," unpublished paper, 1965, referred to by G. Saenger and J. Cumming, "Study of Community Mental Health Clinics," Report I, Mental Health Research Unit, New York State Department of Mental Hygiene, Syracuse, New York, 1966. The category is meaningful to clinics because they prefer such patients and are more likely to accept them for treatment.
3. Eva Mueller, "A Study of Purchase Decisions," in Lincoln H. Clark, ed., *Consumer Behavior* (New York: New York University Press, 1955), p. 79. Despite the attack by social scientists on "economic man" and other rational models of decision-making, most studies of decision-making rarely include measures of the effort made by persons to get information. See Orville G. Brim, Jr., *et al., Personality and Decision Process* (Stanford: Stanford University Press, 1962), pp. 12-13. Brim's own study also finds it more convenient to study the behavior of choosing among alternatives than the behavior involved in the search for alternatives.
4. Elinson, Padilla, and Perkins, *Public Image of Mental Health Services,* Table 80.
5. *Ibid.,* Table 67-0.
6. *Ibid.,* Table 81-1.
7. For example, see Mueller, *op. cit.,* p. 53.
8. This compares to only a 15-percentage-point spread between grade-school and college graduates in the matter of asking for information on durable goods.
9. Eliot Freidson, "Client Control and Medical Practice," *American Journal of Sociology,* 65 (1960), pp. 372-382.
10. *Ibid.* Of course, knowledge is not an unmitigated "good thing." Increased knowledge has negative consequences for the clinics, if not for the individual applicant. Since getting into an analytic clinic is like trying to enter an Ivy League college, those applicants in the know tend to apply to as many clinics as they can, thus creating an administrative nuisance for the clinics.

Hopes and Money:
Cognitions and Evaluations
of Psychotherapy and
Psychiatric Clinics

❖

12

What is psychotherapy? We ourselves have studiously avoided defining psychotherapy, for its definition depends on one's theory of psychiatry, but we doubt that anyone who contemplates entering therapy can so suspend his judgment. Certainly most people who buy a product consider its qualities, so there is no reason to suppose that people who "buy" psychotherapy are any less concerned about the qualities of the product they are deciding about. Once psychotherapy is regarded as a purchase (and it was Freud who first suggested that therapy belonged in this category)[1] it should come as no surprise that there is a "Consumers Union" orientation in psychotherapy, just as in the evaluation of any other service or product. Those who are more expert "customers" know more of what to expect from therapy, and are more concerned about both price and quality.

There are various ways of becoming an expert in psychotherapy. One is, of course, by actually trying it out; another is through membership in the Friends and Supporters of Psychotherapy; and a third, by asking questions about it. As we have pointed out, however, learning about psychotherapy occurs throughout the entire decision process. One's cognitions and evaluations of therapy are therefore constantly shifting. We have captured the applicants' expectations and evaluations of therapy at only one point in time—just about the time of their first visit to a clinic. By sorting many applicants according to their various experiences we can, however, show some of the things that happen to expectations and evaluations during the decision process.

Just how important are the qualities of therapy itself and of psychiatric clinics to the decision process? Studies of consumer decisions suggest that the qualities of products are not always important in the decision to buy.[2] Almost half of durable-goods buyers showed no evidence of choosing with respect to price, and 40 per cent mentioned no specific features they had looked for. On the other hand, brand seems to have been much more important, for over one-third knew from the very beginning what brand they wanted. It is more difficult to evaluate the importance of the attributes of therapy and of various clinics in the decision to go to psychiatric clinics, especially since respondents felt obligated to rate clinics even when they knew of no alternatives. But it is true that almost everyone did expect to be helped and the major differences in evaluation of clinics occurred not between one clinic and another but between types of clinic—an equivalent in psychotherapy to the importance of "brands" in consumer products. Most important is the close match between what applicants expected of clinics and what, in our opinion, the clinics really had to offer. Applicants may not have an exact idea of what the clinics and therapy are like, but many have a very good general idea. In this sense, the entire decision process is a fairly efficient one.

❂ Expectations of Psychotherapy

Hopes for change and some ideas about how it will take place are part of the expectations applicants bring to therapy. Let us first see in what areas of life change is expected, and in whom it is hoped the change will occur. Then we shall analyze how applicants expect this change to come about and how long they think it will take. The most successful predictors of the stand applicants take on these matters are: the type of clinic to which they are applying, their previous experiences with psychotherapy, and their membership in the Friends.

We asked applicants, "In what areas of life do you expect change, should the clinic be able to help you?" The areas listed in Table 30 were offered as checklist alternatives.

A large majority desired three basic changes: changes at home, on

TABLE 30 *"In What Areas of Life Do You Expect Changes, Should the Clinic Be Able to Help You?" (1960 Clinics Only)*

Areas of Life	Analytic Clinics		Religio-Psychiatric Clinics %	Hospital Clinics %
	Members of Friends %	Nonmembers of Friends %		
At home	72	70	77	66
On the job	63	57	62	66
With relatives	39	29	48	43
With children*	–	–	33	36
Social life in general	74	67	62	66
In any area of sexual adjustment	65	45	56	44
With persons of same sex*	–	–	33	27
Regarding my values, religion, and the things I hold most important	46	30	63	42
N†	(549)	(303)	(87)	(98)

*Asked only in interviews at the religio-psychiatric and hospital clinics.

†Of those who answered; adds to more than 100% because more than one goal was usually given.

the job, in social life in general. Another general area, that of "values, religion, and the things I hold most important," was a consideration for the large majority of Religion and Psychiatry Institute applicants as one might expect, but not for those applying to other types of clinics. Changes in one's orientation to relatives are of somewhat less concern than any of these other goals. Sexual adjustment is a primary concern to members of the Friends applying to analytic clinics but not to nonmembers. Members of the Friends are also more interested in change in values, although expectations in this area are not voiced by a majority.

Responses in the area of values and especially in the area of sexual adjustment are much influenced by training and social milieu (presenting problems in these areas are similarly affected by training). Chart XXI shows the percentage of analytic-clinic applicants who hope for change in sexual adjustment, according to both membership in the Friends and the number of previous sessions of psychotherapy.

Both membership in the Friends and previous psychotherapy make applicants more likely to hope for changes in sexual life. But membership in the Friends counts especially among those who had never before experienced psychotherapy, whereas therapy itself has the most effect on nonmembers of the Friends and little effect on the members. Here,

CHART XXI *Per Cent Expecting Change in Sexual Adjustment (Analytic Clinics Only)*

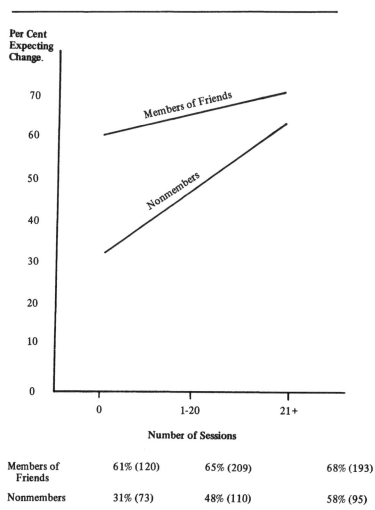

	0	1-20	21+
Members of Friends	61% (120)	65% (209)	68% (193)
Nonmembers	31% (73)	48% (110)	58% (95)

No Answers excluded from base.

again, membership in the Friends and psychotherapy prove to be functional alternatives to "learning" about psychotherapy. Either avenue is a good one (although membership in the Friends is a slightly better one!) and one alone suffices. Not only therapy but even reading serious books on psychology boosts the proportion who hope for change in their sexual relationships, and again the effect is more pronounced among nonmembers of the Friends.

There are many ways to accomplish these changes, only one of which requires the applicant himself to change. Perhaps applicants hoped that the clinic could talk "erring" spouses and relatives into changing. We therefore asked, "In what way can this clinic help you?" and offered five alternatives which elicited the responses indicated in Table 31. The most frequent response is the "correct" one—"Help me understand myself more"—but most respondents also wish for an improvement in their situation.* Few among analytic or religio-psychiatric applicants gave any other responses, but hospital applicants were more likely than others either not to know what the clinic might do or not to believe that it could help. Hospital-clinic applicants are more accustomed to being "pushed around," as well as more likely to come from social classes unfamiliar with psychotherapy. Their greater tendency not to know what might be changed or not to believe that anything could be changed is quite understandable.

TABLE 31   *"In What Way Can This Clinic Help You?" (1960 Clinics Only)*

	Analytic Clinics	Religio-Psychiatric Clinics	Hospital Clinics
	%	%	%
"Help me make specific improvements in my situation"	70	67	53
"Help me change someone else"	3	13	10
"Help me understand myself more"	89	81	63
"I don't think it can help," Other	2	6	17
Don't Know, No Answer	2	5	18
N*	(872)	(99)	(118)

*Adds to more than 100% because more than one way was usually given.

Even though the "correct" response is so frequent, it too can be affected by "learning." Ninety-five per cent of the members of the Friends applying to analytic clinics give this response, but only 71 per cent of nonmembers of the Friends who had not previously had psychotherapy did so. Experience with psychotherapy, however, increases the proportion of non-Friends who want to be helped in this way to about 90 per cent—not quite the level attained by members of the Friends even without psychotherapy.

* This alternative, however, needs some support from authority to become a legitimate response. The first year we conducted the study, this question was left openended. Only one-third of University Psychoanalytic applicants and only one-tenth of Religion and Psychiatry Institute applicants gave change of situation as a free response.

After asking applicants what areas of their life might be changed by psychotherapy, we asked them, "How do you think the clinic will help bring these changes about?" The alternatives listed included, "The therapist will give me suggestions," "The therapist will listen to my problem and let me work it out myself," "I will do most of the talking," and "The therapist will do most of the talking." Sixty-two per cent of analytic-clinic applicants, 72 per cent of religio-psychiatric, but only 51 per cent of hospital-clinic applicants indicated that they expected to work out their own problems or that they would do most of the talking or both. Either of these responses is, of course, the "correct" one. This is one area of expectation in which actual training in psychotherapy is somewhat more effective (among applicants to analytic clinics) in producing "correct" responses than membership in the Friends, and members of the Friends benefit from therapy as much as nonmembers. Prior psychotherapy produces a 15 per cent increase in the proportion who give one or both of the "correct" responses among both members and nonmembers of the Friends; and membership in the Friends alone, regardless of the amount of previous psychotherapy an applicant has had, produces a 10 per cent improvement in "correct" responses. So these two avenues of learning about psychotherapy (membership in the Friends and actual experience of therapy) independently teach about who does the work in therapy. The same sort of effects result from reading serious books about psychotherapy. Both members and nonmembers of the Friends benefit, and the proportion who learn from their reading is about the same for those who learned as a result of previous therapy. How effective is the influence of others who tell a potential applicant to seek therapy? Only among members of the Friends did such influence produce a 15 per cent increase in the proportion of those giving at least one "correct" answer about who does the active work in psychotherapy. The Friends and Supporters of Psychotherapy were able, therefore, not only to influence members to go to a clinic but their suggestions proved instructive as well. Nonmembers had no such increase in knowledge about therapy as a result of their interaction with those who advised them to seek treatment. In general, then, learning about the *processes* of therapy is different from learning about its *goals*. Knowing that one is supposed to do one's own "work" in therapy is not something that one simply acquires from the culture of the Friends and Supporters, although membership in that culture does help. Rather, even if one is a member, actual contact with therapy or specific instruction by other persons through books is helpful in overcoming the usual conception of a professional as someone who prescribes rather than as someone who helps a client do his own work.

Finally, the length of time therapy is expected to take is also sensitive to learning. We asked, "How long do you think it will take you to solve your problem?" We presented a number of alternatives, and with some of the categories collapsed, the frequencies of replies are shown in Chart XXII.

A certain measure of reality is reflected in this chart but here is also some evidence of learning. Analytic clinics, as a rule, do offer longer-

CHART XXII *"How Long Do You Think It Will Take to Solve Your Problem?"*

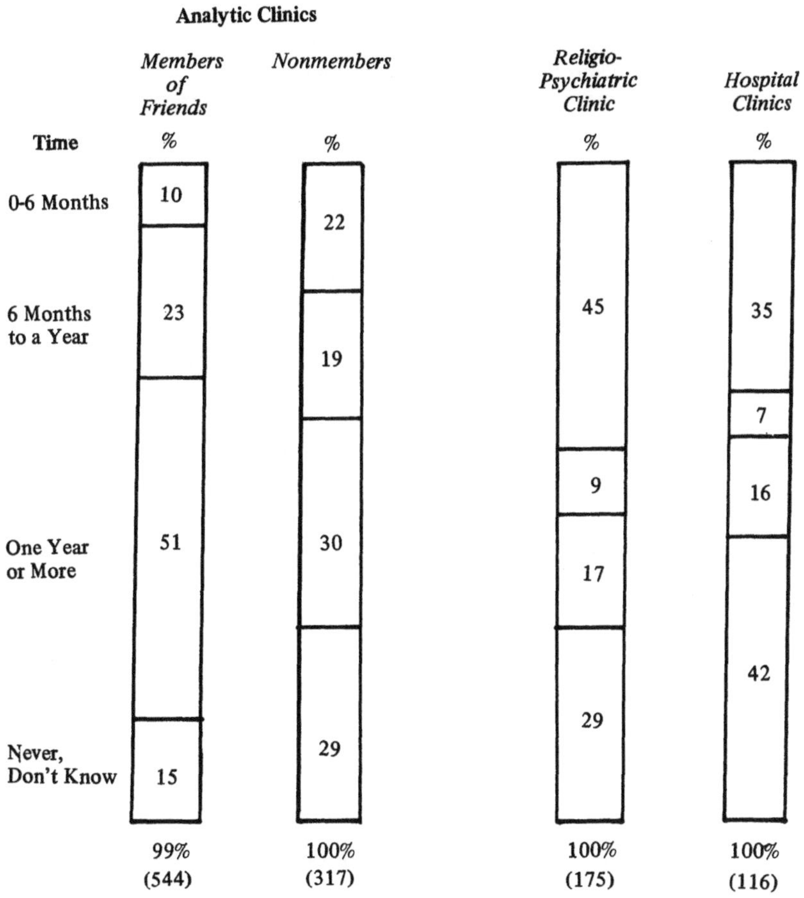

Time	Analytic Clinics		Religio-Psychiatric Clinic	Hospital Clinics
	Members of Friends	*Nonmembers*		
	%	%	%	%
0-6 Months	10	22		
6 Months to a Year	23	19	45	35
				7
			9	16
One Year or More	51	30	17	
				42
			29	
Never, Don't Know	15	29		
	99% (544)	100% (317)	100% (175)	100% (116)

term treatment than either the religio-psychiatric or hospital clinics, and the data show that indeed applicants to analytic clinics are more likely to expect their problems to take longer to solve. On the other hand, the size of the bar showing those who do not know what to expect increases as one's eye moves from members of the Friends to nonmembers applying to analytic clinics, to applicants to a religio-psychiatric clinic and finally over to hospital-clinic applicants. Further, the majority of members of the Friends do expect that their problems will take more than a year to solve. In fact, in Chart XXIII, which includes the effects of both membership in the Friends and previous psychotherapy, expectations about the length of time therapy might take are shown to be more sensitive to learning than are any of the other expectations we have analyzed. In the case of those who have not had previous therapy, membership in the Friends makes for a large increase in accuracy of

CHART XXIII *Per Cent Who Think It Will Take One Year or More to Solve Their Problems (Analytic Clinics Only)*

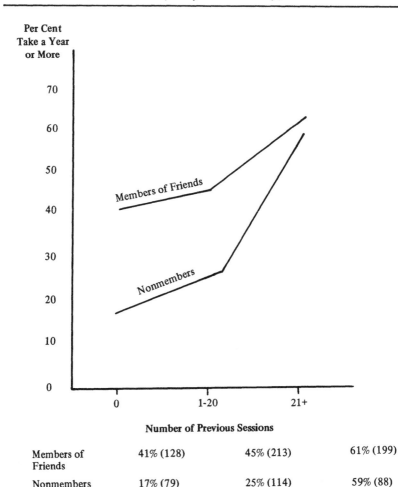

	Number of Previous Sessions		
	0	1-20	21+
Members of Friends	41% (128)	45% (213)	61% (199)
Nonmembers	17% (79)	25% (114)	59% (88)

No Answers included in base.

time-expectation. And while experience with psychotherapy produces a 20-percentage-point increase in accuracy of prediction among members of the Friends, it produces a 42-percentage-point increase among non-members. Experience with actual treatment, then, sharply reduces expectations of a quick cure and drastically cuts down on the proportion who do not even know how long things will take. Those who have already tried therapy know that it will be a long process but with a foreseeable end.

In conclusion, we note that the absolute size of the response to various questions about what will happen in therapy indicates that applicants to analytic clinics have a fairly good idea of what to expect from therapy. Other applicants are not quite as knowledgeable and those applying to hospital clinics are especially uninformed. The best way to learn about the process of therapy is actually to have participated in it. Those who had already tasted therapy knew better who would have to do the work and how long it would take. Membership in the Friends, however, is almost as good a route to learning about therapy. What is more, *either* route produced similar learning. If one was not a member of the Friends, then previous psychotherapy served as a good learning experience. If one had no previous therapy, then membership in the Friends did the trick. But for those who had both, the experiences were not additive. That is what we mean by therapy and membership in the Friends being "functional alternatives." Reading the "right" books was also a functional alternative to actual therapy. The one major exception to these "training" experiences were expectations about who does the work in therapy. Therapy is such a reversal of the common-sense notion that the professional will prescribe that it is impossible to acquire too much training in the idea that the client himself must do the work. Hence, membership in the Friends and psychotherapy itself each independently contributes to a better understanding of this fact.

❁ How Psychiatric Clinics Are Rated by Applicants

One can have high expectations of therapy in general but may still recognize advantages and disadvantages attached to one source of treatment or another. What applicants thought about various sources of therapy and how they rated them is important in understanding their final choices: It becomes clear that money is crucial, but there are also other factors, such as the entire style of therapy one would like. While patients' concerns about money are quite familiar to psychiatrists, we need to document these anxieties in some detail for two reasons. First, the more middle-class and the more medically oriented one is, the less concerned one is about money for such things as operations, on the grounds that health is so important. On the other hand, the cost of psychotherapy is indeed held to be a major deterrent to entering it. Second, the *more* oriented one is to the world of psychotherapy, the *more* one is concerned about money. The most ardent fans of psychiatry are the very ones most concerned about the costs of psychiatry. Let us see how this works out.

REASONS FOR DELAY

We asked our 1960 sample what might have prevented them from seeking help earlier. A list of possible reasons was presented to them. Although not presented in this way, the reasons fell into three major categories: cathectic reasons, which had to do with the emotional cost—shame and denial (and a projection of denial onto others); cognitive reasons—"reality" factors such as financial cost and the absence of therapy from one's very field of vision; and evaluative reasons—weighing the advantages of professional treatment against the nature of one's problem and one's own capacity for dealing with it. Table 32 shows the answers we obtained, according to the type of clinic to which a person applied and his membership in the Friends. The numbers underlined show the modal answer for each type of clinic.

What do these proportions mean? Are not the statements we presented mere rationalizations for not going to therapists earlier? We dealt with this problem earlier by saying there is no such thing as a "mere" rationalization, because any statement assented to by an applicant reveals something about him. Thus, we know from the table of reasons that most people are reluctant to admit that shame or denial of their problems or other fears were reasons for delay, and that applicants are most reluctant to attribute delay to social disapproval. Even so, about 40 per cent mentioned or checked one of these cathectic reasons. We may also accept the fact that the small proportion of those who say their friends or relatives were against it are very likely reflecting reality. Probably, few closely interested persons would overtly object to a friend or relative attempting to do something about the problems that beset him. Hospital-clinic applicants are the *least* likely to report that they refused to admit their problems. This must mean that their predominantly *physical* symptoms served as substitutes for *emotional* problems.

Second, complaints about the costs of therapy were most frequent among analytic-clinic applicants, especially members of the Friends. But these were the applicants who also expected therapy to take a good deal of time. As we have already explained, hospital-clinic applicants, who are in fact the poorest, were least concerned about money, because they are so poor that in our peculiar medical system they do not have to pay at all. Moreover, they do not expect that treatment will last for very long. These findings are similar to those about reasons for leaving thera-

TABLE 32 *"Which of the Following Might Have Prevented You from Seeking Help Earlier?" (1960 Clinics Only)*

Responses	Analytic Clinics		Religio-Psychiatric Clinic	Hospital Clinics
	Members of Friends %	Nonmembers of Friends %	%	%
Cathectic Reasons				
"I was ashamed to talk about it"	20	20	25	19
"I refused to admit I had problems"	25	19	18	11
"My friends or relatives were against it"	12	6	2	4
Other fears, cathectic reasons	3	1	5	6
Cognitive Reasons				
"Psychiatric help was too expensive"	71	57	39	29
"I hadn't thought of it before"	9	12	24	50
Situational or other cognitive reasons	8	8	2	13
Evaluative Reasons				
"I didn't think it would do any good"	18	15	16	14
"I felt I could handle the problem myself"	58	48	68	36
Other evaluative reasons	3	4	3	12
Total number *	(542)	(299)	(89)	(108)

*Of those who answered; adds to more than 100% because more than one reason was usually given.

pists (see p. 218) and evaluations of private psychiatry (see below). Nonetheless, those who had seen psychotherapists were least concerned about money, since of course they did have the experience of meeting their payments.

The most intriguing findings, however, are those responses which most strongly appear to be rationalizations. We offered the alternative, "I hadn't thought of it before," as a way out for those who might be blocked on the other alternatives. It is abundantly clear from all our previous analysis that most hospital-clinic applicants are unlikely to have considered psychotherapy as a way of treating their somatic set of complaints. And they were the very ones who most frequently gave the "hadn't thought of it before" alternative. Indeed, they probably had not. A number of religio-psychiatric clinic applicants also checked this alternative. Again, we know that a considerable proportion of these applicants had never considered psychotherapy and in fact did not perceive that they were even now applying for psychotherapy.

Evaluative reasons were checked almost as frequently as the cognitive ones we have just discussed. Few were willing to admit that applying to a clinic might not do them any good, but a large number evaluated their problem as something they themselves could have handled. The do-it-yourself orientation is concentrated in two groups, and this judgment too reflects social reality. Members of the Friends, who indeed know a good deal about the management of emotional problems, are quite likely to have felt that they could help themselves. But the largest proportion of do-it-yourself advocates are found among religio-psychiatric clinic applicants who follow the ideology of self-help writers such as Norman Vincent Peale.

REASONS FOR GOING TO A CLINIC

The same mixture of concern about money but also about other matters is evident in the reasons applicants gave for going to a clinic rather than to a private psychiatrist. A rather direct question asked, "How would coming here differ from going to a private psychiatrist?" Respondents were asked to check one of the following alternatives (though many checked more than one—it was money *plus* something else).

"I can't afford to go to a private psychiatrist."
"In a clinic you get better care because there are more experts who work together."
"You get less personal attention."
"You get less treatment hours."
"There is no difference between coming here and going to a private psychiatrist."

This all boils down to those who think a clinic is cheaper, those who think it is better in some other way, those who think it worse, and those who think it is about the same as a private psychiatrist.

Money was almost invariably mentioned, but was definitely not the entire story for the applicants to some clinics, as Table 33 shows. While 95 per cent of the applicants to the most "analytic" of the clinics, the University Psychoanalytic Center, say the clinic is cheaper than private psychiatrists, only 35 per cent of Religion and Psychiatry Institute applicants claim this is the main difference. Instead, the majority of them think the clinic is *better* than private psychiatrists. It is the

TABLE 33 *"How Would Coming Here Differ from Going to a Private Psychiatrist?"*

Ways in Which Clinics Differ	University Psychoanalytic Center	Interpersonal Psychiatry Institute	Center for Advanced Psychotherapy	Personal Psychology Institute	Religion and Psychiatry Institute	St. Matthew's Hospital	St. Francis Hospital	Center Hospital
	%	%	%	%	%	%	%	%
Cheaper	95	92	79	82	35	57	80	59
Better	22	9	20	26	55	23	24	31
Worse	5	8	7	13	3	20	24	13
Same	3	9	12	9	7	15	8	0
Don't know	1	9	6	7	29	16	8	16
N*	(143)	(351)	(313)	(54)	(99)	(61)	(25)	(32)

* Adds to more than 100% because more than one difference was usually given.

religion-and-psychiatry orientation, of course, that makes the difference. Private psychiatry does not offer this approach. They are also least likely of all applicants to think the clinic is worse than private psychiatry. A good number of applicants to the Religion and Psychiatry Institute must think the comparison between this clinic and a private psychiatrist is altogether impossible, for almost 30 per cent do not know what to say in response to our question. As we have consistently noted, hospital-clinic applicants have quite a different orientation to money and paying medical fees. They too are less likely than analytic-clinic applicants to emphasize low cost as the difference between a clinic and private psychiatry. Most of them never even hoped to go to a private psychiatrist, and many have their clinic fees paid for them by welfare agencies. St. Francis with its somewhat Bohemian clientele is an exception to the hospital-clinic pattern and closer to that of the analytic clinic. In general, the more an applicant wants psychoanalysis, the more likely he is to find the major difference between a clinic and a private psychiatrist to be a matter of money. But even aside from applicants interested in religion and psychiatry there are quite a few who think clinics are *better* than private psychiatry. Twenty to 25 per cent of applicants to almost all clinics think clinics are better than private therapy. Fear of placing oneself in the hands of a single un-known practitioner must be an important factor for these applicants. Some such fear may explain why some members of the Friends have not previously been to a psychiatrist even though they live in a milieu which encourages attendance. Members of the Friends who have *not* previously been to a psychiatrist are twice as likely as others to think clinics are *better* than private psychiatry.

Through the processes we have described, the various clinics draw upon a clientele which by and large meshes with what each clinic offers —psychoanalysis at clinics whose applicants emphasize low cost, and psychotherapy of limited duration at clinics whose applicants are less likely to emphasize cost. The one major exception is probably the Religion and Psychiatry Institute. Many applicants expect an approach like Norman Vincent Peale's (who is a clergyman associated in the public mind with religion and psychiatry) but instead receive fairly conventional psychotherapy. Another possible exception is found in hospital clinics where applicants with physical symptoms receive psychotherapy, rather than the exclusive ministration of pills and injections which many expect. But all these differences among clinics cannot be explained away in terms of the types of persons who go to them. Even when membership in the Friends is taken into account, there are still differences among clinics in the way their applicants see the difference between *clinics and private psychiatrists*. This can only mean that these differences do explain, in some measure, why applicants choose one clinic over another, or even if they do not know of any other clinics, why they consent to go to the only one they have heard about.

REASONS FOR PREFERRING
ONE CLINIC OVER ANOTHER

This conclusion further suggests that once an applicant has decided to apply to a clinic rather than to go to a private psychiatrist, he makes definite distinctions among them. To ascertain these perceived differences among clinics, we asked, "How would coming here differ from going to some other psychiatric clinic?" Table 34 shows the categories they were asked to check and how applicants to the various clinics responded.

There is a fairly good correspondence between how analytic a clinic is and the proportion of applicants concerned about competence. The outstanding difference, however, is between University Psychoanalytic Center, the only clinic in this study associated with an institute recognized by the American Psychoanalytic Association, and all the other clinics. Apparently, the "imprimatur" of this organization is decisive for those applicants concerned about quality and competence. Theoretical position is of some interest to religio-psychiatric and analytic-clinic applicants but of practically no interest to hospital-clinic applicants. The connection with the medical center and the university is probably also important to University Psychoanalytic Center applicants since "convenience" is more frequently cited by them, as it is by applicants to Center Hospital Clinic—also connected with the medical center. Applicants to analytic clinics were more concerned with the unique quality of the clinic to which they were applying. Only about 6 per cent felt that there was "no difference between this and any other clinic."

The most interesting fact about the response to our request for evaluation of the clinics was the large number who refused to make any evaluation. Except for the applicants to University Psychoanalytic Center, between 40 and 50 per cent of applicants checked the response, "I don't know of any other clinic." When directly asked about other clinics, nearly two-fifths of the analytic-clinic, one-third of religio-psychiatric clinic, and one-half of hospital-clinic applicants repeated that they did not know of any other clinics. But lack of knowledge did not stop persons from evaluating the difference between private psychiatrists and clinics. Although fewer claim not to know of a private psychiatrist, there is still a substantial number who do not know of any psychiatrist or who had not previously visited one. Even in open-ended questions in interviews with hospital-clinic applicants, relatively few refused to make the comparison between private psychiatry and psychiatric

TABLE 34 *"How Would Coming Here Differ from Going to Some Other Psychiatric Clinic?"*

Ways in Which Clinics Differ	University Psychoanalytic Center %	Interpersonal Psychiatry Institute %	Center for Advanced Psychotherapy %	Personal Psychology Institute %	Religion and Psychiatry Institute %	St. Matthew's Hospital %	St. Francis Hospital %	Center Hospital %
Better therapy	71	49	43	28	41	18	26	25
"I like the theoposition of this clinic"	22	19	12	15	23	0	4	0
"I feel this clinic would be more competent"	62	35	31	19	13	18	22	22
Convenience	27	17	18	32	9	20	13	28
"This one is more convenient for me to get to"	21	13	13	13	5	18	13	28
"I applied to others first but this is the first one that would take me"	8	6	7	19	4	3	3	3
Other and "There's no difference between this and any other clinic"	8	9	11	7	25	31	30	22
	6	6	8	6	15	21	22	6
Lack of knowledge, Don't Know, No Answer, "I don't know of any other clinic"	22	42	42	50	40	45	44	41
N*	(143)	(351)	(313)	(54)	(99)	(61)	(23)	(32)

*Adds to more than 100% because more than one advantage was usually given.

clinics. There is a sufficiently widespread image of psychiatrists, at least as far as their cost is concerned, so that everyone has some reaction to them and certainly considers them in deciding to seek psychotherapy. But for many applicants to a clinic, merely hearing about a clinic helped to precipitate the decision, as we shall see in the next chapter. So that for many persons the issue is simply finding a clinic. The decision to seek therapy had already been germinating and the decision actually to go needed just a "clincher" (often from the person giving the information about the clinic). Evaluation of *which* clinic was to the applicant simply irrelevant, *if* the clinic sounded to him like the right kind.

But this does not mean that once he has applied to a clinic a person will not evaluate it against others even though he really knows no others. (The tendency to feel one has made the right choice anyway is sometimes called an attempt to reduce "cognitive dissonance.") While some persons evaluated clinics even though they did not know of any others, some who *did* know of other clinics claimed they really did not know enough about them to make the evaluation. Quite a few checked *both* the "lack of knowledge" and the "better therapy" categories. Hospital-clinic applicants, though they may have heard of Bellevue and hence were counted as knowing about at least one other clinic, often did not have enough information, other than the name, to evaluate the difference between the clinic they were now applying to and some other. Hence, 40 to 50 per cent pleaded lack of knowledge regardless of whether they knew of other clinics or not. Moreover, they may have felt incompetent to evaluate clinics no matter what they knew.

Knowledge of other clinics, therefore, is not the only factor which determines whether a person evaluates clinics. Some of the response is a normative one. That is, some applicants apparently felt they *ought* to have made an evaluation, whether or not they knew anything about clinics. The normatively "correct" response to a question about the difference between clinics was clearly that one clinic offers better therapy than another. Regardless of whether or not an applicant knew of other clinics, the more training he had in psychotherapy, the more likely he was to evaluate clinics in terms of the quality of their therapy. To be sure, training did have more effect if applicants knew of other clinics. In that case, membership in the Friends and previous psychotherapy are once again seen as functional alternatives, for if an applicant had not had previous therapy, then members in the Friends were 30 percentage points more likely than nonmembers to evaluate clinics in terms of quality. And conversely, if an applicant is not a member of the Friends, then twenty-one or more sessions of therapy bring him to the point where he is almost as likely as a member of the Friends to say that better therapy is his reason for choosing the clinic to which he is now applying. If, however, an applicant knew of no other clinics, then it required *both* therapy *and* membership in the Friends before he was likely to assert that he chose this clinic because it has better therapy. In either case, however, membership in the Friends is a somewhat more powerful factor in influencing concern about quality than actual experience in therapy. The Friends are "tough customers" indeed. Evaluating a clinic, then, is not a completely rational act, for whether one evaluates it at all and in what terms is affected by an applicant's psychiatric sophistication.

Looking ahead to the subject of the next chapter, we see that the amount of pressure to go to a clinic also influenced the way applicants evaluated it. Analytic-clinic applicants who indicated they did not know of other clinics and who were influenced to go to a clinic only by other persons were more likely to evaluate a clinic in terms of better therapy. They were also more likely to have added something to the effect that the clinic was recommended as offering good therapy. One of the ways those not knowledgeable about clinics were convinced to go was through having other persons tell them about a *good* clinic. Medical doctors were especially important in this respect. Analytic-clinic applicants who did not know of any other clinics and who were referred by physicians were 11 per cent more likely than others to feel that the clinic they were now applying to offered better therapy. In general, personal influence to go to a psychiatric clinic tends to reduce the proportion of those who say they cannot evaluate a clinic because they do not know of any others. And this is true, especially among hospital-clinic applicants, whether or not they *actually* knew of other clinics. Being pressured by others to go to a clinic, therefore, has, in part, a *reassuring* function.

The one exception is the Religion and Psychiatry Institute. Not integrated into the psychotherapy movement, it relies more on those interested in religion and psychiatry to provide it with enthusiastic applicants. Since such persons more often hear of the clinic through reading, especially through the writings of some self-help writers, personal influence to go to that clinic is not likely to be the factor that sends people to this clinic and therefore those who were not influenced by anyone (i.e. who came without the last personal push) are those who say that the clinic offers better therapy.

There has been a good deal of evidence throughout this section that applicants to the Religion and Psychiatry Institute have a different frame of reference than others. They are especially interested in changing their values; and although they stand between the analytic- and the hospital-clinic applicants in the *amount* of work they are prepared to do in therapy and have a fairly good idea that they will have to work on themselves, they have the shortest time perspective of all—when it comes to reasons for not having entered therapy before (or for leaving their previous therapist) money is not a major factor. Rather, when leaving previous therapists, applicants to the Religion and Psychiatry Institute say more often than others that their problems were not suitable for psychiatrists, and their major reason for not having previously entered therapy was that they tried to help themselves. Their image of the professional world is different, as we saw in Chapter 10, for they group the clergy together with the liberal professions of law and medicine, rather than as relatively adjacent to cultists as do applicants to other clinics. They are unlikely to be referred to the Religion and Psychiatry Institute by orthodox medical sources. Many are attracted by self-help writers associated with the clinic. And their problems are different, for they are much more concerned about family matters than are applicants to other clinics. Finally, they are even ethnically different —middle-class, religious, white Protestants in a city famous for just about every other ethnic group.[3] They seek counseling on family problems that is religiously oriented yet infused with modern psychiatric know-how. The notion of broad-based individual psychotherapy is quite foreign to most of these applicants. This different frame of reference was so apparent in our first administration of questionnaires to University Psychoanalytic Center and to Religion and Psychiatry Institute applicants that we dropped items especially intended to measure this difference as an unnecessary luxury. The most revealing question was, "How would coming here differ from going to a clergyman?" Eighty per cent of Religion and Psychiatry Institute applicants chose the offered alternative, "The people here have more experience and training than do local ministers." In other words, in principle the staff at the clinic was conceived to be the same as local ministers, but better trained. Only 40 per cent of University Psychoanalytic applicants chose this alternative. Instead, more rejected the relevance of ministers to their problems, for 55 per cent chose the alternative, "A minister knows about religion, and this isn't a religious problem." Only 15 per cent of Religion and Psychiatry Institute applicants endorsed this statement. So in one sense, evaluation of clinics is important to Religion and Psychiatry Institute applicants because they reject or are not interested in the usual psychiatric clinic. In another sense, comparative evaluation of clinics is almost irrelevant to them, since most of them had never even considered other types of psychiatric clinics.

✹ Conclusion: The Dilemma of the Sophisticates

The consumer is said to be stupid—"a sucker born every minute." Swayed by his emotions and ignorant of the facts, he chooses blindly, easily influenced by the most recent word he has heard. And although going to a professional such as a doctor or a lawyer is more important in people's lives than buying a TV set, a person is probably better able to judge the quality of his TV set than the ability of the professional to whom he is going. This does not prevent him, of course, from saying that *his* doctor or dentist or lawyer is the best. In fact, his certainty as to the high quality of his own doctor may simply defend him against the possibility that there is no way he can evaluate this person to whom he is entrusting his life. Does this picture also describe the applicant for psychotherapy at a clinic?

In the last chapter we saw that there is a rationality of sorts in attempts to gain information about clinics, especially among members of the Friends. The more one knows about different sources, the more one is likely to hear about a clinic from a source friendly to that clinic. All this is in general terms. What about specific knowledge about *therapy* and about the quality of a specific *clinic*? Does such knowledge swing the decision and make the final difference? These are, of course, two separate but related issues, for one can have definite expectations of therapy without much knowledge about psychiatric clinics. Moreover, in order to enter psychotherapy one need not even have a clear idea of what therapy is like. Other elements might be quite sufficient to force a decision: pain, and the assertion by some authority that therapy will remove the pain. How it will be removed and what the ultimate results of the removal of pain may be are speculations with which potential patients need not be concerned. This simple model of pain and referral does describe the decision processes of most lower-class nonmembers of the Friends applying to hospital clinics. Even money to pay for therapy is no major concern to them because these applicants never expect to pay for the services of any professional.

Pain and referral alone do not describe the decision process of most applicants to other clinics, however, and such a model is especially unfair to the most knowledgeable applicants. For there is a substantial majority who have expectations of change in a series of broad areas and whose expectations of how this change will come about are in fair accord with what clinicians themselves must feel. So there is no question that the qualities of therapy itself are important factors in drawing many persons into therapy. The consumer of therapy in New York City is not so ignorant, although he might have been uninformed just a generation ago. Experience with therapy is increasing and those who have had such experience obviously know better what to expect from it. More important, however, is the ability of those who have never been in therapy before to estimate what it is like. The best avenue for doing so is membership in the Friends and Supporters of Psychotherapy, for in such a circle hearsay and sheer osmosis afford channels for learning about therapy not available to others. Our data therefore showed clear and accurate expectations about therapy among members of the Friends applying to analytic clinics.

But these accurate expectations lead to a serious dilemma. Since they are so knowledgeable about therapy, members of the Friends are more concerned about its quality. If one does not know what to expect, then the grounds for choosing a clinic are mainly fortuitous rather than well founded and such applicants are less concerned with quality. Moreover, this is just what the data did for nonmembers of the Friends. The first hint of the dilemma faced by members of the Friends and those with previous therapy is that even when they do *not* know about other clinics they tend to emphasize quality as the main comparative advantage of the clinic they have chosen. That applicants tend to "whistle by the graveyard" is shown in the way they evaluate money and the relative value of private versus clinic therapy. In their view, clinics are not better than private therapy, they are simply cheaper. And the more knowledgeable the applicant, the more concerned he is about low cost. Although this is the typical "good consumer" orientation, when it comes to one's very life the double concern about quality and low cost is likely to lead to a serious dilemma. For like good consumers, these applicants also know that you generally "get what you pay for." Hence, the statement that the clinic to which they are applying is better than other clinics, regardless of what they know about other clinics, may simply be a *hope* that the clinic is better.

Another bit of analysis also tends to downgrade the importance of applicants' evaluation of clinics. Many came shortly after they had heard about a clinic simply *because* they heard it was good and were apparently waiting for just this sort of information. The "word" is important, and the entire matter of personal influence as the last straw will be more thoroughly investigated in the next chapter.

The combination of an accurate expectation about the process of therapy and wishful evaluation of the quality of a clinic can be very important to future decisions the applicant may make. For the fact is that many (the overwhelming majority, in some clinics) will not be accepted by the clinic to which they have applied. We dared not ask applicants, "What do you think are your chances of being accepted by this clinic?" It is reasonable to suppose that applicants knowledgeable about other matters would also know that their chances of acceptance were fairly small. We do know that the more knowledgeable applied to other clinics as well. It seems most likely, then, that the sophisticates about therapy will eventually solve their dilemma of quality versus cost by going to a private psychotherapist after the clinic rejects them. They hope to get by with less cost, but if necessary they will pay more for the therapy they feel they need. Nonmembers of the Friends, less concerned about either quality or costs, are simply less interested in therapy in general and if rejected may not go elsewhere. Curiously, then, the weighing of cost versus quality may be less important for the immediate decision than for one which may take place in the future.

NOTES

1. "Further Recommendations in the Technique of Psychoanalysis," first published in *Zeitschrift*, Bd. I, 1913.
2. Eva Mueller, "A Study of Purchase Decisions," in Lincoln H. Clark, ed., *Consumer Behavior* (New York: New York University Press, 1955), pp. 47-49.
3. Lest the reader assume that there is something "wrong" with these applicants, he should be reassured that they are just like the rest of the United States. In earlier work, we were able to reproduce many of the findings of a national sample as reported in G. Gurin, J. Veroff, and S. Feld, *Americans View Their Mental Health* (New York: Basic Books, 1960). The sample of the present study is sufficiently different from the rest of the United States to make such replication, except for special instances, much less possible.

Personal Influence
and the Last Straw

☀

13

A referral to a clinic has two aspects: information and pressure. Information consists in telling a person where he can get treatment, and this function of a referral was just analyzed in Chapter 11. But contacts between human beings are rarely neutral. In addition to mere information, many referrals carry an emotional charge—suggestion, persuasion, or influence to go to a clinic. This chapter describes the nature, extent, and consequence of personal influence upon applicants to go to a clinic.* In particular, we are interested in personal influence as the

* Throughout this chapter we shall be concerned mainly with the decision to go to the clinic to which a respondent is now applying. Logically, there are two separate decisions: the decision to undertake psychotherapy, and the decision to go to a specific clinic. Although these two decisions were unraveled in interviews, it was impractical to do so in a questionnaire so that the two decisions will be somewhat intertwined throughout our discussion. But exploratory interviews showed that in most people's minds *finding* a place to go is so linked with the actual decision to undertake therapy that linking a decision about a clinic and a decision about therapy is not unreasonable. Moreover, later we shall analyze differences between start-

"last straw" which sends a person to a clinic, for the time to talk about last straws has arrived. Until now we have been dealing with an almost infinite regression of reasons for entering therapy—having a problem (and why one has a problem), discussions about problems with friends, reading books, getting information about sources of therapy, trying out various other sources of treatment, and evaluating differences between one clinic and another. But there must be some last crisis, thought, or occasion which serves as the final propellent into therapy at a clinic. Though personal influence has previously appeared in our analysis at a number of points, especially in the discussion of problems, the influence of other people is a key last straw for a number of reasons.

Popular understanding of the decision to go to a psychiatrist often includes a vision of people being dragged off screaming, against their will. We will show that this image is wrong, but still, it must be faced and dealt with. How, then, is the decision really clinched? There is a considerable literature on decision-making which shows that personal influence is an important factor in various types of decision ranging from the act of juvenile delinquency, to adopting new agricultural techniques, to brand-changing in consumer product-buying.[1] Studies in the area of personal influence on decision-making have shown that even in a mass society characterized by heavy mass-media promotion of every sort of thing from political opinion to soap, a major factor in individual decision-making is the influence of other people. The flow of influence is viewed as stemming from mass media, but mediated through several stages of "opinion leaders," that is, persons who are looked to for advice on various matters. In fashion, for example, some younger, more interested and more gregarious women may read such journals as Vogue and pass new fashion information on to other women who themselves may never read these journals. And this flow of influence typically passes through several steps—from woman A to woman B and so on.

Personal influence in the decision to undertake psychotherapy is potentially more important than it is in other decisions. As a rule, mass media do not afford much information about specific clinics, but it is possible to come across a clinic more or less accidentally, as one would encounter a new product on the shelves of a supermarket. For one may see a hospital as he walks by in the street, or might even have previously used its medical clinic. And if one is affiliated with an organization which sponsors a psychiatric clinic, then its name is already familiar. But for analytic clinics and certainly for private psychotherapy personal contact is overwhelmingly the most frequent source of infor-

---

ers and those with previous experience in therapy which will reveal some differences (not many) between first deciding upon therapy and deciding upon a clinic this time.

mation. Ninety-five per cent of analytic-clinic applicants heard of the clinic to which they are now applying from other persons. In general, because of the social structure of psychiatry, the likelihood of a personal influencer serving as the "last straw" in the decision to undertake psychotherapy is considerably greater than in the case of most other decisions, for in the field of psychotherapy there are professionals who exert such influence in addition to the "amateurs." Doctors, psychiatrists, social workers, clergymen, and other professionals are important "opinion leaders" and the major source of information about clinics. This is in sharp distinction to discussions about problems, earlier in the decision, when even among unsolicited advice-givers, professionals were a distinct minority. Thus the presence of professional influencers, especially in the last stage of the decision, changes the entire pattern of personal influence in the decision to undertake therapy, and we shall have to study the relative impact not only of mass media as opposed to personal influence, but of laymen as opposed to professionals.

Influence in the decision to undertake psychotherapy is clearly separable into influence on a person to make him feel that he has emotional problems, which we discussed in Chapter 8, and influence upon him to go to a particular clinic, which is analyzed here. Not only is this division a theoretical possibility but our data will show it to be the most usual pattern. Those who first influenced a person about his problem are usually not the same ones who later told him to go to a clinic.

Finally, in the decision to undertake psychotherapy, the entire relationship to opinion leaders is somewhat different from what it is in other, more casual decisions. We have been stressing throughout this book that not only is there a set of opinion leaders about psychiatric problems but that this set is "organized" as a circle of Friends and Supporters of Psychotherapy. True, this organization is a very loose one, but it is a real one, nevertheless. Such circles no doubt exist in the other areas of personal influence that have been studied, but since they have not been so conceptualized, there is no systematic evidence about them. The Friends and Supporters of Psychotherapy have a symbiotic relationship to the professionals in the field. They give them business, echo their values, and provide an alternate way for persons to learn about emotional problems and about therapy itself. Now one might suspect that members of the Friends, surrounded as they are by this circle of psychiatric opinion leaders, would garner many suggestions to go to psychiatrists. Indeed, in a previous chapter we showed that no matter what the extent to which they searched for knowledge or the actual amount of their knowledge of alternative sources of treatment, members of the Friends were *more likely* to hear of psychiatric clinics through their friends and relatives. However, and this is crucial, we shall show that personal influence is *less likely* to be the last straw which sends members of the Friends to a psychiatric clinic. They are, instead, much more liable to be "self-starters" when it comes to the final decision to go to a clinic. The influence of friends occurs earlier in the decision process for them—while they are considering their problems, not while they are finally deciding to go to a clinic. And this is to be expected since we saw that members of the Friends are much more apt to seek out sources of information about treatment on their own. Since self-initiated search is the opposite of being pressured, members of the Friends may, as a result of their search, get a good deal of *information* from laymen, but this information is not usually in the form of pressure, or at least it was not crucial to the final decision to go to a clinic.

The situation for nonmembers of the Friends is the opposite. Since they are less likely to engage in supportive interactions with laymen early in their decision to go to a clinic, know less about sources of treatment and about therapy itself, and even have the "wrong" problems for therapy, if they are at all to enter psychotherapy they *must* have some pressure placed upon them from the outside. Thus, personal influence is *more* likely to be a last straw in their case. Moreover, because they are not enmeshed in a lay circle of psychiatric opinion leaders, this influence must more frequently come from professionals such as doctors, social workers, and even previous psychotherapists. All this holds true for those persons who are in a position to receive influence from lay or professional sources. There are those who are totally removed from such contacts, either because they are alienated from standard medical and psychiatric practice, as in the case of many applicants to the religio-psychiatric clinic, or as is true for hospital-clinic applicants, because they belong to the lower class and share a culture which has very different attitudes to professionals in general and psychiatrists in particular. Accident and happenstance contact are important in their case.

In this chapter, then, we shall first examine the extent of personal influence upon applicants and the circumstances in which it occurred. We shall show that the structure of psychiatry and the effectiveness of different sources of information explain why influence and pressure are fairly low. Then we shall divide applicants into those for whom personal influence was the sole last straw, those for whom it was a contributing factor in their final decision, and those for whom it played no part. We shall want to know in what way these types of applicants differ and what the differences indicate. A brief inquiry into differences between applicants with varying histories of previous consultations with professionals will complete our analysis.

❀ *The Amount of Influence and the Structure of Psychiatry*

The amount of pressure placed upon applicants to apply to a clinic is a great deal less than most persons might imagine. We asked our coders to note whether respondents were subjected to "heavy pressure," which we defined as "urging to go to this clinic; direct order; prediction of dire consequences if the person did not go; glowing picture of the consequences of treatment." In contrast, "moderate pressure" was defined as "suggesting a clinic but not urging a person to go." Here are three cases, one subjected to a great deal of pressure, one to only moderate pressure, and the third to no pressure at all.

HEAVY PRESSURE

A thirty-year-old restaurant worker studying for religious orders applied to St. Matthew:

> "Originally I was supposed to go to St. Francis. They told me my district was Lincoln Hospital and they told me my district was here. The priest told me to go to St. Francis. They sent me." His problem is that "I'm going into religious orders—I'm a convert. Before, I experienced overt periods of homosexuality. The Church is concerned. They want to see that I'm mentally acceptable as well as physically. . . . After coming into the Church I would still lapse into an affair. . . . A priest in confession mentioned St. Francis a year and one half ago—my spiritual advisor mentioned it one and one-half weeks ago." When asked about any special incident that made him decide to come now he said, "Well, I decided a year ago. It was just my nature of putting it off." He did *not* assent to our final question that the reason he came was that things got so bad he "could not handle it himself." Rather, after his last ritual in January he was approached by his advisor who indicated that he would have to go for evaluation if he wished to take orders. It was easy for him to decide now to come "because I'm directed to do it by my superior," although "the business of writing a letter [required by St. Francis] is terrible." It is obvious that without heavy pressure, this person, who had not previously been to a psychiatrist, would not have now come.

MODERATE PRESSURE

A thirty-four-year-old Negro social worker applying to an analytic clinic wrote:

> "Part of my problem is around self-assertion and expressing anger directly. A second portion comes from my need for external work pres-

sures. Even under such pressures there is always a part which is left undone."

His supervisor and his wife who is also a psychiatric social worker "have both itemized in great detail (his problems) in the last few months." His supervisor suggested the clinic without being invited to do so. He also checked "things got so bad. . . ." Yet the incident which precipitated his coming was not direct personal influence. "I felt deeply inadequate in job, community, and family situations. I was also displacing my anger onto my family inappropriately." In contrast to the case with heavy pressure, this person was not practically forced to go or face the loss of his career. Moreover the last straw was experienced as an internal state, rather than external pressure.

NO PRESSURE

A forty-two-year-old TV repairman applied to an analytic clinic, stating:

"I am a stutterer." The main things about his problem that bother him are, "Stuttering prevents a normal association with people through the exchange of ideas. It prevents my trying an occupation requiring 'talk' in its course." In response to our checklist about problems he notes about physical well being that "I do get headaches but I attribute these to too much coffee, or, at times tension on the job." He also writes, "I'm classed as a good repairman and tend to be 'too critical' (that is, too exact). No one has given him unsolicited comments about his problem and when he discusses it with his wife she says "that my affliction was not noticeable," but this was not helpful. His reasons for not going into therapy before were shame, denial and a feeling he could handle it himself.

His decision to go to the clinic is typical of personal influence without pressure. He checked that a friend had suggested it without being asked, but also that the friend mentioned the clinic without knowing he was interested. "In the course of conversation my friend would mention of his visits to the Personal Psychology Institute and I suddenly decided to also do so." He first heard about the clinic six months before his application. He knows of no other clinic, but what appeals to him about this one is that "the cost is within my range of income."

Only 3 per cent of analytic, 6 per cent of hospital-clinic, and 15 per cent of religio-psychiatric applicants were classified as having been subjected to heavy pressure. These results are not peculiar to our method or our sample of outpatients. In another study of outpatient service in all of New York State, using somewhat different methods of assessment, investigators found that only 9 per cent of clinic applicants "came because they were told 'to go or else.' "[2] Now these figures are in fact not radically different from those reported in *Personal Influence* for brand shifting (15 per cent), motion-picture selection (14 per cent), or fashion change (8 per cent).[3] These percentages, arrived at after a detailed reason analysis, represent the number of persons in each area who (in answer to a direct question) said that personal influence was the most important factor in their decision. In contrast, our procedure depended upon *coders* to make the assessment. Nevertheless, the figures in our study are roughly the same as in the New York State study of decision to enter therapy, as well as in the study of more casual decisions. Why should this be so?

At first blush we might expect the extent of personal influence in casual decisions and in a depth decision to be different for these reasons: First, as we said, the sheer *opportunity* for personal influence to be the crucial one is greater in the decision to undertake psychotherapy, since exposure to impersonal sources (such as the mass media) is much less frequent than in decisions to buy consumer products or to go to the movies. There is, it is true, considerable exposure to "theoretical" (impersonal) material about psychotherapy, as shown in our chapter about reading, but this source of information rarely mentions specific places where one can be given therapy and certainly does not extol them. But that is the difference between advertising and simply giving information. Second, one would expect that a decision which is essentially much more difficult to make might require more personal pressure by others.

While these suppositions are reasonable, in fact there is shown to be *no more* personal influence operating in the decision to undertake psychotherapy in a particular clinic than in the decision to go to a particular movie. These facts substantiate our previously stated findings that much of the distance from the feeling that one does not need psychiatric treatment to the decision to apply for such treatment has been traversed *before* the stage of deciding to go to a clinic. Moreover, and this is extremely important, a person entering outpatient treatment is rarely *forced* into treatment, in contrast to the fate of many mental hospital patients. Except for applicants to hospital clinics, almost all of our sample came to treatment because they wanted to; and the extent of their volition differs in no substantial way from the free choice made in going to a movie or buying soap.

The applicants' own reports support and substantiate our coders' judgment that influence brought to bear upon most applicants was fairly mild. These reports cover two related areas. The first deals with the circumstances under which other people happened to tell the applicant about a clinic. The second covers an account of who did the telling and under what circumstances. From the first set of data it will be apparent that, for the most part, unlike discussions at an earlier phase about problems, *the applicants themselves asked to be told about therapy.* If one asks to be influenced, the pressure applied cannot be altogether incongruent with a person's own desires. The second set of data shows in particular that professionals, the bulk of those who gave information about clinics, usually did so in response to a request from their client for information about treatment sources. Rarely was this advice unsolicited, except among hospital-clinic applicants.

Applicants to clinics were quite well able to tell us about the circumstances which surrounded their receipt of information about a clinic. Only 10 per cent (mostly those who heard from mass media or the environment) did not answer our five questions.

First we ascertained who received unsolicited influence by asking, "What made you decide to come to this clinic now?" Those choosing the alternative, "Someone suggested it without my having asked them," were classified as unsolicited influence. Then, after respondents indicated who told them about the clinic, we asked, "How did they happen to tell you about this clinic?" The following alternatives were available:

I was just asking about how to get treatment.

I was just discussing my problem.

I was asking for advice in general.

They just mentioned the clinic without knowing I was interested.

These alternatives were added to the one on unsolicited advice to give a list of possible circumstances in which applicants were told about a clinic. Since one or all of these could have occurred together or in conversations with different persons, the responses add to more than 100 per cent.

Purely unsolicited influence formed only a small proportion (5 per cent) of the occasions upon which religio-psychiatric and analytic-clinic applicants were told about a clinic. On the other hand, 27 per cent of hospital-clinic applicants were given unsolicited suggestions to go to the psychiatric clinic to which they were now applying—usually by physicians at a hospital clinic to which they had applied for purely medical treatment. (At the stage of discussing problems with laymen, 66 per cent of analytic, 52 per cent of religio-psychiatric, and 51 per cent of hospital-clinic applicants who talked with others received some unsolicited advice.) The greater frequency of unsolicited referrals occurs in the case of hospital-clinic applicants because most of them had not gone through the first stage of decision—getting the "right" problem. Most continued to feel they had physical symptoms whose appropriateness for psychiatry might be questionable. Of course, once one is concerned about getting treatment, one's problems do come in for discussion, so about 30 per cent of all applicants were told to go to a clinic during a discussion of their problems—and this is somewhat like being given unsolicited advice one has in fact asked for. (These discussions, however, were generally *not* the ones earlier analyzed in Chapter 8.) All the rest of the applicants either openly solicited the information or received it quite casually in the course of other events. Directly asking for treatment sources was the occasion for almost half of the analytic-clinic applicants (but only 20 to 30 per cent of the time for applicants to other clinics). Asking for advice in general accounted for another 10 per cent. Finally, a mention of the clinic in casual conversation or some nonpersonal way of acquiring information occurred for 20 per cent of the analytic- and hospital-clinic applicants, but for almost half of the applicants to the religio-psychiatric clinic. At most, only one-third of all applicants received some form of unsolicited directive to go to a clinic. That is why coders so rarely assigned the category of "heavy influence." Even the hospital-clinic applicants who were told to go to a psychiatric clinic often expected such influence. Since they lacked psychiatric sophistication, the only way they knew to get emotional relief was to go to a hospital medical clinic, and then let the authoritative medical system take its course. They would in this way be absolved of the responsibility of deciding to go to a psychiatrist.

The social structure of psychiatry itself insures that heavy pressure on outpatients will be quite rare. Though laymen are more frequently consulted about problems (see Chapter 8), professionals are the most frequent sources of influence about psychiatric clinics. Excluding cases in which *no* personal influence was apparent in the decision to go to a clinic, 85 per cent of hospital-clinic applicants, 66 per cent of analytic-clinic applicants, and even 47 per cent of religio-psychiatric clinic applicants were told about the clinic to which they were applying by professionals. Hence the opportunity for professionals to exert strong influence at this stage of the decision is considerably greater than it is for laymen. Yet the entire ethos of professionals when it comes to out-patient psychiatric treatment is that patients must go voluntarily. Hence, Table 35, which shows the occasions upon which different types of influencers told applicants about a clinic, indicates that professionals most frequently gave their information only when they were *asked* for sources of treatment, and this holds true whether the professional is a friend ("Oh, you're a doctor, I just happen . . .") or is seen in formal conference. These figures are for analytic-clinic applicants only (where we have enough cases to be able to include friends and relatives). The different situation in hospital clinics is reflected by the fact that psychotherapeutic ethos or not, almost 30 per cent of professionals who gave information gave it unsolicited. But then, since their clients were simply not involved in the culture of psychotherapy, these professionals must have felt no other choice was possible.

Laymen have a different relationship to this entire process of influencing others to go to a psychiatric clinic. Their information was typically given earlier in the decision process, during a discussion of the problem. Because of the prevalence of so many members of the Friends

TABLE 35 *Occasions in Which Various Influencers Told Analytic-Clinic Applicants about the Clinic**

Influencer	Unsolicited	Discussion of problem	Request for Advice	Source of Treatment	Mentioned	N
Parent	0	44	0	22	33	(9)
Spouse	15	62	0	8	23	(13)
Close friend	6	47	18	34	24	(71)
Casual friend	2	32	8	44	20	(93)
Friend who is a professional	0	28	16	56	16	(25)
Professional in conference	6	29	12	57	8	(449)

*For applicants receiving influence from one source only, for specified influencer only. Rows may add to more than 100% since some persons checked more than one occasion.

in the social environment of analytic-clinic applicants, however, the Friends and Supporters themselves often serve in place of professionals as a source of referral. Many laymen, therefore, were asked about places for treatment. The few spouses who were the source of information were, not surprisingly, both the most likely to give *unsolicited* suggestions and the most likely to do so during the course of a discussion about problems. Yet there is no doubt that, except for spouses, the ethos of the professionals pervades the efforts of laymen since it has become rather widely known that office psychotherapy has little value if patients are unwilling to go.

Because professionals are unlikely to give unsolicited advice, however, does not mean that when they do inform a patient about a clinic their advice is unimportant or unheeded. One of the reasons professionals appear to exert so little direct pressure is that merely telling a patient about a clinic is sufficient, in most cases, to send him there without any other significant event occurring in his emotional life. Professionals, especially psychotherapists, do not make referrals unless they think their clients are ready for it. Our coders estimated whether, when information about a clinic was given to one of our respondents, he then immediately applied to a clinic or delayed his application until something else happened. For example, suppose that a physician suggested to a patient that he go to a psychiatrist but he did not actually go until he was faced with the loss of his job. That threatened loss is then the immediate precipitating event, and the suggestion of the physician, while ultimately important, cannot be said to be the precipitating event or the last straw. The over-all effectiveness of different types of information givers can be rated by noting the proportion of times, after hearing about a clinic from a given source, an applicant went directly to the clinic without some other event intervening.* Table 36 shows these proportions for various types of influencers and clinics.

The most striking fact the table makes clear is that personal sources of information are more effective than impersonal ones; and this is the general finding for all decisions, whether to buy groceries, get married, or go to the movies. For example, Table 36 indicates that in 62 per cent

TABLE 36 *Proportion of Information Sources That Triggered the Decision to Go to a Clinic*

Information Source	Analytic Clinics		Religio-Psychiatric Clinic		Hospital Clinics	
	%	N	%	N	%	N
Mass media	62	(29)	30	(94)	–	–
Environment	50	(18)	41	(17)	87	(60)
Therapist	95	(213)	100	(3)	100	(6)
Psychiatric clinic	92	(83)	–	–	92	(13)
Social agency	92	(120)	100	(5)	71	(7)
Private doctor	79	(43)	–	–	100	(7)
Other medical	83	(12)	–	–	–	–
Other agency	83	(89)	–	–	–	–
Clergy	63	(8)	87	(15)	33	(3)
Friends, relatives	73	(364)	62	(37)	63	(24)

of the cases in which an analytic-clinic applicant heard of a clinic through mass media, he went there without some other event intervening in his life; in contrast, in 95 per cent of cases in which a person heard about a clinic from a therapist he applied directly. Mass media are even less effective among religio-psychiatric clinic applicants, despite their frequent use by these applicants. Among the professionals, private psychotherapists are the most effective, and psychiatric clinics and social agencies only slightly less so. For after all, those who have been to such professionals have already determined, at least once, that they need some form of psychotherapy. Hence they are the ones most ready for a referral. Physicians who are not psychiatrists are more than 10 points *less* effective than psychotherapeutic sources, and this may be caused partly by the

* In measuring "effectiveness" we always have the problem of self-selection; that is, persons tend to expose themselves to media which are likely to tell them what they wish to hear. Those who talk to others about problems may be more ready to go to a clinic than those who merely read.

greater psychological distance *their* patients must travel before they are ready for therapy, but may also be caused by the previously noted general ineffectiveness of physicians in the mental health area. Connections count, of course, and physicians generally have poor contacts with psychiatrists. Where they do have better relations, as in hospital clinics, their rate of effectiveness is higher ("environment" in the hospital situation also includes referrals by medical clinic physicians in the hospital itself). Similarly, clergymen have lower effectiveness than any other personal source except among religio-psychiatric clinic applicants, for with the exception of that one clinic, clergymen have fewer connections with the world of psychiatry. Laymen, in general, stand between therapists and the mass media in effectiveness. Their general rate of effective referral is surprisingly high for analytic-clinic applicants, perhaps because so many of them are members of the Friends.

The effectiveness of professionals and even of laymen, coupled with the ineffectiveness of mass media and its relative unimportance in sending people to psychiatrists, may be responsible for the popular conception that people go to psychiatrists as a result of heavy pressure. Perhaps also, except for those familiar with the culture of psychotherapy through membership in the Friends, most people think of the encounter with a therapist as a terrifying experience and imagine that only the most severe pressure could induce a person to go through with it. But every bit of evidence at our command suggests that although personal contact is vital in sending persons to psychiatric clinics, and may often be the last straw, the pressure to go is rarely stronger than that placed upon people to go to a movie. Before most applicants for psychotherapy expose themselves to the influence of other people they are already ready to go for help.

❈ Influence as the Last Straw

Usually information received about clinics or influence exerted to go to one did not precede actual application by a very long period. In fact, over half such applications were made during the month after receiving the information or influence. The short length of time between these two events suggests that personal influence often had a "last straw" effect. For by the time they received information about a particular clinic many persons were really ready to go. Previous conversations with laymen about problems, previous attempts at receiving professional help, and the various attempts on the part of applicants to gain information about treatment sources had all contributed to the decision to go to a clinic. Nonetheless, there is considerable variation among applicants in the extent to which personal influence alone was sufficient to send them to a clinic, even at this final stage of the decision. The sources of this variation indicate the real role of personal influence in the decision.

To measure this variation we turn to a more objective classification of the responses concerning the role of personal influence in the final decision to go to a clinic. On the basis of answers to the question, "What made you decide to come to this clinic now?" as well as to the other questions about personal influence, we classified respondents into three groups: those who checked nothing but personal influence in response to this question and who reported no special incidents involving some other propelling event than personal influence; those who did note personal influence but also reported other events or some unusual symptoms that suddenly appeared; and those who, even if they did hear about a clinic from other persons, did not give a response suggesting that personal influence had anything to do with their ultimate decision.* We cite three illustrative cases, the first showing only personal influence, the second both personal influence and other events, and the third other events only.

PERSONAL INFLUENCE ONLY

The following case shows how personal influence alone can trigger going to a psychiatrist yet not be exceptionally heavy pressure.

A twenty-two-year-old girl who is a college student applied to an analytic clinic complaining that "I seem to be reacting like a typical hysterical case. Constant headaches and the inability to initiate action." Her boyfriend (who is a psychology major) had been going to the clinic for about a year and one-half. A few weeks before her application, he spoke to her about her problems without being asked to do so. He said "that I have the inability to initiate action. He was also very sympathetic about my headaches, and recommended getting help from you." He said, "Why don't you try Interpersonal Psychiatry Institute, it's a very good place." When we probed the reasons (she was among the subsample who both filled out questionnaires and were later interviewed) she explained why she did not check the item that she came because things were getting so bad she could not handle them. "If I had felt that way I would have tried faster to find help. Things have been about on an even keel. I would have done it earlier—except that I have this inability to initiate action. I didn't go out searching." This girl clearly would not have come without personal

* Note that this assessment of the over-all final decision is much more mechanical than that made in relation to particular sources of information. Moreover, it does not attempt to measure *how much* influence, but merely whether or not it was present. It therefore depends much less on coder-judgment than any of the other indicators of personal influence; yet findings using other indicators are similar to those reported here.

influence, yet it is also fairly clear that this influence cannot be considered heavy pressure.

PERSONAL INFLUENCE AND OTHER

A nineteen-year-old girl studying to be an actress applied to an analytic clinic and wrote,

"My problem is concerned generally with finding out *who* I am, why I do certain things, and how to channel creative energy. . . ." A month before she applied for treatment both her parents and a close friend suggested "that I should try to get professional help." But a special incident seems to have triggered her decision to come for help now. "An old family friend (a married man) visited our house for an evening—without having any previous relationship or cause, I slept with him—and the distress after kept me from concentrating on school." The previous summer she had seen a private psychiatrist for three or four sessions. Now, "I told him my problem" and he recommended the clinic to which she is now applying.

In this case, laymen suggested psychiatric help and a professional made a referral but a specific event triggered the decision to apply now. Hence both personal influence and other matters were present.

OTHER THINGS ONLY: NO PERSONAL INFLUENCE

A thirty-eight-year-old retail shoe salesman, who is a high school dropout applied to an analytic clinic.

His problem is: "intense anxiety—feeling of worthlessness, failure, inadequacy, hopelessness—physically manifested by sleeplessness, indigestion, dizziness—shortness of breath, chest pains, obsessive thoughts." How did you first notice. . . . "It was a gradual process—avoiding intellectual contact with people, shying away from problems, judging people severely and finding them lacking in intelligence, sensitivity, etc.—and most recently awakening in the middle of the nite with feelings of utter inadequacy and despondency."

In 1949 he had three sessions of therapy—one at a clinic and two with a private psychiatrist. A month ago he asked the mental health association to recommend a clinic. "Things got so bad I couldn't handle it myself." He did not continue before because of the expense. The incident that precipitated going for help was "waking in a panic of uncontrollable anxiety every nite and continuing that way." This man's panic seems responsible for his search for treatment. His referral was obtained because he himself initiated the quest.

When such cases are added together, personal influence is found to be the sole last straw for 29 per cent of analytic-clinic applicants, 24 per cent of hospital-clinic applicants, but only 8 per cent of religio-psychiatric clinic applicants. At the other extreme—being completely free from personal influence as a last straw—there are 43 per cent of religio-psychiatric clinic applicants, 30 per cent of those going to analytic clinics, and only 16 per cent of hospital-clinic patients. Between 40 and 50 per cent of all cases at all the different clinic types showed both personal influence and other events.

The most important characteristics of those for whom personal influence was the single last straw is that they are *less* likely to be members of the Friends (by about 12 percentage points with education controlled). On the other hand, with membership in the Friends taken into account, better educated persons are *more* likely (by about 8 percentage points) to report personal influence alone as the last straw. As we shall show, members of the Friends need this last push much less than do others despite the fact that the higher education and social class of the Friends frequently expose them to professionals who are more effective than laymen in sending people to psychiatrists; besides, they come in contact with a more knowledgeable group of lay experts in psychiatry.

The activities a person engaged in early in his decision to undertake psychotherapy explain why, at the final step, he is less likely to be precipitated into therapy by others and more likely to go solely on his own initiative. First, those who either had no contact with laymen at the earlier stage of discussing problems or who had received *un*solicited advice from them about their problems were the very ones who at the final stage of decision needed to be pushed into therapy by others.*
Now these "others," these final influencers are, as we know, most frequently professionals rather than laymen. Hence, if a person did not discuss his problems with laymen he was more likely (by 15 percentage points) to be sent to a clinic by a professional. And there is an important difference between merely discussing one's problems and finally making the decision to go to a clinic. The persons consulted about *problems* were rarely the ones who told applicants about *clinics.* For the most part laymen led in the discussion about problems, and professionals, in referring to clinics. Only when professionals gave unsolicited advice about problems did they also (80 per cent) make a referral to a clinic. There is thus considerable "division of labor" in the process of sending persons to seek psychiatric help. The stage of discussion of problems has quite different significance from that of impelling a person to take action—to go to a clinic or a psychiatrist. In the former stage, discussion with

---

* The differences are 37 percentage points for hospital and 20 percentage points for analytic-clinic applicants. Religio-psychiatric clinic applicants, with their reliance on mass media, present a different picture.

knowledgeable and understanding laymen can have, as we have seen, a supportive function, and thus may be more easily engaged in by persons who themselves are knowledgeable about therapy. But once the introspective process is started, the more knowledgeable are much less prone to rely on others to get them into therapy.

The stage of reading about emotional problems reflects the different nature and social setting of self-analysis as compared to the ultimate decision to seek therapy. Almost 40 per cent of analytic-clinic applicants who only read for help with their problems and who normally do not read much of anything were, in their decision to go to a clinic, propelled *only* by personal influence; this compares with about 25 per cent of readers of serious or popular mental health literature who were otherwise regular readers. Persons who are not usually introspective and who read only when faced with an emotional calamity need the forcefulness of others to clinch their decision to seek therapy.

The extent to which one searched for knowledge makes a great deal of difference in the amount of personal influence necessary to clinch the final decision. Those who did *not* make inquiries were much *more* likely to have decided to come to a clinic *only* on the basis of personal influence. Applicants who knew of alternative sources of therapy were, however, slightly more likely to have come entirely as a result of personal influence. But this is true simply because most influence at this stage comes from professionals, and one of the best ways to discover another source for therapy is actually to have tried it.

This raises the question as to the validity of our findings for the choice of a private psychiatrist rather than a clinic. Much of our argument has been based on the effect of previous professionals on the decision to enter therapy. Though there may be differences between private practice and analytic clinics in the extent to which their patients had previously been to other professionals, I doubt it. Informal interviews with a number of private therapists in New York show, upon probing, that a great number of their patients had previously been to other professionals—not necessarily to psychotherapists, of course. (No formal statistics are available.) So the key question becomes: what is the effect of the various paths taken to psychiatry upon the amount of pressure and influence that must be exerted on an applicant to enter or re-enter therapy.

The principal differences are between those who have never been to a psychiatrist and those who have been at least once before. Members of the Friends who had never been to psychiatrists and who are now applying to analytic clinics are the real self-starters when it comes to entering therapy. Personal influence was the last straw for only 20 per cent of them, as compared to 30 per cent of those who had already been to psychiatrists. The additional 10 per cent is due chiefly to the force of the recommendation of a clinic by a previous therapist. As for non-members of the Friends, it matters not whether they had been to a psychiatrist before or not. For 35 per cent of them, personal influence was the last straw in their decision. Apparently, it takes a certain amount of influence to get a nonmember of the Friends into therapy whether or not he has tried before. In short, the tendencies we have described are simply intensified for beginners in therapy, and direct personal influence may be even less important compared to the influence of one's entire milieu.

❂ Conclusion

To sum up, the decision to seek psychiatric care can be represented as a balanced distribution of the effects of personal and social influence. In any decision the influence of others is a key factor even if, as we saw earlier in this chapter, the influence does not represent severe pressure. For the crucial questions are (1) at what phase in the decision is personal influence most important; (2) is this influence the result of single opinion leaders or is it the result of an entire climate or circle of influencers; (3) is this influence something which confirms and supports a person in a decision he might have reached by himself or is influence a factor which converts a person to a position or action which he might not otherwise have taken. For the decision to undertake psychotherapy, the answers to all these questions depend on whether or not a person is a member of the Friends and Supporters of Psychotherapy. If he is a member, then he is already immersed in a circle of influencers whose effect on his decision is more subtle than overt influence. In the first place he tends, by participating in their culture to have the "right" problems for therapy. Some of this wisdom is obtained from reading the "right" books. When he discusses his problems with others, they tend to support and confirm his feelings about himself and his problems. He is more likely to initiate a quest for information about sources of therapy and is more likely to know what to expect from it. Finally, as we have just seen, with all of this social support, his final decision to enter or re-enter therapy is more likely to appear to be his own decision. It is his own only in the sense that he is less likely, in the end, to need someone else to push him over the precipice into therapy. It is *not* his own in another sense, however, because the entire decision has been supported by his circle of Friends and Supporters of Psychotherapy.

For those who are not members of the Friends, their entrance into therapy is much more dependent on the specific social control of individual others. They do not have the "right" problems, and if they read at all, they read the "wrong" books. They are less likely to discuss their problems with others to begin with, and if they do, they are more likely to receive controlling and converting pressure. They are less likely to ask about therapy and know less about it. No wonder, then, that their final decision is more dependent on the direct influence of others. Moreover, these others are typically professional influencers—the equivalent of single opinion leaders, rather than an entire circle of supporters. They are not part of the daily life of the applicant. Yet even for nonmembers of the Friends, the structure of psychiatric outpatient service and its unwillingness to accept persons who have not voluntarily decided to come means that the amount of absolute force, pressure, or influence to go is not likely to be greater than in many casual or trivial decisions.

NOTES

1. E. Katz and P. F. Lazarsfeld, *Personal Influence* (New York: The Free Press, 1955).
2. Gerhart Saenger and John Cumming, "Study of Community Mental Health Clinics, Report I, Characteristics of Patients Applying for Service and Factors Determining Acceptance for Treatment" (Syracuse, New York: Mental Health Research Unit, New York State Department of Mental Hygiene, October 1965), Table VI-1 and pp. 104-106.
3. Katz and Lazarsfeld, *op. cit.*

TOWARD BETTER COMMUNITY MENTAL-HEALTH PROGRAMS

V

Summary of Findings

✸

14

The decision to go to a psychiatrist or a psychiatric clinic is most complex. In this book we have discussed three types of clinics, basically two types of patients, and four main stages in the decision to seek help. To put matters in perspective, we shall review some of our major findings. The implications of these findings for community mental health will be stated in the next chapter.

✸ Types of Clinics

There are basically three types of psychiatric clinics: analytic, religio-psychiatric, and hospital. Each has a different organizational perspective and a different type of clientele. Analytic clinics are mainly devoted to training new psychoanalysts, although those that are more "psycho-therapeutic" than "psychoanalytic" tend to concentrate more on a group practice with middle-income patients. Analytic clinics are usually operated by some form of collegial rather than bureaucratic organization and are usually independent rather than part of a hospital. The trainees or "candidates" generally do almost all the therapy under the supervision of graduate psychiatrists. In the more traditional psychoanalytic institutes the trainees are M.D. graduates of an approved psychiatric residency program. The less traditional clinics also have Ph.D. psychologists and graduate social workers as trainees. In addition to supervising, the graduate, attending, or supervisory therapists direct the clinic and have the final word on who is admitted as a patient. Most analytic clinics admit relatively few applicants. More analytic-clinic applicants tend to be referred by friends or by psychiatrists than do applicants of other clinics, and they tend to be young, single, sophisticated, and Jewish, and from professional or student occupations.

A religio-psychiatric clinic is much like a psychotherapy-oriented analytic clinic except that the trainees are ministers. Applicants tend to hear of this type of clinic from the mass media, from ministers, and from friends. Most are Protestant, and many are businessmen (or their wives) and married.

As their name implies, hospital psychiatric clinics are outpatient services connected with hospitals. As such they fall in line with other services of urban voluntary hospitals: they have a chief of service, residents, interns, a few social workers, attending physicians, and a somewhat tighter bureaucratic structure than the other clinics, even though key professionals usually serve part time. Receiving greater public support and accepting for short-term therapy a greater proportion of applicants, hospital clinics cater to the urban working class and poor, many of whom were referred by other medical services or physicians. Considerably more women than men apply.

To understand the role of psychiatric clinics in community mental health, a matter that will occupy us in the next chapter, we must understand what clinics produce for the community and for professional organizations. The process by which patients become an "input" into the system is of course the major concern of this book and will be summarized in some detail in this chapter. As for the other partners in the operation of clinics, the community gives money and patients in the hope that the latter will be socially controlled. Trainees and supervisors give their time, rarely at rates commensurate with the professional market, in order to receive training and to have some opportunity of working with other professionals rather than only with patients in isolated offices. Then too, through an affiliation with a hospital, psychiatrists can more easily place patients needing emergency hospitalization. In some situations, therapists can gain a supply of private patients. The institutes and hospitals with which the clinics are affiliated supply supervision, organization, and funds in return for a supply of training cases. Some clinics with less public support depend on patient fees to finance part of the training program. The benefits which professionals and their organizations receive, coupled with the fairly loose organization of most clinics which makes abstract and distant demands more difficult to enforce, tend to make most clinics more responsive to the training needs of future psychotherapists and less responsive to community needs for the treatment (or social control) and rehabilitation of low- and middle-income patients. The newly perceived need to train experts in community action and organization is only beginning to be noted by clinics.

☸ *Types of Patients*

There are two distinct types of patients, each of which is in turn divided into two types. Those applicants who knew others who had problems like their own, knew others in therapy, asked their friends for a referral, and who told their friends that they were applying to a clinic belong to a social circle to which we give the name of "Friends and Supporters of Psychotherapy." There are two types of Friends and Supporters: the vast majority are not only psychiatrically but culturally sophisticated; on the other hand, some are only psychiatrically oriented. Similarly, the large majority of nonmembers of the circle are not culturally sophisticated. Since entrance into the circle is dependent on meeting other knowledgeable laymen, having already been to a psychotherapist is not correlated with circle membership except among the less educated whom previous therapy recruits into the ranks of the psychiatrically but not culturally sophisticated. Compared to other clinic applicants, members of the Friends and Supporters of Psychotherapy are better educated and come from professions in the arts, communication, teaching, and medicine rather than from engineering, law, or business. They tend to be less religious, though among analytic-clinic applicants, Protestants are slightly more likely than Jews to belong to the Friends and Supporters. Members of the Friends and Supporters also tend to be younger and not to live with families.

☸ *Steps in Going to a Psychiatric Clinic*

The decision to go to a psychotherapist or to a psychiatric clinic is composed of four steps or stages: the realization of a problem, consultation with laymen, choice of type of healer, and choice of an individual practitioner. The same factors are not equally important in all stages or steps, although the type of clinic and the type of applicant are important in all stages.

STEP 1: REALIZATION OF A PROBLEM

The first and perhaps foremost reason people give for going to a psychotherapist is that they have problems. Stress can create problems, but whether or not problems actually result in going to a psychotherapist depends more upon people's feelings about the psychiatric relevance of their problems than on the presence of a stressful environment. The process of channeling people to psychiatrists also affects the type of problems psychiatrists see. In short, people do not go to psychiatrists merely because they are sick. The best measure of "sickness," diagnosis, is generally unrelated to anything in this study except the acceptance or rejection of some patients by some clinics.

Physical Symptoms. Although supposedly clearcut indications of the need for a doctor, physical symptoms show that knowledge and an understanding of psychiatric symptoms affect the decision to seek psychiatric care. Unlike other persons, lower-class applicants for psychotherapy tend to come because of their physical symptoms. Yet in the age range of applicants to psychiatric clinics, there is *no* clear relation in the general population between physical conditions and social class. Rather, lower-class persons tend to interpret their psychological distress in physical terms. Working-class applicants to psychiatric clinics who are psychologically sophisticated do *not* present physical symptoms more frequently than applicants of higher-class background. It is also true that unsophisticated lower-class persons find it easier to go to a "doctor" if they can tell him about physical pain.

Psychoanalytic Syndrome. At the other end of the scale, there are the special problems of sophisticated people. These are the traditional psychoanalytic problems of feelings of lack of self-worth, inadequate interpersonal relationships, and various sexual problems. These people do not seem, by and large, to be the products of stressful social environments (though sexual problems seem to be related to possible social stress). Rather, problems belonging to the psychoanalytic syndrome are brought to psychotherapists mainly by patients who have been trained to recognize and evaluate such difficulties. Training overcomes the reluctance of women to talk about sexual problems and the tendency of lower-class persons to be less overtly concerned about feelings of self-worth. Training occurs through reading the right books, actually going to a psychotherapist, or through membership in the Friends and Supporters of Psychotherapy.

Psychiatric Syndrome. People who bring physical symptoms to psychotherapists also often bring other problems that belong to the traditional psychiatric syndrome: lack of orientation, or hysteria, tantrums, phobias, diffuse anxiety, immobility and depression. Except for inability to think or to orient oneself, problems which are more common among students or the upwardly mobile, traditional psychiatric problems are seldom occasioned by any specific events, are not especially prevalent in one group or another of applicants, and generally are unaffected by whatever previous training in psychiatry an applicant may have had. For these reasons, we conclude that the traditional psychiatric problems are probably harder for a person himself to recognize or to bring to an outpatient psychiatrist, although when they become unusually pronounced and bizarre, others may recognize them as indicating the need for hospitalization. So despite the pervasiveness of "psychiatric" problems among applicants, they are probably not as effective in getting people to outpatient psychotherapy as are the "psychoanalytic" type of problem.

Projective Problems. Another group of problems—marital, family, and situational difficulties—are called projective problems because those who present them tend to say that *other* people caused them. Family and marital problems have a peculiar relationship to psychiatric sophistication. Whether or not they are seen as fit problems for psychiatric treatment depends on the level of a person's general and psychiatric sophistication. Those who have neither a good general education nor psychiatric sophistication do not see family and marital problems as suitable reasons for going to a psychotherapist. Those with little general education but some psychiatric knowledge find family problems a good reason for going to a psychotherapist. Persons of good education but who are middle-class Protestants of an engineering, law, or business background and who are not especially psychiatrically sophisticated are also especially likely to seek help for such problems, but they bring them to a religio-psychiatric clinic in which family counseling by ministers seems especially appropriate. Finally, those who are both well educated and psychiatrically knowledgeable do not find family or marital problems especially good material for psychotherapists; they view such problems as merely indicative of other more basic personal difficulties.

STEP 2: DISCUSSION OF PROBLEMS WITH LAYMEN

People recognize problems not only because of pain but because other people have told them they have problems. The force of lay influencers and amateur psychotherapists (including nonpsychiatric doctors, ministers, and so on) is expended in two directions: first to get potential applicants for psychotherapy to realize that they have problems, and second, to get them to a psychotherapist. While these actions may occur simultaneously, they are analytically separate and, in fact, empirically distinct. The people who discuss an applicant's problems with him are generally not the same ones who influenced him to come to a particular clinic. Laymen tend to dominate the discussion of problems and to do so earlier in the process of seeking help, but professionals tend to suggest a particular source of treatment. Talk is apparently almost a prerequisite for going to a psychotherapist, for 80 to 90 per cent have talked with others.

Social Control. Discussion can take place because a person has asked for it or because others feel impelled to intervene. Purely unsolicited comments offer something new to an applicant and are a form of social control, but those comments he has apparently asked for serve to confirm what he already knows. Those who have interpersonal or marital problems are of course more likely to annoy others and so are more liable to receive unsolicited remarks. Those who are annoyed are not necessarily those whom the disturbed person would himself have sought out. They therefore tend to tell him things he does not want to hear and exert moderately heavy pressure. As a result, clinic applicants evaluate their remarks as not too helpful. Those who received purely unsolicited comments tend to come from strata that are not predisposed to recognize problems on their own. Nonmembers of the Friends and Supporters, upwardly mobile Catholics, Negroes, Puerto Ricans, and men were all more likely to be told they had problems. In our evaluation, between 15 and 20 per cent of clinic applicants might not have recognized their problems had others not intervened.

Confirmation and Support. For the majority of those who eventually go to psychotherapists, conversations about their problems have a confirming effect. They already know they have problems but need others to bolster this feeling. The support of others operates much the way conversations about politics do in election campaigns. Voters are kept from wandering from their normal affiliation through contacts with others who share their opinions. Similarly, conversation with the Friends and Supporters of Psychotherapy keeps potential patients aware of the psychological dynamics of their difficulties. This is especially important for such persons as working-class patients whose environment might not otherwise give much support for "psychologizing." On the other hand, some few people in election campaigns do get "converted" when they happen to run into others of an opposed view. Overt influence on prospective patients to convince them that they have problems when they do not already know this is also fairly rare. But like the importance of the few who are converted in an election campaign, influence from unexpected sources can have a decided effect on the total social distribution of psychiatric patients.

STEP 3: CHOOSING THE TYPE
OF HELPING PROFESSION

Because a person thinks he has problems does not mean he will seek professional help for them. In logical sequence, the next decision a prospective patient faces is to decide upon professional help. He then must decide what sort of professional to see. Should he try a doctor or a psychologist, or both? Should he try a psychoanalyst or a supportive, short-term therapist? Whether or not patients consciously make such decisions, the consequences of their choices are very evident in the type of problems presented to different types of psychiatric clinics. Clinics which were most like the private practice of psychotherapy and psychoanalysis—the analytic clinics—received the psychoanalytic problems brought by members of the Friends and Supporters of Psychotherapy and other middle-class people. Clinics associated with general hospitals seemed to specialize in the physical problems of lower-class applicants. And as noted, a religio-psychiatric clinic received the marital and family problems normally brought to ministers. Analysis of how patients choose professionals explains a good part of these findings.

Previous Choices. Only in a complex metropolis such as New York City can there be such an extensive division of labor in psychiatric services. The variety of available choices does lay bare some processes of decision and channeling that might otherwise remain hidden. It is apparent in such a city that clinics are a second choice, for almost all the applicants to almost all clinics had previously been to other professionals. Most had seen a psychiatrist or other psychotherapist at least once. Almost three-quarters of those applying for a hospital clinic had seen a physician (not a psychiatrist); almost half of applicants to other clinics had been to a physician. Over one-third of those applying to a religio-psychiatric clinic had consulted a clergyman. Moreover, the revolving door will continue to spin since most of those now applying to the clinics will not be accepted for treatment, will drop out, or will be scheduled for only a few sessions. They will have to try elsewhere. The process of choosing professionals is a continuous one for many patients. But shuttling from one professional to another is a constantly selective filter, and occurs according to discernible rules. The first professional seen is the key to later choices. The choice of the first professional, however, has little to do with the specific problems a patient now presents to a clinic. Rather, the selection is made according to the person's usual mode of operation and follows the lines of his social circle, social class, and his motivation to pay for private psychotherapy. So the channeling of different problems to different clinics takes place *after* the first professional and is in part the result of that experience, as well as the impact of the entire referral process. In referral, each profession tends to closely affiliated sources. Psychiatrists tend to refer to the more psychoanalytic clinics, social-service agencies to the more psychotherapeutic clinics, doctors to hospital clinics, and ministers to religio-psychiatric clinics.

Referral hardly accounts for most of the movement from one professional to another, so that many subtle processes are also involved. The majority left previous psychotherapists and physicians without a referral because they were dissatisfied. Cost was the chief dissatisfaction among those who eventually applied to an analytic clinic. Less than a third of those who left psychotherapists said they were referred elsewhere, and only one-sixth of those who had seen physicians (except those going to hospital medical services) had actually been given the name of a psychiatrist.

We judged continuity of care as important in determining whether a clinic received the outright failures of other professionals or people who wished to expand the goals of their treatment. By this criterion, only some analytic-clinic patients but a majority of those applying to other clinics were failures. Patients with good motivation who are continuing their therapy tend to have high education; on the other hand, among patients who are not continuing their previous treatment, and who are poorly motivated, a great deal of therapy is *not* accompanied by high education. So when analytic clinics take in the wash of other therapists they generally get the more desirable patients; when hospital and religio-psychiatric clinics get applicants with a good deal of previous psychotherapy, they tend to receive less desirable patients. Nonetheless, all clinics tend not to accept patients who have had a good deal of previous treatment.

Images of the Professions. The choice of one type of professional or another is not influenced merely by drift and referral. The images applicants to different types of clinics have of the different professionals are quite distinct. Applicants to analytic clinics grant psychiatrists greater legitimacy in dealing with their problems. Though psychiatry in their collective view does share something in common with such helping professions as the clergy and counseling, it differs in being much more nondirective. From the point of view of applicants to hospital clinics, medicine is almost as appropriate for their problems as psychiatry. In their view both medicine and psychiatry seem instrumental and concerned with getting specific things accomplished. But the main difference between medicine and psychiatry, in the collective judgment of hospital-clinic applicants, is that psychiatry, together with religious healing, deals more with internal than external matters. Religio-psychiatric applicants also grant legitimacy to psychiatry but give the clergy a much higher rating than do applicants to other types of clinics. The clergy are grouped together with the other two liberal professions— law and medicine. Psychiatry is off in "left field" and quite different from everything else. Applicants to all clinics tend to see the offbeat professions as similar: social improvement, cultism, religious healing, and mass-media advice columns are grouped together. But analytic-clinic applicants see these offbeat professions as similar to the clergy and quite distant from psychiatry, while applicants to other clinics see them as nearer to psychiatry and further from the clergy. The choices applicants have actually made fairly well match the way they see the professions. In part, these views are the result of their experiences; in part, they must have influenced the paths which applicants had taken.

STEP 4: CHOOSING A PARTICULAR CLINIC

Once the decision has been made to seek professional help and a general type of professional chosen, a person must choose a specific individual professional. The study has concentrated on the choice of a particular clinic. There are three elements in choosing a clinic: gathering information, evaluating the attributes of the clinic and the advantages of therapy itself, and getting a referral or a push into therapy.

Knowledge. Information-gathering may be the most crucial element in the final stage. Individual psychotherapists and psychiatric clinics are quite unknown to the general public, and merely finding a good therapist (or any therapist) is a serious problem for potential psychiatric patients. The result is that there is an enormous difference between those applicants who took steps to gain information about psychiatrists and psychiatric facilities and those who did not. Those who did ask for the names of clinics or private psychotherapists are much more liable eventually to apply to analytic clinics. Official information sources, such as doctors and other professions, are used much less often than are laymen. The Friends and Supporters of Psychotherapy are of course the ones who ask their friends for help. Also, those who have "sicker" problems and who read mental health books only because they were looking for help are more likely to ask others for information. Not surprisingly, asking is related to getting answers. Those who went to psychiatrists before coming to a clinic and who now know many alternative sources of treatment are much more apt to have asked for information. Asking for information is likely to lead a person to an analytic clinic because the very process of asking as well as the resulting answers lead a person to become part of the "psychoanalytic system," and this system considers analytic clinics better than other kinds. So asking questions is not simply an act of gathering information—it leads potential patients into becoming more involved with psychotherapy and into changing their self-concepts even before actually beginning treatment. In fact, asking questions puts people in touch with *any* system (depending on whom one asks) so that those who ask ministers for information are more likely to go to a religio-psychiatric clinic and those who ask doctors are apt to go to a hospital clinic.

Expectation and Evaluation. To apply to a clinic one must know of its existence, but knowledge is obviously not the whole story, for most people must be motivated by their hopes of cure and their expectations and evaluations of the clinics. Evaluation and expectation of treatment are less important elements, however, in the decisions of lower-class persons who are not members of the Friends and Supporters of Psychotherapy and who are applicants to hospital clinics. Key elements in their decision are the pain they feel and a recommendation by an authority that they go to a psychiatric clinic. On the other hand, most applicants to other types of clinics, especially if they are members of the Friends and Supporters of Psychotherapy, have a fairly good idea of what to expect from therapy, how change will take place, and what they would like a clinic to be. Despite the basically high level of consensus about expectations of therapy, membership in the Friends and Supporters of Psychotherapy, reading books about psychotherapy, and actual previous therapy all increase the proportion of applicants who express an opinion in accord with the notions of therapists themselves. Applicants who are thus already inducted into the world of therapy are more likely to hope for changes in their sexual lives and their basic values, and to hope for greater self-understanding. They also expect to do the work in therapy themselves and expect that it will take a year or more to work out their problems. Membership in the Friends and Supporters and actual previous psychotherapy are functional alternatives when it comes to training in knowing the *goals* of therapy, but therapy itself is a better teacher about the *process* of therapy. Regardless of what they know about therapy or other clinics, members of the Friends and Supporters of Psychotherapy and applicants to psychoanalytic clinics are very concerned about both the quality and cost of a clinic. Even if their concern with quality represents a wish and a hope rather than an actual consideration in the decision to go to a particular clinic, a "Consumer Union" orientation to psychotherapy—getting the most for the least— can lead to serious problems for community psychiatry.

Personal Influence to Go to a Clinic. The final element in the decision to go to a clinic is often a referral or push by other people. This is quite distinct from merely talking about problems (Step 2, discussed above). When problems in general were discussed, only a minority suggested a professional psychotherapist, and only a tiny minority actually named some one or some place. Now, in the final step, everyone got the name of a clinic to which he might go. Yet the amount of pressure that is placed upon people to go to a particular psychiatric *clinic* is a great deal less than most observers might imagine, and less than the pressure to recognize *problems*. Only about 5 per cent of clinic applicants were subjected to heavy pressure to go to a clinic, and only 5 per cent of applicants to analytic and religio-psychiatric clinics had not themselves actually asked to be sent to a psychiatric clinic. In contrast, over 25 per cent of hospital-clinic applicants were given unsolicited referrals to the clinic. Once told about a clinic, however, most applicants went quite promptly, indicating a suggestion to go to a *particular* clinic indeed comes at the end of the decision process and is often a "last straw." But personal contact is a much more effective last straw than reading about a clinic or merely picking up information about it. Professionals, especially psychiatrists, are the most effective, although medical doctors who are not psychiatrists are barely more effective than laymen.

Personal influence to go to a particular clinic, alone and without any specific event, circumstance, or sudden flash of insight, is a force which is more important in the decisions of people who were not members of the Friends and Supporters of Psychotherapy, who did not have the "right" problems, who did not read the right books, who had not voluntarily discussed their problems with others, and who did not search for information about psychiatrists and psychiatric clinics. In other words, persons who were surrounded by a milieu favorable to psychotherapy and who had previously prepared themselves to go to a psychiatric clinic generally do not need the *direct* intervention of others to make them go to a clinic. The final act in the sequence which leads to a psychiatrist is for the initiated a matter long ago determined by their entire social network, and so, when the last step is taken, it appears to be more autonomous than it really is. Although all such decisions are individual, the decision to go to a psychiatrist, involving as it does such a radical change in a person's self-concept, is *less* internalized and *less* seemingly independent when strong group support is *not* available. Social support tends to take place early in the decision and is especially important at the stage of realizing that one has a problem which could be alleviated through psychoanalytic or psychotherapeutic intervention.

❁ Decision-Making and the Friends and Supporters of Psychotherapy

A common strand runs through all the decisions that must be made before a person applies for psychotherapy at a clinic. At each level of decision-making, members of the Friends and Supporters of Psychotherapy differ from nonmembers in important ways. They realize their problems in a different fashion. The Friends tend to be more sensitive to problems of self-value, sex, and interpersonal difficulties. Members of the Friends are somewhat more likely to take the next step and talk to laymen about their problems. More important, at this second stage of decision-making, they are liable to receive support in their self-recognition of problems whereas nonmembers of the Friends and Supporters are more likely to be goaded into problem recognition. When it comes to the choice of type of professional to see first, members of the Friends are more likely to try psychiatrists, and this is in part responsible for their overwhelming choice of analytic clinics when they decide to seek help from a clinic. This last decision is dependent upon knowledge about clinics and sources of treatment, knowledge about treatment itself, expectations of psychotherapy, and finally, upon the kind and strength of the last push. Friends and Supporters of Psychotherapy more often seek knowledge actively and get answers, are more likely to know what to expect from therapy, and are less likely to be pushed into it. Since a great deal of therapy takes place *before* the beginning of formal treatment, members of the Friends, when they do apply to clinics, tend to feel differently about treatment and to have different needs from others. The Friends and Supporters of Psychotherapy form a clientele and a community quite different from the nonmembers, and the existence of these two sets of potential patients poses serious problems for community psychiatry, matters to be taken up in the next chapter.

Community Psychiatry and the Friends and Supporters of Psychotherapy: Some Recommendations for Action

❀

15

Although psychotherapy seeks to change individuals, the decision to go to a psychotherapist has community implications, for it is the community, directly or indirectly, which supplies the psychiatric facilities. In the United States, many of these facilities have been publicly maintained for generations as community-wide resources for both practical and moral reasons. Persons who are mentally disturbed have lower productivity and their discontent is a potential source of energy for antisocial activity. Misery is not only functionally disruptive, however, but antithetical to the Jewish and Christian traditions of charity and justice as expressed in the historic institutions of the Anglo-Saxon community. Because of these traditions, control of the criminal and aid to the orphaned, the poor and the distressed, as well as the treatment and control of the mentally disordered and incompetent have all been community-wide responsibilities. And because all these conditions have one thing in common—their deviation from the norms of the community—all forms of deviance have on occasion been uniformly treated by the same social institution. As late as the eighteenth century, American and British jails contained not only the criminal, but the poor, the orphaned, the illegitimate, and the mentally disturbed and deficient as well, all lumped together.

Poor relief in the Anglo-American tradition was originally a parish responsibility, but dissatisfaction with local efforts led first to township then to county and then to statewide relief.[1] Since the New Deal, the Federal government has been contributing most of the money and much of the policy to all kinds of welfare activities. Mental disorder has increasingly been dealt with on a more nearly national basis, but before the 1840's, the mentally disturbed in the United States were incarcerated in a variety of local institutions—almshouses, jails, and county workhouses. The "solution" to an inhumane situation was the creation of the state hospital system. Although the limitations of this system have been evident for over fifty years, the nation as a whole has turned its collective attention to the problems of the mentally or emotionally ill only recently. A variety of circumstances, some of which we will later discuss, led to this national concern expressed in President Kennedy's 1963 message to Congress on mental health and mental retardation. In it he noted the responsibility of the Public Health Service of the United States for a concerted attack on the nation's health problems and advocated "a new type of health facility, one which will return mental-health care to the mainstream of American medicine, and at the same time upgrade mental-health services."[2] This message resulted in the appropriation of $150 million to aid the states in constructing mental-health centers. Even more recently, under President Johnson, Congress has authorized the expenditure of additional funds to help staff these centers. A state cannot receive Federal support unless its plans are approved by the Surgeon General. To this end, the National Institute of Mental Health has formulated criteria which conform to the highest standards of community mental-health services.[3]

New York State's plan, developed by many regional and state committees, is one of the more sophisticated attempts to meet criteria set down by The National Institute of Mental Health. In brief, it will provide for central registries, systematic districting, and central coordination in the form of local mental-health agencies or departments covering both mental hospitals and outpatient services. In adult services, the sector discussed in this book, the plans call for the integration of all services: outpatient, inpatient, partial hospitalization rehabilitation, twenty-four-hour emergency, and other services. Though these will not necessarily be housed in the same location, an attempt will be made to insure continuity of care. The state hospital system will be utilized as a resource, especially by creating within the system units with a maximum of 1,000 beds to provide medium-length intensive care along modern lines. These units will in turn be related to community mental-health centers, to be located usually in connection with general hospitals. The local centers will provide short-term inpatient service, as well as outpatient, aftercare, precare, and consulting services to other care-giving agencies as well as to schools and the like. Private physicians may be allowed to follow their patients through the mental-health system just as they may now do in general hospitals. The plan also calls for increased training programs and increased financial aid from government, insurance, and voluntary sources. All this will indeed "return mental-health care to the mainstream of American medicine."

Yet despite the theoretical excellence of the plan, serious difficulties face its implementation, and indeed the implementation of any community mental-health plan. An examination of the structure and ideology of the mental-health field together with a review of our findings on the social system which sends people to psychiatrists show that many deep-seated contradictions must be resolved before any encompassing mental-health system can be made to work.

The growth of the community mental-health concept underscores two fundamental developments in modern psychiatry.[4] First, modern experts do *not* feel that mental hospitals ought to be *asylums*, placed away from and outside the community. Emphasis is now placed on the treatment of mental patients *within* the community, in facilities ranging from office and outpatient treatment to "halfway houses" and recreation centers, day hospitals, and night hospitals. Second, the nature and degree of the emotional disturbances in which psychiatrists are interested have changed. Since Freud, there has been increasing concern not only with psychoses and gross overt disturbances in functioning, but in unhappiness and in problems of living. Both treatment within the community and concern with the less dramatic disorders of everyday living have focused attention on outpatient psychiatry in the community mental-health movement.

Each of these two trends has been championed, by and large, by a different movement in the mental-health field. The more traditional mental-health or mental-hygiene movement has been particularly concerned with mental hospitals. Founded in 1908 by Clifford Beers, a former mental-hospital patient, the mental-hygiene movement stressed the humane treatment of persons suffering from obvious psychotic disorders.[5] The lay members of this movement often espoused a middle-class "Protestant Ethic" morality and felt that the unfortunate ought to become better adjusted.[6] Interested in improving facilities as well as in developing more tolerant attitudes toward present and former mental patients, leaders of the mental-hygiene movement give the impression that their concern is for *other persons* who have problems, not for themselves. Professionals in this movement, psychiatrists interested in developing new methods of treatment and in raising professional standards, founded such famous hospitals as the State Psychopathic Hospital at the University of Michigan (1907) and the Boston Psychopathic Hospital (1912); discovered the connection between syphilis and paresis (1913); pioneered in various forms of shock therapy; and developed tranquilizers and antidepressants (1950's). They also became increasingly interested in social psychiatry—in viewing the mental hospital as a "therapeutic community" and in developing psychiatry as an effective factor in the community outside the walls of the hospital. Unlocked wards, home visits, and concern with the families of patients are all part of these newer trends, many of which were first developed in England. The type of psychiatry we have just described was called "directive and organic" by Hollingshead and Redlich,[7] although perhaps it should now be called "directive-organic-social." The impression remains, however, that the mental-hygiene or health group is generally concerned with the more disruptive, bizarre, and antisocial mental disorders.

The second movement within the mental-health field was described in this book as the Friends and Supporters of Psychotherapy. The name is our own invention, for unlike the mental-hygiene group which is a self-defined, conscious group with a formal name and a formal membership, the Friends and Supporters of Psychotherapy is an informal social circle noticed by us but not necessarily by its members, with no official name or official membership list. Initiated by Freud, and interested primarily in the psychodynamics of office patients, this movement recruits laymen of quite a different type from those attracted by the mental-hygiene movement. As we have shown, these people tend to be intellectuals, artists, and professionals, often of a literary bent, and frequently Jewish, whereas the Protestant businessman is more characteristic of the lay leadership in the mental-hygiene group. Most important, the Friends and Supporters of Psychotherapy almost invariably see *themselves* as suffering from the types of mental disorder recognized by their movement, and these disorders tend to be less bizarre and more like the tensions experienced at one time or another by almost everybody.* They are therefore not offering benevolent help to unfortunate others, but like converts wish to spread the story of their own cure. The requirement that the professional psychotherapists themselves undergo treatment institutionalizes this point of view. Self-involvement also allows the Friends and Supporters of Psychotherapy to function in a less formal fashion than the mental hygiene group. Perhaps because of their proselitizing they form a social circle rather than a formally con-

* To be sure, the founder of the mental-hygiene movement had been himself a psychiatric patient, but as the movement grew, this type of self-involvement became fairly rare.

stituted group, and rather than being limited to the single profession of psychiatrist many diverse professionals such as ministers, psychologists, and social workers first undergo and then come to practice psychoanalysis and psychotherapy.

Although the type of patient seen by most psychotherapists is different from the type dealt with by traditional psychiatrists, this situation is changing. Originally concerned only with neuroses, professional psychoanalysts and analytically trained psychotherapists have increasingly expanded their interests and techniques to include working with schizophrenics and other psychotics. Like the directive organic group, they have become more interested in social systems and group processes, and especially in group and family therapy. They have also entered the domain of psychiatric hospitals, once the exclusive province of the directive-organic psychiatrists; every inpatient unit associated with the outpatient facilities we have studied is dominated by the ideology of the psychoanalytic movement. This trend is not unique to New York City. A study of twenty-two psychiatric clinics all over New York State found that over 60 per cent of the patients in treatment were given psychotherapy which emphasized analytic or depth approaches.[8] And despite the fact that at least three-quarters of the therapists who answered questionnaires stated that the treatment of choice with schizophrenia was "supportive,"[9] in actual fact over half the schizophrenic patients studied were given analytic therapy.[10] Further, ten of the eleven best community mental-health centers in the United States consider psychotherapy to be the treatment of choice.[11] Nonetheless, despite the pervasiveness of psychotherapy, most of the patients treated by therapists associated with the Friends and Supporters of Psychotherapy probably are less noticeably disturbed than those whom psychiatrists of the mental-health movement work with.

The mental-hygiene movement and the circle of Friends and Supporters of Psychotherapy have both contributed to the concept of a community mental-health center. The interest of the mental-hygiene group in continuous, community-related care for the severely disturbed, as well as in preventive community psychiatry, meets the interest of the Friends and Supporters in extending the principles of psychodynamics to cover the severely disturbed as well as those without overt psychiatric symptoms. They have both become interested in group processes in treatment. And modern training of residents in psychiatry in the United States almost universally offers a combination of psychodynamic theory with social management of groups of patients, although a few programs train community psychiatrists.

Despite this growing rapprochement between mental hygiene and psychotherapy, unresolved tensions exist between the two orientations which are reflected in many aspects of the mental-health field. These areas are (1) the present organizations and facilities for mental-patient care; (2) the "medical model" implied by Kennedy's message and which necessarily stems from the investment in current facilities; (3) the modalities of treatment and of professional roles which result from the medical model; (4) the way in which public facilities for outpatient care actually work; (5) and perhaps most important, the expectations of the clients and constituents of mental-health services. All these facets of the mental-health field are inevitably interlocked.

❋ Why Outpatient Programs in Community Mental Health Will Not Work

The relationship between community psychiatry and the community at large appears at first glance to be a relationship between an organized professional minority and an unorganized mass of potential clients. But nothing could be further from the truth. As we have just pointed out, the professionals themselves are organized into two somewhat distinct circles: the psychiatric mental-health circle and the circle of psychotherapists and psychoanalysts. But less obvious and even more important to the community relations of mental-health programs, some laymen and potential clients of mental-health services are also organized into two groups. The first group is organized as a formal voluntary association and is the lay counterpart of the mental-health circle of psychiatrists. The second group, the one we have called the Friends and Supporters of Psychotherapy, is just as viable, but less organized, since it is a social circle, not a formal organization. Because social sets and circles are unorganized and so have no "public relations" staff, mental-health planning tends to ignore them in favor of the better organized.

The consequence of failure to recognize the difference between the mental-health movement and the Friends and Supporters of Psychotherapy is an excessive reliance on the existing system of mental-patient care, which at its best was geared to meet the ideology of mental hygiene alone. An editorial entitled "A Sensible Approach" which appeared in the October 1964 issue of New York State's *Mental Hygiene News* explained why the existing system has to be utilized.

> In New York State, as we address ourselves to the future, we begin with an assessment of our present resources—the bulk of which consists of a two-billion-dollar investment with a vast unrealized potential. As (the late) Commissioner Hoch has pointed out, the state hospitals are more than a farflung collection of brick and steel. They are an efficient operating organization of 32,000 trained people. With many handicaps and only minimal support this organization is now dealing effectively with

the great mass of major mental illness. It would be wasteful, irresponsible and utterly foolish to consign it to the scrap heap.

The state hospital system is not, of course, the only vested interest—there are many others including child guidance and family service agencies, corrective institutions and general hospitals. Most of these existing systems, insofar as they deal with outpatients, are more like hospital psychiatric clinics than like analytic or religio-psychiatric clinics. And as Schwartz and Schwartz comment, "The difficulty of course is that attempts at solution are generally made by using the very organization that gave rise to the problem."[12] Yet any other approach is, by definition, unrealistic.

Part of the problem, which reliance on existing organizations engenders, is that the mental-health movement tends to regard mental problems as *medical* illnesses. As a leader in mental-health planning has pointed out, "Control of mental disorders is a public-health problem."[13] He believes that the standards of the public-health field should be applied to the mental-health field. He noted four levels of public-health concern: mortality, serious morbidity, minor morbidity such as common colds, and finally positive health.

> The Joint Commission on Mental Illness and Health recommended top priority for level 2, serious morbidity. Available data amply demonstrate that except for public mental hospitals psychiatric resources are preoccupied with caseloads that correspond to level 3, minor morbidity, and limit their treatment armamentarium to procedures and techniques suitable for illnesses at the lower level of morbidity.[14]

In our terms, what is being said is that analytic clinics and private psychotherapy are treating the "psychoanalytic syndrome" of interest to the Friends and Supporters rather than true psychiatric problems of interest to mental-health experts. In addition, the structural arrangements of medicare and medicaid confirm the commitment to a medical model.

The medical model contains at least two incorrect assumptions from which a dangerous conclusion logically follows: It assumes that physicians can distinguish between those who are mentally well and those who have varying degrees of mental illness and that specific disease entities can be expressed in a standardized diagnostic vocabulary. Second, the medical model assumes that the sick person's own actions roughly correspond to the physician's diagnosis of his state of illness, that is, that persons who are more sick are more likely to seek medical help. The implied conclusion is that public psychiatric facilities should turn away those who are not very sick if they do apply and instead seek out those who are more ill who might not have even considered applying.

Why are these assumptions and the conclusions which follow in-correct or misleading? Our analysis of diagnoses in Chapter 6 shows that psychiatrists do not at present have an adequate means for sorting patients into any set of categories, much less deciding who is sick and who is not. As Glasscote and others observe in their review of criteria for evaluating community mental-health programs, what is missing is "a consensus about the cutoff point that differentiates the 'mentally ill' from the 'mentally well' since otherwise all those who seek help pre-sumably have to be taken into treatment."[15]

The second assumption, that the more medically ill are more likely to seek treatment, is also wrong. The Friends and Supporters of Psy-chotherapy are more likely to seek treatment than others. They go mainly for help with "psychoanalytic" problems, which tend to be less bizarre and less obvious than other psychiatric symptoms. And to average Americans, the most significant personal problems are family problems, not the traditional medically noted psychoses. Neither of these groups tends to select psychiatric facilities in mental or general hospitals where working-class outpatients do come with the more "medical" types of problems. When alternatives are available, the Friends and Supporters of Psychotherapy tend to choose independent analytic clinics, and the average middle-class American Protestant tends to prefer religio-psychiatric counseling or family guidance agencies. Both groups find these facilities more suitable for their problems and more competent than others. So the bulk of the actively interested "public" of psychiatric clinics rejects the medical model. The New York State Psychological Association, which for its own reasons rejects the medical model, is actually more in tune with its public when it states that com-munity mental health should be more concerned with "individuals who in one degree or another have reached a 'stalemate in living' or who have had a 'breakdown in living.' The goal should be that of actualizing our human resources."[16]

Realizing humanity's potential is obviously too broad a concern to serve as an effective guide for public policy. Moreover, the inadequacy of psychiatric diagnosis as a screening device accentuates some of the built-in biases of public outpatient clinics alluded to by the New York State planners. If public-health experts advocate programs which lead indirectly to the rejection of the Friends and Supporters of Psycho-therapy, it is only because at present most clinics outside of central New York City tend to reject unsophisticated, less educated appli-cants.[17] The effect of such a policy is to cause moral and political embarrassment to community psychiatry. However, a policy which in reaction *systematically* rejects the Friends and Supporters of Psycho-therapy is politically unwise, since the Friends and Supporters are the real constituency of community psychiatry. Because of their own

personal involvement, in contrast to the concern of the mental hygien-
ists for the problems of *other* people, the Friends are much more likely
to give active support to programs that meet their approval. After all,
the late President Kennedy was probably himself a member, and so
it was no accident that he was the first President to be actively concerned about the Federal role in community mental health.

Community psychiatry is faced with a dilemma largely because regardless of the criteria for acceptance or rejection of applicants, public
facilities cannot now give sufficient treatment to all who apply. The
"revolving door" effect described in Chapter 9 is a consequence at
least in part of the lack of adequate treatment facilities. The net result
of several attempts at therapy is not necessarily bad, since we have
shown throughout that people learn a good deal from their first efforts
and can begin anew, and perhaps even more wisely, with a new therapist. Yet the new starts are often poorly articulated with earlier treat-
ments, so the less sophisticated and less educated tend to pile up in
hospital clinics as failures of previous treatment, while the better
educated are the ones who achieve some continuity. In any case, because they are said to be poor training cases, clinics discriminate against
persons with previous therapy, so that the ultimate consequence of
inadequate facilities is that money becomes the filter. Poor people who
do have the more "medical" problems tend to apply to hospital clinics
and are often rejected, especially if they have had previous treatment.
They may not seek further help unless they become very sick and
hence an even greater public charge. The Friends and Supporters of
Psychotherapy, however, are quite likely to seek private therapy if
their clinic application is rejected, especially since they are more concerned about the quality of low-cost clinic treatment to begin with.
Yet most of them could not have afforded long-term private treatment.
One obvious reason for the log jam in treatment facilities is the lack
of sufficient personnel, especially if the only qualified personnel are
medically trained psychiatrists. The New York State Department of
Mental Hygiene took note of the problem in the following way:

> The ratio of manpower in the mental-health field to persons in need
> of care and treatment virtually eliminates as a significant element of
> treatment traditional one-to-one psychotherapeutic modalities—at least in
> publicly supported programs. Major reliance must be placed on psycho-
> pharmacological, somatic, and therapeutic community efforts.[18]

The implications of offering one form of treatment in *public* facilities and another form in private care are most profound. In the first
place, this distinction destroys the medical model that public-health
officials advocate. In medicine, poor people and rich people, when they

suffer from the same illness, are presumably treated in the same fashion; for the same physical condition, the same form of operation is generally effective for both rich and poor people. In psychiatry, however, this may not be true. Although they may have received the same diagnosis as wealthier persons, lower-class applicants to psychiatric clinics tend to have quite different problems, and more limited expectations of treatment, as we have seen. It may very well be, therefore, that unique forms of treatment more suited to their nonpsychodynamic orientation will be more effective with poorer persons.[19]

Whether new therapies are developed for the nonmember of the Friends, or a division of labor among existing psychiatric clinics in New York City is expanded and perpetuated, the ultimate result will be to reinforce that tendency in the treatment of the mentally disturbed which has been the most criticized—namely, the two-track system. The two-track system has been a notable characteristic of mental health facilities since Bethlehem Hospital was publicly investigated in eighteenth-century England. There has always been one form of treatment for the rich and another for the poor. Now the rich have by no means always had the best of it, since in eighteenth-century England, for example, the rich in private madhouses seemed relatively worse off than the poor in county workhouses.[20] Nevertheless, whether they are kept in attics, bled, beaten, or given psychotherapy, whatever the rich get is generally deemed better than what the poor receive. And so, if those who can afford private treatment obtain psychoanalysis and if those who cannot pay for it are given something else, then psychoanalysis is, *ipso facto*, thought "better" than any other form of treatment. Moreover, we have shown that an entire social system exists, centered around the Friends and Supporters of Psychotherapy, which exalts this form of treatment. If public facilities are to be used to give an "inferior" form of treatment to the poor and the culturally deprived, these facilities will, in this day and age, be subject to vigorous attack, for the canons of evaluation are at least, in part, social. In fact, the present trend to extend psychotherapy to some state hospital patients is a response to the felt injustice of depriving them of this "better" treatment.

The facts about outpatient psychiatry are such, however, that even if the planners wanted public facilities to be more community-mental-health-oriented, it would be very difficult to accomplish such a goal. We saw in Chapter 3 that every good clinic, and every clinic that wants to become better, initiates a training program. Whether those who are being trained are psychiatrists or nonmedical trainees, both types generally wish to enter the private practice of individual psychotherapy which promises greater rewards than public service. And for reasons we have mentioned, the ideology of even medical psychiatry in the United

States is today becoming psychoanalytically tinged. There are few good residency training programs today that do not emphasize a psycho-dynamic point of view, so that clinics perforce must stress training in psychotherapy if their trainees are to enter the lucrative mainstream of treatment. Anything else is strongly resisted by trainees, as well as by their mentors.

❀ Some Incomplete Solutions

Exactly what community psychiatry is or is not is very difficult to say, but certainly the difference between private and community psychiatry is that the latter is committed to help the entire community, rather than just those who desire to come for treatment and who can afford to pay for it. As our analysis suggested, however, public outpatient services in psychiatry are indeed placed in a most difficult situation, one which almost guarantees that whatever they do will seriously wrong a good part of the community. As matters now stand, there is probably no complete solution to this unsatisfactory situation. But several partial adjustments seem dictated by our findings.

DIVERSIFIED BUT RESPONSIBLE OUTPATIENT SERVICES

The first lesson is learned from the flaws as well as the advantages of New York City's division of psychiatric labor. The flaws are obvious. The poor who have medical symptoms with a psychiatric basis apply to hospital clinics which may give them, on the average, a few interviews but which are not equipped to give them any real support, much less long-term treatment. Waiting lists are often so long that over a year may elapse after intake before a patient can get treatment—at which point he may no longer be interested, even though from a medical or psychodynamic point of view he is just as "sick" as he ever was.[21] Only a very specialized and atypical population with marital problems uses the facilities of a religio-psychiatric clinic (though they might be less atypical outside New York City). Analytic clinics promise relatively long-term treatment to the few who are chosen—but except at one "middle-income" clinic very few indeed *are* chosen and given treatment. Moreover, doctors, clergymen, and even psychiatrists are notoriously inefficient in their referrals. The clinics tend to refer to one another without ascertaining whether another clinic really will accept a patient they themselves have just rejected. Coordination is certainly badly needed. But so is diversification.

Our study and many others as well have demonstrated the relatively poor channels to mental-health organizations possessed by the very professions—the clergy and nonpsychiatrist physicians—who are usually the first to be consulted by mentally distressed individuals.[22] The solution usually proposed is to appeal to individual doctors and clergymen in a variety of ways designed to make them better acquainted with mental-health facilities. It is a truism, however, that appeals to individuals are rarely effective over a long run. The proper solution is an institutional one, and has already been indicated by the division of psychiatric labor in New York City. Doctors do have good connections with hospitals, and the new community mental-health plans aim to take advantage of that connection. But clergymen have good connections with a religio-psychiatric clinic, and teachers, with child-guidance clinics (an institution ruled out of our study by our emphasis on individual decisions by adults). *Community* mental health should be just that and take advantage of counseling facilities wherever they may be, rather than concentrating on a medical model. *Only* in this fashion can all types of potential patients be quickly channeled into treatment.

Diversification imposes a serious organizational strain on community mental-health leaders. The directors of a community mental-health program must have considerable ability and willingness to work with a wide range of facilities which are not housed under the same roof. The individual organizations themselves must be prepared to give up some of their autonomy. The power of the public purse, when properly used, however, is an excellent means of insuring cooperation and coordination. Federal and state grants must be given to all sorts of counseling organizations, but with explicit conditions and with clear rules of procedure more rigorously enforced than at present. *E pluribus unum* is a slogan which has had no small success in the past; it promises much in the case of a well-organized community mental-health program.

Such a program tranfers the dilemma and the battle from one of designing the right single community mental-health center attached to a hospital to that of creating rules under which a variety of therapy organizations can operate in unity through diversity. Though diversification does recruit for mental-health treatment a wider variety of patients than any other device, it also tends to limit any given treatment unit's responsibility for its applicants. The single most important concept medical psychiatry can extend to the psychotherapy movement is the value concept of "responsibility."

Psychotherapy tends to emphasize the importance of individual patient volition rather than the therapist's responsibility for his patient. Should a patient fail to keep his appointment, the analytically oriented therapist will rarely attempt to discover why, to call the patient on the telephone or even, in a drastic step, to send an investigator to the patient's home. When the therapist refers a patient, he generally makes no attempt to insure that the patient actually arrives at another therapist's office or is properly taken care of by the new therapist. Nor does a new therapist usually talk at length to the previous one about his former patient. The reasons for this behavior on the part of therapists are rooted in psychoanalytic theory. We suggest that the theory is in turn rooted in the conditions under which patients come to office therapy to begin with. As we have shown, office patients or hospital outpatients generally come under very little coercion, in contrast to many mental-hospital inpatients. Hence the office or outpatient is held to be individually responsible for his behavior. This theory also coincides with the liberal economic theory of the customers of a private enterprise as originally defined by Freud.[23] Such a theory is also congruent with the requirements of maximum civil liberties for patients. In contrast, public-health and mental-hospital theory have stressed the social need for coercive control over populations and patients. Individuals in most American localities have no say about whether or not their milk is pasteurized; mental patients who wish to leave a mental hospital are frequently not permitted to do so, and many are interned who did not wish to enter in the first place.[24] Needless to say, coercive control of populations and patients, although congruent with the value concept of medical responsibility, contradicts the value concept of civil liberties.[25]

At present, one of the encouraging results of some rapprochement between the mental-hygiene and psychotherapy traditions is increasing freedom for mental-hospital patients.* At the same time, the medical concept of responsibility is not being sufficiently applied to outpatient treatment. Diversified outpatient treatment can work as a community facility only if each treatment center assumes much more obligation to follow through on patients than is now the practice. The community rules should therefore center on this problem without dictating style of therapy or the nature of therapists. A central organization of these units with some power of control can insure the visibility of all the resources and all the places available to treat a patient so that clinics cannot assume a "let George do it" attitude. Further, many clinics now have no connection with inpatient facilities. Through the proper organization of community mental health, presently isolated clinics can be articulated into other treatment facilities. At the same time, inpatient units may be able to use the facilities of even analytic clinics for certain types of discharged patients.

---

* In New York State, almost all new admissions are now on a voluntary basis, and stay is subject to periodic review.

THE FRIENDS AND SUPPORTERS
OF PSYCHOTHERAPY AS
AGITATORS AND THERAPISTS

Even assuming coordination, problems remain. Although the clinics we studied in New York City are among the very few who do not individually discriminate against unsophisticated patients, the system *as a whole* is discriminatory. Because of the referral system we have described, lower-income patients are more likely to apply to hospital clinics where they have very limited chances for long-term therapy. Further, they do not understand the basis of their problems to begin with. So although the psychiatric division of labor gets patients to therapy, it cannot handle them once they have arrived. The problem can be completely solved only with more resources, something we shall discuss very shortly. But part of the problem is that low-income patients in general are not interested in long-term treatment or in an intro-spective view of their problems. In short, they are just not likely to be members of the Friends and Supporters of Psychotherapy. The family-oriented businessmen, lawyers, and engineers who apply to a religio-psychiatric clinic also are not members of the Friends nor are they likely to become members. Except for unusual circumstances, mem-bership in the Friends is like an ethnic or ascribed status. It cannot be acquired for the asking. Yet despite the individual nature of psycho-therapy, lower-class persons who have had a good deal of therapy are more likely to be members than other lower-class applicants without therapy. We therefore suggest building an *artificial circle* of Friends and Supporters of Psychotherapy by encouraging group activities of all sorts in hospital and religio-psychiatric clinics. By mingling in social activities, group therapy, and other forms of group activities, led or conducted in an atmosphere conducive to talking about problems, pa-tients can observe that there are others like themselves. The distribution of the right kinds of books about therapy and psychology seems also surprisingly helpful. Relatives and friends can also be included in these activities. Volunteers who are members of Friends and Supporters of Psychotherapy (rather than the mental-hygiene-oriented Junior League volunteers who now give time to mental hospitals) could also join these group activities. Such activities are indeed already advocated by many mental-health experts for a variety of reasons. We suggest that their helpfulness is mainly based on their contribution to creating an arti-ficial circle of Friends and Supporters of Psychotherapy. If this latent function is made manifest, at least in the eyes of the professionals involved in organizing these activities, the goal can be more efficiently reached.

The possible use of Friends and Supporters of Psychotherapy in the creation of artificial circles who understand modern analytic psychiatry suggests that the Friends are important not only in their role as psychiatric patients but in their relationships to psychiatric institutions and to potential patients and other disturbed individuals.[26] We have shown that although they are not formal organizations, the circles and sets of Friends and Supporters of Psychotherapy have definite traits, for example, the fact that they know others who have been in treatment and that they are likely also to belong to culturally sophisticated circles. Both these traits suggest that the Friends are politically accessible. They are not an amorphous mass but have a structured existence. Community organizers can therefore both locate them and influence them to support local community mental-health activities that are analytically oriented.[27] Just as some New York City reform leaders have relied on a wedge into social circles of the culturally sophisticated in order to enlist them in political activity, so community psychiatrists can meet with similar groups to engage them in mental-health activities. It is important to realize that these communities of Friends and Supporters of Psychotherapy are *not* neighborhood but interest groups and so traditional neighborhood means of recruitment (through neighbors, libraries, supermarkets, churches, property associations and the like) are not the best methods. Rather, professional groups and social groups are better sources. The mailing lists of certain book clubs are better sources than the list of registered voters of a given party.

We have also seen that the most effective influencers of the mental-health activities of individuals are these very same Friends and Supporters. They are the ones, collectively, who help support people in the realization that they have problems and who give them information about mental-health facilities. Mental-health campaigns directed at teachers, policemen, doctors, and clergymen are important, but those directed toward making the role of the Friends and Supporters of Psychotherapy more manifest than latent may be even more useful.

There are many ways in which the Friends and Supporters can be enlisted and better organized to support others in mental distress. Here we suggest one important way which is based on some of our findings. There is no doubt that even among the Friends and Supporters there is some feeling of stigma attached to going to a psychotherapist (see above p. 248). Nonetheless, the most salient characteristic of members of the Friends is that they asked their acquaintances for the name of a clinic or a psychiatrist (above, p. 254). Finding the name of a reputable clinic or psychotherapist is one of the key problems of a person who wishes to enter therapy (above, p. 252). And despite the fact that members of the Friends and Supporters were more likely than others to have heard of the clinic to which they applied through a friend, professionals remained the most important source of information (above, p. 295). Putting all these facts together means that the Friends and Supporters of Psychotherapy are insufficiently linked to actual treatment sources, especially to public clinics. These laymen could be in the position of serving as very effective referral sources. A major reason they are not more effective is that after they complete their own therapy they tend to have no further contact with their therapist. For those who have completed a successful therapy, shame is probably not the major reason for this lack of further association. Both the relief at "graduation" and the ideology of psychoanalysis which limits social contact between patient and therapist are probably responsible. Yet satisfied "customers" are the best source for new customers, as any businessman knows. Despite the squeamishness of some clinics and some therapists about relating to former patients, there is every good community mental-health reason for periodic contacts with former patients. Renewing the old relationship even in a less therapeutic guise can aid former patients personally, but even more important, could allow them to serve as more effective referral sources for others. This is especially true of former patients of psychiatric clinics, some of whom are occasionally contacted for donations, but all of whom could form an "alumni association" which like all good "boosters" could recruit for "alma mater."

The chief difficulty with all our proposals for community psychiatry is that they will increase the demand for psychiatric service. This holds true even for state hospital use. "Experience of the last ten years has shown that any increase in community services in the field of mental illness stimulates the demand for the utilization of state hospitals."[28] The only way to reduce this demand is to alter our entire society and its notions of welfare, deviant behavior, and individualistic family life. And though changes in these areas may be desirable, the means to accomplish such change is well outside the ability of mental-health organizations or, for that matter, of any others. So the means must be found to increase facilities which are even now inadequate without disproportionately appropriating society's scarce resources for what is after all not a production but a maintenance function.

As a natural outgrowth of our consideration of the role of the Friends and Supporters of Psychotherapy as a mental-health lobby and amateur referral system, one must raise the question of their utility in the therapy as well as the support of mentally disturbed persons. The issue of whether laymen (nonmedical doctors) could ever become psychotherapists was one "which most keenly engaged Freud's interest, and indeed emotions, during the last phase of his life. It was associated with a central dilemma in the psychoanalytical movement, one for which no solution has yet been found."[29] As is well known, Freud held that under suitable conditions and with adequate training, laymen could and

should become psychoanalysts and certainly could become psychotherapists. Other experts, including the recent Joint Commission, have suggested the use of nonmedical analysts.[30] American psychoanalysts, led by
A. A. Brill, were always officially opposed to this view. The shortage
of personnel in the mental-health field is even greater now than in the
1930's when there were fewer members of the Friends and Supporters
of Psychotherapy and hence less pressure on mental-health facilities.
In fact, the demand for service has so far outstripped the supply that
Freud's prediction that laymen were going to practice psychoanalysis
with or without the consent of the American Psychoanalytic Association[31] has come true with a vengeance. The ultimate irony of the
growth in popularity of analytic psychotherapy is that many *psychiatrists*
practice psychoanalysis or analytically oriented psychotherapy without
ever having attended a psychoanalytic institute of whatever persuasion
and without a personal psychoanalysis. One aspect of "the return of
mental health to the mainstream of American medicine" is to take
definite sides in this controversy and insure that only psychiatrists will
engage in therapy. It is true that the "team approach" is increasingly
popular in community mental-health theory, but however it works out
in practice, the theory of the team still holds that psychologists be
limited to diagnosis—an area, in view of our findings, which is even
more difficult than therapy—and that social workers or clergy be limited
to the even more difficult task of dealing with the patient's social environment. The logic of assigning the most difficult tasks to those members of the team who are supposedly least trained is rather hard to
follow. This division of labor therefore falls apart and lay members of
clinic teams are in fact usually engaged in even more treatment than
are staff psychiatrists who generally supervise both the lay therapists
and the resident psychiatrists. And no one seems involved with diagnosis
or the social environment.

We are not mainly concerned, however, with the present division of
labor in psychiatric clinics or with the issue of whether professionals
with a nonmedical background should be permitted to engage in therapy,
though in our own opinion the last issue is entirely academic. These
facts were introduced to give some background to the question of
whether persons who are not mental-health professionals of any kind
be recruited to give some types of therapy in public facilities. We feel
that members of the Friends and Supporters of Psychotherapy who
have had a personal analysis could make excellent therapists if properly
trained and would perform exceedingly well as volunteer aids even with
minimal training and indoctrination. One might even argue that precisely because their own therapy was in response to their emotional needs
and was not disguised as a so-called training analysis the Friends and
Supporters might be even more sensitive to the needs of a patient than

career-minded therapists. Better than some current therapists, even if less qualified, the Friends and Supporters of Psychotherapy can help to alleviate the very shortage of personnel that they themselves have created.

Two categories of Friends and Supporters can be well utilized. The first group consists of persons who are fully employed professionals in other fields and who could be persuaded to give some volunteer time to mental-health centers. Such volunteers might be among those who have already been reached to aid the mental-health lobby and who constitute an active "alumni association" interested in referring patients. These persons could help to organize the social activities which would build the artificial community of Friends and Supporters of Psychotherapy so necessary to successful treatment of lower-class applicants. In fact, these are really the only persons who could successfully organize such activities. The writers, actors, publicists and other such media-oriented persons and teachers would be especially useful, but so would those professionals less often found among the Friends—engineers and lawyers. Job counseling might be another suitable role for lay volunteers. These persons with middle-class ideologies would differ in one crucial respect from the middle-class mental hygienist volunteers—they would all have "been there themselves." The problems that current patients face are their problems as well.

The persons recruited as lay volunteers may have limited loyalty and interest, since those we have in mind for such work are already *over*employed. But there are many Friends and Supporters of Psychotherapy who are *under*employed, and they might be put to use, even more effectively, as part-time semi-professional therapists. In the underemployed categories are housewives, artists of one kind or another, and clericals or even some of the few working-class persons who are members of the Friends. Many persons in all these categories we have called underemployed are women who hold relatively unskilled jobs merely because they need the extra money or want something to do, or who, because of family obligations and the general position of women, cannot take the time to acquire the professional training they would like to have. In the United States, women are the "natural" Friends and Supporters even without formal induction. Many housewives would be delighted to find a part-time job—say of twenty hours a week—which together with on-the-job training would allow them to engage in counseling and supportive psychotherapy under the supervision of full-fledged professionals in the mental-health field.[32] Those who are now employed but are what we have called underemployed might want full-time work in the mental-health field even if it pays no more than their current job. All these persons would have to be trained, so that the desire of every clinic to be a training center would thus be easily met—even if with expanded facilities there are not enough residents in psychiatry and interns in social work or psychology to go around. The general interest in and understanding of emotional problems as well as formal therapy and prior active reading in the field of psychology possessed by almost all members of the Friends and Supporters of Psychotherapy makes them far better candidates for such jobs than their formal qualifications might indicate, yet they are not as costly to the institutions as are fully trained mental-health professionals.

Some of our proposals have been individually made before, but the common thread that runs through our suggestions and which makes them a potentially useful contribution is the basic idea of turning an informal social set or circle into an organization with some viable formal aspects. There are many such circles in our population, yet their existence is barely recognized much less exploited for the benefit of society. While a more formal function for the Friends and Supporters of Psychotherapy will not revolutionize mental-health care, it will certainly help to alleviate some of its most pressing problems. Nor need those who look to the perpetuation of informal circles be overly concerned that our calling attention to them will thereby destroy them or their informal nature. The Friends and Supporters of Psychotherapy have sufficient strength to survive even the best intentions of sociologists and mental-health experts.

NOTE

1. For a history of the emergence of a national mental health system in England, see Kathleen Jones, *Lunacy, Law and Conscience* (London: Routledge & Kegan Paul, 1959), and *Mental Health and Social Policy* (London: Routledge & Kegan Paul, 1960). For the American experience see Albert Deutsch, *The Mentally Ill in America* (New York: Columbia University Press, 1946). See also Norman Dain, *Concepts of Insanity in the United States, 1789-1865* (New Brunswick, N.J.: Rutgers University Press, 1964).
2. Eighty-eighth Congress, 1st Session, House of Representatives, Document No. 58, Message from the President of the United States Relative to Mental Illness and Mental Retardation, p. 4.
3. Community Mental Health Centers Act of 1963, Title II, Public Law 88-164. Regulations, *Federal Register*, May 6, 1964, pp. 5951-5956.
4. For a review of recent developments see Morris S. Schwartz and Charlotte Green Schwartz, *Social Approaches to Mental Patient Care* (New York: Columbia University Press, 1964); R. M. Glasscote, D. S. Sanders, H. R. Forstenzer, and A. R. Foley, *The Community Mental Health Center* (Washington, D.C.: Joint Information Service of the American Psychiatric Association and the National Association for Mental Health, 1964); Ernest M. Gruenberg, ed., "Evaluating the Effectiveness of Mental Health Services," *The Milbank Memorial Fund Quarterly*, XLIV (January 1966, part 2); Hugh Freeman and James Farndale, *Trends in Mental Health Services* (New York: Macmillan, 1963).

5. For a history of this movement see Nina Ridenour, *Mental Health in the United States* (Cambridge: Harvard University Press, 1961).

6. Kingsley Davis, "Mental Hygiene and the Class Structure," *Psychiatry*, 1 (1938), pp. 55-65.

7. *Social Class and Mental Illness* (New York: Wiley, 1958), pp. 155-161.

8. Gerhart Saenger and John Cumming, "Study of Community Mental Health Clinics, Report II: Treatment Provided for Patients," Mental Health Research Unit, New York State Department of Mental Hygiene, Syracuse, July 1966 (duplicated), Table II-5.

9. *Ibid.*, Table 1-8.

10. *Ibid.*, Table II-11. And, in general, the authors remark, on page 39, that although "treatment approaches used in individual therapy did vary to some extent among the different illnesses . . . observed differences are smaller than would be consistent with the responses obtained on the opinion questionnaire."

11. Glasscote, *et al.*, *op. cit.*, p. 22. (The outpatient clinic of one of the centers in this survey is also included in our study.)

12. *Op. cit.*, p. 97.

13. Hyman M. Forstenzer, Assistant Commissioner for Mental Health Resources and Policy Planning, New York State Department of Mental Hygiene, "Planning and Evaluation of Community Mental Health Programs," address presented at Institute for Training in Community Psychiatry, Arden House, Harriman, New York, February 25-29, 1964, pp. 7-8.

14. *Ibid.*

15. Glasscote, Sanders, Forstenzer, and Foley, *The Community Mental Health Center*, *op. cit.*, p. 28.

16. Memo to the Members of the Executive Committee, State Mental Planning Committee, from B. F. Riess, Isidor Chein, and Allen V. Williams, n.d.

17. Saenger *et al.*, *op. cit.*, Chapter VII.

18. Department of Mental Hygiene, "Statement on Long-Range Plans in Mental Health," June 15, 1964, p. 11.

19. Frank Riessman, Jerome Cohen, and Arthur Pearl, eds., *Mental Health of the Poor* (New York: The Free Press, 1964), Part 3, "Psychotherapeutic Approaches for Low-Income People."

20. Kathleen Jones, *op. cit.*, p. 32.

21. Some observers think this is all to the good, since people can be sick only when their residual deviant behavior becomes organized into sickness through the labeling by other people. See Thomas J. Scheff, *Being Mentally Ill: A Sociological Theory* (Chicago: Aldine, 1966), *passim*, but especially pp. 117-121.

22. For example, Raymond Fink and Sam Shapiro, "Methodological Considerations in Studying Patterns of Medical Care Related to Mental Illness," *Milbank Memorial Fund Quarterly*, Vol. 41, No. 4, Part I, October 1963. Elaine Cumming and Charles Harrington, "Clergyman as Counselor," *American Journal of Sociology*, LXIX (November 1963), pp. 234-243.

23. Freud, "Further Recommendations in the Technique of Psychoanalysis," first published in *Zeitschrift*, Bd. I, 1913, *passim*. Current psychoanalysis also operates under these assumptions of private contract. See Karl Menninger, *Theory of Psychoanalytic Technique* (New York: Basic Books, 1958), Chapter II, "The Contract."

24. Thomas J. Scheff, *Being Mentally Ill*, op. cit., Part II.

25. Our British cousins have for historical reasons been more sensitive to the concept of civil liberties than to medical responsibility. So milk need not be pasteurized and mental-hospital patients can generally not be detained against their will. Thomas S. Szasz in many publications has crusaded for greater civil liberties for mental patients in the United States.

26. See Eugene Litwak and Henry J. Meyer, "A Balance Theory of Coordination Between Bureaucratic Organizations and Community Primary Groups," *Administrative Science Quarterly*, 11 (1966), pp. 31-58, for a discussion of the types

of informal groups which function best with different organizations and some general mechanisms of coordination.

27. For a description of a situation exactly opposite to the one we have in mind, see Ray H. Elling and Ollie J. Lee, "Formal Connections of Community Leadership to the Health System," *Milbank Memorial Fund Quarterly*, XLIV, No. 3, Part I (1966), pp. 294-306.

28. New York State Department of Mental Hygiene, *op. cit.*, p. 26.

29. Ernest Jones, *The Life and Work of Sigmund Freud*, Volume III (New York: Basic Books, 1957), pp. 287ff.

30. Joint Commission on Mental Illness and Health, *Action for Mental Health* (New York: Basic Books, 1961), pp. 244-252, 256-260.

31. In his "Postscript to a Discussion on Lay Analysis," first published in English in the *International Journal of Psycho-Analysis* 8 (1937).

32. See for example the NIMH project described in M. J. Rioch *et al.*, "Pilot Project in Training Mental Health Counselors," Publ. No. 1254, Bethesda, Md., U.S. Public Health Service, 1965.

Appendix

Sample Cover Letter

Clinic Letterhead

Dear

Thank you for returning the application form. We further ask you to aid us by filling out the enclosed opinionnaire which is part of our research program. A stamped self-addressed envelope is enclosed for your convenience.

The results of this study will aid us to plan our program so that we may be better able to serve the community. Everything you say will of course be confidential.

The success of this research is dependent on the return of every questionnaire. We would therefore like you to return it within one week. Thank you for your cooperation.

Sincerely,

Clinic Director

Sample Second Letter

Clinic Letterhead

Dear

Sometime ago we mailed to you an opinionnaire about mental health problems. We have not yet received your reply, however. Your responses are most important since they may affect the way this clinic can best serve the community. We expect to have answers from all persons to whom the opinionnaire was mailed, for only in this way can our research be successful. In case you may have mislaid the opinionnaire we are enclosing another one for your convenience. Please help us by returning it as soon as possible, since we normally expect to receive the replies within ten days of the first mailing. Thank you for your cooperation.

Sincerely,

Clinic Director

MENTAL HEALTH OPINIONNAIRE

PLEASE READ THE FOLLOWING CAREFULLY

By completing this questionnaire you can help us to help you and others. This clinic needs help in planning its program to serve the community better. THIS IS NOT A TEST: WE WANT YOUR HONEST OPINIONS. EVERYTHING YOU SAY WILL BE STRICTLY CONFIDENTIAL. WHAT YOU SAY WILL NOT AFFECT THE QUESTION OF YOUR ACCEPTANCE AT THE CLINIC. For most of the answers in this questionnaire you will not have to write. JUST PLACE A CHECK MARK NEXT TO THE ANSWER YOU MOST AGREE WITH. Do not spend too much time on any one question. THERE ARE NO "RIGHT" ANSWERS and your first reaction is what counts.

THANK YOU VERY MUCH

344

Please write a general description of your problem.

What seem to be the main things about your problem that are bothering you now? Please list them in order of their importance to you.

About how long has the most important problem been troubling you? (Check one)

Less than a year _____
Between one and five years _____
More than five years but not dating
 back to childhood _____
From the time I was 15 years
 old or even younger _____

How did you first notice the problem or become aware of it? What was it like then? When did it occur? Write a brief description.

Here is a list of things that bother some persons. Check those that are disturbing to you. Indicate when they began to bother you.

Physical Well Being	When?	
	Month	Year
Headaches _____	_____	
Fatigue _____	_____	
Ulcers _____	_____	
Heart Palpitation _____	_____	
Drug Addiction _____	_____	
Alcoholism _____	_____	
Other — What? _____	_____	

Relationships on your job or other major activity   When?
                                                        Month   Year

    Can't get enough work done _____   _____
    Not creative enough _____   _____
    Have troubles with people on the job_____   _____
    Other — What? _____   _____

Relationships with people in general

    Afraid to meet and talk with people_____   _____
    Lose your temper too often _____   _____
    Feel people don't agree with you _____   _____
    Other — What? _____   _____

Inner Emotions

    Feel generally unhappy_____   _____
    Feel guilty and sinful _____   _____
    Feel unsatisfied with yourself_____   _____
    Nervous breakdown _____   _____
    Other — What? _____   _____

Sex Life

    Frigidity _____   _____
    Impotence_____   _____
    Homosexuality_____   _____
    Masturbation_____   _____
    Can't get along with opposite sex _____   _____
    Other — What? _____   _____

Which of the following describe how you feel about the cause of your problem? (check all that apply)

If I could only change my surroundings or the situation I find myself in, everything would be all right _____
If I could only feel well physically, things would be fine _____
It's all due to my unhappy childhood or unfortunate family background_____
The main thing is that other people are causing most of the trouble I now have _____
My troubles are mainly of my own making _____
Something else (Please explain) _____

Did anyone ever notice your problem or mention it to you without your ever mentioning it to them?

                                                        When?
Yes   Month   Year

    A close friend _____   _____
    A parent _____   _____
    Husband or Wife _____   _____
    A professional (Who?)_____   _____
    Someone else (Who?)_____   _____

346

What did he (she) say?

Was this helpful?

    Yes _____
    So So _____
    No _____

Have you ever brought your problem yourself to a friend   Yes _____
or relative and discussed it with him (her)?   No _____

	When?	
Yes	Month	Year
A close friend _____	_____	
A parent _____	_____	
Husband or wife _____	_____	
A professional (Who?) _____	_____	
Someone else (Who?) _____	_____	
What did he (she) say? _____		
Was this helpful? _____		

Do you know anyone with the same or similar problem   Yes _____
to your own?   No _____

Yes	Month	Year
A close friend _____	_____	
A parent _____	_____	
Husband or Wife _____	_____	
A professional (Who?) _____	_____	
Someone else (Who?) _____	_____	

What is his (her) problem?

What did they do about it?
   Talk it over with friends _____
   Take a vacation _____
   See
      A doctor _____
      A psychiatrist or psychologist _____
      A clergyman (Minister) _____
      Someone else (Who?) _____
   Something else (Please explain) _____
   Nothing _____

In comparison with most of the people with problems similar to your own, you feel that you are (check one)

   Better off _____
   About the same _____
   Worse off _____
   Don't know anybody with
      a similar problem _____

Check below those things which you have seen or read in search of help with your problems, or about your problems.

Radio or TV_____   Books_____
Movies_____   Lectures_____
Newspaper articles_____   Courses_____
Magazine articles_____   Church Services_____
                             Something else (Please explain)___

Which did you find most useful?

IF YOU READ SOMETHING IN SEARCH OF HELP WITH YOUR PROBLEM, What things about your problem have you read, and when did you read them?

book or article	author	when?
book or article	author	when?
book or article	author	when?

Which books did you find the most useful?

Here is a list of places people sometimes go to with problems. Check below those places you have ever <u>considered</u> going to yourself? – whether or not you actually went there.

Newspaper advice column _____   Friendship club _____
Alcoholics Anonymous _____   Yoga _____
Psychoanalyst _____   Hypnotism _____
Bartender _____   Psychiatric clinic_____
Welfare department_____   General hospital_____
Christian Science practitioner_____ Marriage broker or
Other religious practitioner_____   introduction center_____
Social service agency_____ Psychologist _____
Minister, priest, or rabbi _____ Spiritualist_____
Social dance studio_____   Police _____
Psychiatrist_____   Chiropracter_____
Fortune teller _____   Dale Carnegie or other
Astrologist _____   personality training program___
Theosophist _____   Mental hygiene clinic_____
Lawyer_____   Radio or TV program _____
Mental hospital _____   Doctor _____
                                    Vocational guidance center_____
                                    Other (please explain) _____

Now looking over the list above, which three places do you think can do the most good for people with problems like your own?

Which three places can do the least good for people with problems like yours?

List below the various people and places that you have <u>actually</u> visited in the past in search of help with your problems, and when you visited them. Try to be as specific as possible.

WHO?	WHEN?		HOW MANY VISITS?
For example:			
Minister of local church	March to June 1956		5
	Months	Years	
Psychologist	October	1957	1
	Months	Years	
Doctor	November & Dec. 1957		2
	Months	Years	
	Months	Years	
	Months	Years	
	Months	Years	

Others:

Now here are ways some persons get information about psychiatrists and psychologists and psychiatric clinics. Have you ever done anything of the following?

	When?	Month	Year
Ask your friends if they knew of any:	(1) private psychiatrists		
	(2) clinics		
Ask your doctor if he could recommend a:	(1) private psychiatrist		
	(2) clinic		
Ask some other professional – minister, nurse, etc.			
Ask the local mental health association to refer you to a psychiatrist			
Look up the names of: psychiatrists in a directory, clinics			

Other (please explain)

In what areas of life do you expect changes, should the clinic be able to help you? (check all that apply)

At home _____   In any area of sexual adjustment _____
On the job_____   Regarding my values, religion, and
With relatives_____   the things I hold most important__
Social life in general_____   Other (please explain)_____

How do you think the clinic will help bring these changes about? Check all that apply.

The therapist will give me   I will do most of the talking_____
  suggestions _____   The therapist will do most of
The therapist will listen to my   the talking_____
  problem and let me work   Other (please explain) _____
  it out myself_____

IF YOU HAD SEEN A MEDICAL DOCTOR:
Did any doctor prescribe   (Check   Did any doctor recommend a
  medicine?   one)   psychiatrist?
  Yes: tranquilizers_____   Yes: Gave you the name of
      something else__   a psychiatrist_____
  No _____   Just said to see one_____
                   No _____

IF YOU HAD SEEN A PSYCHIATRIST OR PSYCHOLOGIST:
Why did you leave (or why do you want to leave) the (last) psychiatrist or psychologist? (Check all that apply)

He referred me elsewhere__   My problem was no longer suitable
He said I no longer needed   for a psychiatrist or psychologist__
  treatment_____   It was too expensive_____
He moved or I moved _____   He didn't help the problem _____
My problem got better_____   He didn't answer my questions_____
                 Something else (please explain)_____

How long has it been since you left the (last) psychiatrist or psychologist?

Am still with him_____   6 months to a year_____
Less than a month_____   A year to 2 years_____
More than a month but   More than 2 years_____
  less than six months_____

FOR ALL:
Which of the following might have prevented you from seeking help earlier? (Check all that apply)

Psychiatric help was too expensive_____ I refused to admit I had
I was ashamed to talk about it_____   problems_____
I didn't think it would do any good__ I hadn't thought of it before_____
My friends or relatives were   I just left my previous
  against it _____   therapist (or am still with
I felt I could handle the   him)_____
  problem myself _____   Something else (please explain)__

350

What made you decide to come to this clinic now? (Check all that apply)

Someone suggested it without my having asked them
A friend _____
A parent _____
A wife or husband _____
A doctor _____
Someone else (Who?) _____

Things got so bad I couldn't handle it myself _____
I just had to have someone to talk to _____
My previous therapist recommended it (Why?) _____

Can you recall any particular incident or series of incidents which directly influenced your decision to come to this clinic? Please describe.

Who referred you to this clinic?

Clergyman (Minister, Rabbi, Priest) __ Court _____
Private psychiatrist _____ Department of public health __
Other private doctor _____ Department of welfare _____
General hospital, psychiatric dep't __ Department of correction (police) __
General hospital, other dep'ts _____ Friends or relatives _____
Psychiatric hospital _____ Other agency _____
School _____ Nobody referred me, I came myself _____
Other (please explain) _____

Who first told you about this clinic and when did they tell you? (Check all that apply)

		Month	Year
The person who referred me here.	When?		
Somebody who is a patient here.	When?		
Friends (who are not coming here).	When?		
I read about it. Where? _____	When?		
I just heard about it.	When?		
Other (please explain)			

How did they happen to tell you about this clinic?

I was asking how to get treatment __ I was asking for advice in general _____
I was just discussing my problem _____ They just mentioned the clinic without knowing I was interested _____

Do you know of any other psychiatric clinics?

Yes:___   No:___

    Which ones?

Have you applied to any of them?

Yes:_____ Which ones?

_____ when?_____

_____ when?_____

    What results:

        Accepted and left_____

        Accepted for waiting list _____

        Not accepted_____

        Don't know_____

    No:_____

Do you know of any private psychiatrists or psychologists?

    None_____

    One _____

    Two_____

    3-5_____

    More than 5_____

What kinds of people do you think come here for help?

Draw a picture of the kind of person you think comes here for help.

How long have you been thinking about coming here? (Check one)

I didn't think about it, an   Between a month and six months__
    appointment was made for me_ Between six months and a year_____
Less than a week_____ More than a year _____
Between a week and one month _

How easy would you say it was to get yourself to come here? (Check
                                                one)

      Nothing to it _____
      Not too hard _____
      Very hard _____
      I never thought I'd be able to do it_____

What is it about this clinic that most appeals to you? (Explain briefly)

In what way can this clinic help you? (Check all that apply)

Help me make specific improve-   I don't think it can really
    ments in my situation _____   help _____
Help me change someone else _____ Something else
Help me understand myself more_   (please explain)_____

How long do you think it will take to solve your problem? (Check
                                                one)

Less than a month _____ A year or two_____
Between a month and six months_ More than two years_____
Between six months and a year___ It can never be solved _____

Whom have you known who was going to a psychiatrist, a guidance
clinic, or a mental hygiene clinic? When did you find out about it?

     A friend _____ When? _____
                                     month   year
     A relative _____ When? _____
                                     month   year

     Someone you didn't know very well __ When? _____
                                               month   year
     Nobody _____

If you did know someone getting psychiatric treatment, how do you
think the treatment turned out? (Check one)

It solved the problem completely___ It didn't help_____
It was very helpful _____ It did more harm than good_____
It did some good _____

How would coming here differ from going to some other psychiatric clinic? (Check all that apply)

I like the theoretical position of this clinic _____

I feel this clinic would be more competent _____

This one is more convenient for me to get to _____

I don't know of any other clinic _____

I applied to others but this is the first one that would take me _____

There's no difference between this clinic and any other clinic _____

Other (please explain) _____

How would coming here differ from going to a private psychiatrist? (Check one)

I can't afford to go to a private psychiatrist _____

In a clinic you get better care because there are more experts who work together_____

You get less personal attention _____

You get less treatment hours_____

There is no difference between coming here and going to a private psychiatrist _____

Other (please explain) _____

About how many patients in this clinic do you think have the same problems that you have?

        Almost all _____
        About 2/3 _____
        About 1/2 _____
        About 1/3 _____
        Very few _____

Whom have you told about coming here? (Check all that apply)

    Almost everyone I know_____ A few people _____
    My family_____ Nobody _____

Do you feel that some persons think there is something wrong with a person who goes to a psychiatrist?

Do you feel that a psychiatrist of your own religion can best understand you?

        Yes _____
        No _____
        Don't know _____

Do you think there are too many Jewish psychiatrists?

        Yes _____
        No _____
        Don't know_____

What is the maximum fee you could possibly afford per week for treatment? (Remember these answers <u>will not</u> affect your fee at this clinic.)

0 - .99 _____	6.00 - 6.99 _____	20.00 - 24.99 _____
1.00 - 1.99 _____	7.00 - 9.99 _____	25.00 - 29.99 _____
2.00 - 3.99 _____	10.00 - 14.99 _____	30.00+ _____
4.00 - 5.99 _____	15.00 - 19.99 _____	

Which of the following would you consider doing to help pay for treatment? (Check all that apply)

—use your savings or loans _____
—forego family expenditures such as for clothing and vacations _____
—make major changes in your life such as changing jobs, or moving
   your place of residence _____
—ask for financial help from others (friend or relative) _____
—expect the clinic to alter its policy of fees in order to take you _____

We should now like to know a bit more about the way you spend
   your leisure time.
How often do you go to the movies: (Check one)

Almost every day _____	A few times a year_____
About once a week _____	Hardly ever _____
About once a month_____	Never_____

How often do you go to the theatre to see plays:
About once a week ____ Hardly ever _____
About once a month___ Never_____
A few times a year____

How often do you go to musical concerts:
About once a week ____ Hardly ever_____
About once a month___ Never _____
A few times a year____

How often do you go to cocktail parties:
About once a week ____ Hardly ever_____
About once a month ___ Never_____
A few times a year____

How often do you visit art museums or galleries:
About once a week ____ Hardly ever_____
About once a month___ Never _____
A few times a year ____

How often do you attend religious services:
Almost every day _____ A few times a year_
About once a week_____ Hardly ever_____
About once a month___ Never_____

Which of the following is a regular part of your life? (Check all that apply)

Reading books _____	Sewing _____
Going bowling _____	Bible reading at home _____
Grace at meals_____	Going to sporting events such as
"Do it yourself" hobbies _____	baseball and basketball games _____
Going fishing _____	Observance of all religious
Daily prayer_____	holidays _____
Knitting _____	Going camping _____
	Other hobbies (What?) _____

What is your religious affiliation?

Protestant _____   Jewish _____
Catholic _____   None _____
Greek Orthodox _____   Other (What?) _____

If Protestant: What is your denomination?

Episcopalian _____   Methodist _____
Lutheran _____   Christian Science _____
Congregational _____   Dutch Reformed _____
Baptist _____   Unitarian _____
Presbyterian _____   Other (What?) _____

If Jewish: Do you consider yourself orthodox, conservative, or reformed?

Orthodox _____   Reformed _____
Conservative _____   None _____

What is your wife's (husband's) religious affiliation?

Protestant _____   Jewish _____
Catholic _____   None _____
Greek Orthodox _____   Other (What?) _____

If Protestant: What is his (her) denomination?

Episcopalian _____   Methodist _____
Lutheran _____   Christian Science _____
Congregational _____   Dutch Reformed _____
Baptist _____   Unitarian _____
Presbyterian _____   Other (What?) _____

If Jewish: Does he (she) consider himself (herself) orthodox, conservative, or reformed?

Orthodox _____   Reformed _____
Conservative _____   None _____

What is your father's religious affiliation?

Protestant _____   Jewish _____
Catholic _____   None _____
Greek Orthodox _____   Other (What?) _____

If Protestant: What is his denomination?

Episcopalian _____   Methodist _____
Lutheran _____   Christian Science _____
Congregational _____   Dutch Reformed _____
Baptist _____   Unitarian _____
Presbyterian _____   Other (What?) _____

If Jewish: Does he consider himself orthodox, conservative, or reformed?

Orthodox _____   Reformed _____
Conservative _____   None _____

What is your mother's religious affiliation?

Protestant _____ Jewish _____
Catholic_____ None _____
Greek Orthodox _____ Other (What?) _____

If Protestant: What is her denomination?

Episcopalian _____ Methodist _____
Lutheran _____ Christian Science _____
Congregational _____ Dutch Reformed _____
Baptist _____ Unitarian _____
Presbyterian_____ Other (What?) _____

If Jewish: Does she consider herself orthodox, conservative or reformed?

Orthodox _____ Reformed _____
Conservative_____ None _____

Here are some things people believe about God. Which do you agree with?

I believe in a Divine and personal God, Creator of the Universe and of
man, my Redeemer to whom I shall one day be accountable _____
I trust in a merciful and loving God, King of the Universe, who softens
justice with charity and who listens to man's prayers _____
I believe in God as a Supreme but impersonal Being, who expresses His
power and goodness through natural laws _____
There is no such thing as a personal Creator or a Supreme being; there
are only the laws of nature _____

Here are some things people believe about Jesus. Which do you agree with?

I believe in a Divine Jesus, Son of God, our Savior and Redeemer_____
Jesus was not Divine, but one of God's chosen prophets _____
Jesus was just a man _____

If one parent was Catholic: How often do you receive communion?

Almost every day_____ Several times a year_____
About once a week _____ Once a year _____
About once a month_____ Hardly ever_____
Never _____

If one parent was Jewish: To what extent do you observe Jewish dietary
laws?

Not at all _____ Only at home _____
Generally not, but don't   Both at home and when
eat pork or bacon _____   not at home _____

Here are some opinions people sometimes have. Put a check mark under
"strongly agree" if you strongly agree. Put a check mark under "moderately agree" if you agree only somewhat. Put a check under "moderately disagree" if you disagree only somewhat. Put a check under
"strongly disagree" if you strongly disagree. Make only one check for each
opinion.

	Strongly Agree	Moderately Agree	Moderately Disagree	Strongly Disagree
Doctors will tell you quite frankly when they don't know what the trouble is	_____	_____	_____	_____
Only severely disturbed people go to psychiatrists	_____	_____	_____	_____
Scientific notions and religious notions are in conflict	_____	_____	_____	_____
Doctors will tell you there's nothing much wrong with you when you know there is	_____	_____	_____	_____
Clergymen (Ministers, Priests, Rabbis) have the most important opinions on questions of religion	_____	_____	_____	_____
Persons who feel tired all the time should see a doctor right away	_____	_____	_____	_____
When you have a personal problem a psychiatrist is better to talk to than anyone else	_____	_____	_____	_____
Every child should study mathematics and science for at least ten years	_____	_____	_____	_____
Doctors give quite a bit of their time free to people who need it	_____	_____	_____	_____
The opinions of scientists should guide our thinking on social and political matters	_____	_____	_____	_____
The trouble with clergymen is that they are always preaching	_____	_____	_____	_____

	Strongly Agree	Moderately Agree	Moderately Disagree	Strongly Disagree
Persons who have a cough for several weeks should see a doctor right away	———	———	———	———
Religion is now becoming scientific	———	———	———	———
Clergymen don't really understand people's personal problems	———	———	———	———
Psychiatrists charge too much	———	———	———	———
Scientists will be able to put a space ship, carrying human beings, on Mars in less than 15 years	———	———	———	———
The opinions of psychiatrists should guide our thinking on social and political matters	———	———	———	———
Psychiatrists and psychologists are the only ones who can help people with serious emotional difficulties	———	———	———	———
Nobody should go to a hospital unless there's just no other way to take care of him properly	———	———	———	———
The opinion of clergymen should guide our thinking on social and political matters	———	———	———	———
Being sick in bed for a week has a lot of advantages	———	———	———	———
Psychiatrists can make people feel worse	———	———	———	———

	Strongly Agree	Moderately Agree	Moderately Disagree	Strongly Disagree
Science will eventually be able to solve almost all problems	_____	_____	_____	_____
When you have a personal problem a clergyman is better to talk to than anyone else	_____	_____	_____	_____
A person understands his own health better than most doctors do	_____	_____	_____	_____
Psychiatrists don't really understand people's personal problems	_____	_____	_____	_____
Persons who have a backache fairly frequently should see a doctor right away	_____	_____	_____	_____
Modern advances in science have done some harm	_____	_____	_____	_____
Doctors charge too much	_____	_____	_____	_____

Complete the following sentences in whatsoever way you wish. Write the first thing that comes to your mind. Do not spend too much time on these sentences.

Families with problems _____

_____

Most friends _____

_____

Most people I know _____

_____

Keeping trouble to yourself _____

Now we should like to ask a bit about your background.

Male _____   Female _____

Race: Negro _____   Asiatic _____

White _____   Other _____

360

When were you born?_____

                   Month   Day   Year

Where?   USA _____

                 City   State

          Not USA _____

                     Country

Where was your husband (wife) born?

         USA _____

               City   State

          Not USA _____

                     Country

And where were your parents born?

    Mother – USA _____

               City   State

          Not USA _____

                     Country

    Father – USA _____

               City   State

          Not USA _____

                     Country

Are you: Single _____ Divorced but single _____

            Married_____ Separated _____

            Divorced but remarried___ Widowed _____

Do you have children?   Yes _____

                          No _____

              If yes: How old are they?

Are you a veteran?   Yes _____ World War I _____

                     No_____ World War II _____

                                Korean _____

How many years of school have you completed?_____
(Does not include business, trade or secretarial school)

How much school did your wife (husband) have? _____

How much school did your father have?
Eighth grade or less _____   Some college _____
Some high school _____   College graduate _____
High school graduate _____   Post graduate _____

How much school did your mother have?
Eighth grade or less _____   Some college _____
Some high school _____   College graduate _____
High school graduate _____   Post graduate _____

What is your present occupation? (Please be as specific as you can)

_____

In what industry? _____

Are you an employer, an employee, or self-employed?
Self-employed _____   Employer _____
Employee _____   How many people do you employ_____

What kind of occupation would you like to have?_____

In what industry?_____

What is your wife's (husband's) occupation? _____

In what industry?_____

What is (was) your father's usual occupation?_____

In what industry? _____

Is (was) he an employer, an employee, or self-employed?
Self-employed _____   Employer _____
Employee_____   How many people does (did) he employ____

What is (was) your mother's usual occupation?_____

In what industry? _____

Is (was) she an employer, an employee, or self-employed?
Self-employed _____   Employer _____
Employee_____   How many people does (did) she employ____

Are you now living in your parent's home?   Yes _____
                                                 No_____

Income: What was your (family) income before taxes last year?
              If you do not know, how much do you make per week?

Amount per week _____

Amount per year

    Less than $2,000 _____
    $2,000 to $3,000 _____
    $3,000 to $4,000 _____
    $4,000 to $5,000 _____
    $5,000 to $6,000 _____
    $6,000 to $7,000 _____
    $7,000 to $9,000 _____
    $9,000 to $15,000_____
    Over $15,000   _____

DATE _____

Thank you for your help. You have advanced the cause of research in mental health and have helped many people.

Bibliography

Anderson, T. W. "Some scaling models and estimation procedures in the latent class model." In U. Grenander (ed.), *Probability and Statistics*. New York: Wiley, 1959.

Asheim, Lester. "A survey of recent research." Conference on the Undergraduate and Lifetime Reading Interest: *Reading for Life*. Ann Arbor: University of Michigan Press, 1959.

Avnet, Helen. *Psychiatric Insurance*. New York: GHI, 1952.

Berelson, B., P. Lazarsfeld, and W. McPhee. *Voting*. Chicago: University of Chicago Press, 1954.

Bieber, Irving, *et al*. *Homosexuality*. New York: Basic Books, 1962.

Blum, Richard H. "Case identification in psychiatric epidemiology: methods and problems." *Milbank Memorial Fund Quarterly*, 40, 1962: 253-288.

Bradburn, Norman M., and David Caplovitz. *Reports on Happiness*. Chicago: Aldine, 1965.

Brim, Orville G., Jr., *et al*. *Personality and the Decision Process*. Stanford: Stanford University Press, 1962.

Cantor, Morton B. "Karen Horney on the psychoanalytic technique: the initial interview." *American Journal of Psychoanalysis* (Part II), 17, 1957.

Coleman, James C. *Introduction to Mathematical Sociology*. New York: The Free Press, 1964.

Committee on Nomenclature and Statistics of the American Psychiatric Association. Washington, D.C.: American Psychiatric Association Mental Hospital Service, 1952.

Community Mental Health Centers Act of 1963, Title II, Public Law 88-164. Regulations, *Federal Register*, May 6, 1964: 5951-5956.

Cooley, William W., and Paul R. Lohnes. *Multivariate Procedures for the Behavioral Sciences*. New York: Wiley, 1962.

Crowley, Ralph M. "A low cost psychoanalytic service: first year." *Psychiatric Quarterly*, 24, 1960: 462-482.

Cumming, Elaine, and Charles Harrington. "Clergyman as Counselor." *American Journal of Sociology*. LXIX, November 1963: 234-243.

Cunliffe, Marcus. "The history of our friends: on Paul Goodman." *Encounter*. June 1962: 58-62.

Dain, Norman. *Concepts of Insanity in the United States*. New Brunswick, N.J.: Rutgers University Press, 1964.

Davis, Kingsley. "Mental hygiene and the class structure." *Psychiatry*, 1, 1938: 55-65.

Deutsch, Albert. *The Mentally Ill in America*. New York: Columbia University Press, 1946.

Dibble, Ursula. "Social factors in attitudes towards health and the medical profession." Unpublished Columbia University master's essay, 1965.

Dibble, Vernon. "Occupations and ideologies." *American Journal of Sociology*, 68, 1962: 229-242.

Dohrenwend, Barbara S., and Bruce P. Dohrenwend. "The problem of validity in field studies." *Journal of Abnormal Psychology*, 70, 1965: 52-59.

Dohrenwend, Bruce. "Social status and psychological disorder." *American Sociological Review*, 31, 1966: 14-34.

————, and D. Crandell. "Some relations among psychiatric symptoms, organic illness and social class." *American Journal of Psychiatry*, 123, 1967: 1527-1538.

Durkheim, Emile. *The Division of Labor*. New York: The Free Press, 1947.

Eighty-eighth Congress, First Session, House of Representatives, Document No. 58, Message from the President of the United States Relative to Mental Illness and Mental Retardation.

Eilson, J., E. Padilla, and M. E. Perkins. *The Public Image of Mental Health Services in New York City*, Columbia University School of Public Health and the New York City Community Health Board, 1965.

Elling, Ray H., and Ollie J. Lee. "Formal connections of community leadership to the health system." *Milbank Memorial Fund Quarterly*, 44, No. 3, Part I, 1966: 294-306.

Fenichel, Otto. *The Psychoanalytic Theory of Neurosis*. New York: W. W. Norton, 1945.

Fink, Raymond, and Sam Shapiro. "Methodological considerations in studying patterns of medical care related to mental illness." *Milbank Memorial Fund Quarterly*, Vol. 41, No. 4, Part I, October 1963: 377-399.

Flusser, Susan E. "The not so secret consultation: the role of reading mental health literature in the decision to seek psychotherapy." Unpublished Columbia University master's essay, 1966.

Forstenzer, Hyman M., Assistant Commissioner for Mental Health Resources and Policy Planning, New York State Department of Mental Hygiene. "Planning and evaluation of community mental health programs." Address presented at Institute for Training in Community Psychiatry, Arden House, Harriman, New York, February 25-29, 1964.

Fox, Renée C. "Training for uncertainty." In Robert K. Merton, George G. Reader, and Patricia L. Kendall, *The Student Physician*. Cambridge: Harvard University Press, 1957, pp. 207-241.

Freeman, Hugh, and James Farndale. *Trends in Mental Health Services*. New York: Macmillan, 1963.

Freidson, Eliot. "Client control and medical practice." *American Journal of Sociology*, 65, 1960: 372-382.

Freud, Sigmund. "Further recommendations in the technique of psychoanalysis." First published in *Zeitschrift*, B. 1, 1913.

Glasscote, R. M., D. S. Saunders, H. R. Forstenzer, and A. R. Foley. *The Community Mental Health Center*. Washington, D.C.: Joint Information Service of the American Psychiatric Association and the National Association for Mental Health, 1964.

Goodman, Paul. *The Empire City*. New York: Bobbs-Merrill, 1959.

Gruenberg, Ernest M. (ed). "Evaluating the effectiveness of mental health services." *Milbank Memorial Fund Quarterly*, 44, January 1966: Part II.

Gurin, Gerald, Joseph Veroff, and Sheila Feld. *Americans View Their Mental Health*. New York: Basic Books, 1960.

Hollingshead, A., and F. C. Redlich. *Social Class and Mental Illness*. New York: Wiley, 1958.

Horney, Karen. *Our Inner Conflicts: A Constructive Theory of Neurosis*. New York: W. W. Norton, 1945.

Jacob, Norma. "Referral sources and methods in community psychiatric clinics in New York State." Unpublished paper, 1965.

Joint Commission on Mental Illness and Health. *Action for Mental Health*. New York: Basic Books, 1961.

Jones, Ernest. *The Life and Work of Sigmund Freud*. Volumes I-III. New York: Basic Books, 1953-1957.

Jones, Kathleen. *Lunacy, Law and Conscience*. London: Routledge & Kegan Paul, 1960.

———. *Mental Health and Social Policy*. London: Routledge & Kegan Paul, 1960.

Kadushin, Charles. "The friends and supporters of psychotherapy: on social circles in urban life." *American Sociological Review*, 31, December 1966: 786-802.

———. "Individual decisions to undertake psychotherapy." *Administrative Science Quarterly*, 3, 1958: 379-411.

———. "Reason analysis." In the *International Encyclopedia of the Social Sciences*, Volume 13, Second Edition. New York: Macmillan and The Free Press, 1968, pp. 338-343.

———. "Social class and the experience of ill health." *Sociological Inquiry*, 24, 1964: 67-80.

———. "Social distance between client and professional." *American Journal of Sociology*, 68, 1962: 517-531.

———. "Steps on the way to a psychiatric clinic." Unpublished Columbia University doctoral dissertation, 1960.

Katz, Elihu, and Paul F. Lazarsfeld. *Personal Influence*. New York: The Free Press, 1955.

Kazin, Alfred. "The language of pundits." In *Contemporaries*. New York: Knopf, 1961.

Kinsey, Alfred C., et al. *Sexual Behavior in the Human Female*. Philadelphia: Saunders, 1953.

———. *Sexual Behavior in the Human Male*. Philadelphia: Saunders, 1953.

Klausner, Samuel Z. *Psychiatry and Religion*. New York: The Free Press, 1964.

Kruskal, J. B. "Multidimensional scaling by optimizing goodness of fit to a nonmetric hypothesis." *Psychometrika*, 29, 1964: 1-27.

———. "How to use MDSCAL, a multidimensional scaling program." Bell Telephone Laboratories, Inc., Murray Hill, N.J., n.d., multilith.

———. "Nonmetric multidimensional scaling: a numerical method." *Psychometrika*, 29, 1964: 115-129.

Kubie, Lawrence S. "Social forces and the neurotic process." In A. H. Leighton, J. A. Clausen, and R. N. Wilson (eds.), *Exploration in Social Psychiatry*. New York: Basic Books, 1957, pp. 77-97.

Langner, Thomas S., and Stanley T. Michael. *Life Stress and Mental Health*. New York: The Free Press, 1963.

Lawrence, P. S. "Chronic illness and socio-economic status." In E. Gartly Jaco (ed.), *Patients, Physicians and Illness*. New York: The Free Press, 1958, pp. 37-49.

Lazarsfeld, Paul F. "A conceptual introduction to latent structure analysis." In *Mathematical Thinking in the Social Sciences*. New York: The Free Press, 1954, pp. 378-379.

———. "Latent structure analysis." In Sigmond Koch (ed.), *Psychology: A Study of a Science*. New York: McGraw-Hill, 1959, pp. 476-543.

———. "The statistical analysis of reasons as a research operation." *Sociometry*, 5, 1942: 29-47.

———, and N. W. Henry. *Latent Structure Analysis*. Boston: Houghton Mifflin, 1968.

———, and Morris Rosenberg. *The Language of Social Research*. New York: The Free Press, 1955.

Lemkau, Paul V., and Guido M. Crocetti. "An urban population's opinion and knowledge about mental illness." *American Journal of Psychiatry*, 118, February 1962: 692-700.

Litwak, Eugene, and Henry J. Meyer. "A balance theory of coordination between bureaucratic organizations and community primary groups." *Administrative Science Quarterly*, 11, 1966: 31-68.

Lorenzen, Irma J. "Acceptance or rejection by psychiatric clinics." Unpublished Columbia University master's essay, 1967.

Lowe, Edmund G. *Subways Are for Sleeping*. New York: Harcourt, Brace, 1957.

Maccoby, Eleanor E. "Pitfalls in the analysis of panel data: a research note on some technical aspects of voting." *American Journal of Sociology*, 61, 1956: 359-362.

McHugh, R. B. "Efficient estimation and local identification in latent class analysis." *Psychometrika*, 21, 1956: 331-347.

Mechanic, David. "The concept of illness behavior." *Journal of Chronic Disease*, 15, 1962: 189-194.

Memo to the Members of the Executive Committee, State Mental Planning Committee, from B. F. Riess, Isidor Chein, and Allen V. Williams, n.d.

Menninger, Karl. *Theory of Psychoanalytic Technique.* New York: Basic Books, 1958.

Merton, Robert. *Social Theory and Social Structure* (second edition). New York: The Free Press, 1957.

Miller, Daniel R., and Guy E. Swanson. *Inner Conflict and Defense.* New York: Holt, 1960.

Moses, R., and J. Shanan. "Psychiatric outpatient clinic." *Archives of General Psychiatry,* 4, 1961: 60-73.

Mueller, Eva. "A study of purchase decisions." In Lincoln H. Clark (ed.), *Consumer Behavior.* New York: New York University Press, 1965.

New York State Department of Mental Hygiene. "Statement on long-range plans in mental health," June 15, 1964.

Park, R. E., E. W. Burgess, and R. D. McKenzie. *The City.* Chicago: University of Chicago Press, 1925.

Parsons, Talcott. "Definitions of health and illness in the light of American values and social structure. In E. Gartly Jaco (ed.), *Patients, Physicians and Illness.* New York: The Free Press, 1958.

———. "General theory in sociology." In Robert K. Merton, *et al., Sociology Today.* New York: Basic Books, 1959, pp. 3-38.

———. *The Social System.* New York: The Free Press, 1951.

———, and E. A. Shils (eds.). *Toward a General Theory of Action.* Cambridge: Harvard University Press, 1951.

Reissman, Frank, Jerome Cohen, and Arthur Pearl (eds.). *Mental Health of the Poor.* New York: The Free Press, 1964.

Report of the Subcommittee on Manpower of the New York City Regional Mental Health Planning Committee, October 1964.

Ridenour, Nina. *Mental Health in the United States.* Cambridge: Harvard University Press, 1961.

Rosenstock, Irwin M. "Why people use health services." *Milbank Memorial Fund Quarterly,* 44, Part II, July 1966: 94-127.

Saenger, Gerhart, and John Cumming. "Study of community mental health clinics, Report I and II." Mental Health Research Unit, New York State Department of Mental Hygiene, Syracuse, New York, 1965 and 1966.

Schaie, K. Warner, Lois R. Chatham, and James M. A. Weiss. "The multiprofessional intake assessment of older psychiatric patients." *Journal of Psychiatric Research,* Volume I, 1962: 92-100.

Scheff, Thomas J. *Being Mentally Ill: A Sociological Theory.* Chicago: Aldine, 1966.

Schwartz, Morris S., and Charlotte Green Schwartz. *Social Approaches to Mental Patient Care.* New York: Columbia University Press, 1964.

Srole, Leo, Thomas S. Langner, Stanley T. Michael, Marvin K. Opler, and Thomas A. C. Rennie. *Mental Health in the Metropolis: The Midtown Manhattan Study.* New York: McGraw-Hill, 1962.

Statistical Report of Psychiatric Clinics in New York State for the Year Ended March 31, 1960. State of New York Department of Mental Hygiene, January 1961.

Steiner, Lee. *Where Do People Take Their Troubles?* Boston: Houghton Mifflin, 1945.

Stoeckle, J. D., *et al.* "On going to see the doctor: the contributions of the patient to the decision to seek medical aid." *Journal of Chronic Disease,* 16, 1963: 975-989.

Suchman, Edward A. "Sociocultural variations in illness and medical care." *American Journal of Sociology*, 70, November 1964: 319-331.
————. "Stages of illness and medical care." *Journal of Health and Human Behavior*, 6, 1965: 114-128.
Szasz, Thomas S. "A questionnaire study of psychoanalytic practices and opinions." *Journal of Nervous and Mental Disease*, 137, 1963: 209-221.
————. "The myth of mental illness." *American Psychologist*, 15, 1960: 113-118.
Tietze, C., P. Lemkau, and M. Cooper. "Schizophrenic, manic-depressive psychosis, and social-economic status." *American Journal of Sociology*, 47, 1941: 167-175.
U.S. Department of Health, Education and Welfare, Public Health Service. *Health Manpower Source Book*, Section 14, Medical Specialists, Public Health Service Publication No. 263, 1962.
Vernon, Raymond. *Metropolis 1985*. New York: Doubleday Anchor Books, 1963.
Wing, J. K. "A simple and reliable subclassification of chronic schizophrenia." *Journal of Mental Science*, 107, 1961: 862-875.
Zetterberg, H. L. "Compliant actions." *Acta Sociologica*, 2, 1957: 179-201.
Zola, I. K. "Culture and symptoms—an analysis of patients' presenting complaints." *American Sociological Review*, 31, 1966: 615-630.

Index

The notes at the end of each chapter have not been indexed. See the Bibliography for further listings.

Milton Keynes UK
Ingram Content Group UK Ltd.
UKHW040013071024
449327UK00011B/215